T0306032

Masterclass in Medicine

Nearly every medical school around the world teaches a class about the clinical foundations of medicine and how to start the process of becoming a skilled and caring physician. However, there has never been a book on it—until now. This premier text brings together talented and renowned physicians from across the globe in order to discuss important topics related to clinical excellence, including humility, empathy, and ingenuity in medicine. Students, physicians-in-training, and health care professionals will gain tremendous knowledge by hearing the stories of what these master clinicians have learned from their patients and colleagues, thereby providing a foundation in how to achieve greatness as a clinician.

KEY FEATURES:

- Features engaging patient stories and personal reflections from a diverse set of authors
- Explores successes, failures, and lessons learned that cut across all fields of medicine
- Serves as a comprehensive meditation on master clinicianship that is ideal for courses in clinical foundations of medicine

Masterclass in Medicine
Lessons from the Experts

Edited by

Marcy B. Bolster, MD

Professor of Medicine, Harvard Medical School
Division of Rheumatology, Allergy and Immunology
Director, Rheumatology Fellowship Training Program
Boston, MA

Jason E. Liebowitz, MD

Assistant Professor of Medicine
Columbia University Vagelos College of Physicians and Surgeons
New York, NY

Philip Seo, MD, MHS

Associate Professor of Medicine
Johns Hopkins University School of Medicine
Baltimore, MD

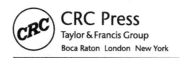

CRC Press
Taylor & Francis Group
Boca Raton London New York

CRC Press is an imprint of the
Taylor & Francis Group, an **informa** business

Designed cover image: shutterstock.com/image-photo/small-plastic-bonsai-tree-isolated-on-399492055

First edition published 2025
by CRC Press
2385 NW Executive Center Drive, Suite 320, Boca Raton FL 33431

and by CRC Press
4 Park Square, Milton Park, Abingdon, Oxon, OX14 4RN

CRC Press is an imprint of Taylor & Francis Group, LLC

ISBN: 978-1-032-52951-6 (hbk)
ISBN: 978-1-032-52949-3 (pbk)
ISBN: 978-1-003-40937-3 (ebk)

DOI: 10.1201/9781003409373

Typeset in Palatino LT Std
by Apex CoVantage, LLC

I would like to dedicate this book to my father, Victor Behar, a retired cardiologist, lifelong mentor, and the first and most steadfast person in guiding me toward excellence in the pursuit of patient rapport and care.
Marcy B. Bolster

I would like to dedicate this book to my wife, Anat Chemerinski, the most brilliant and caring physician that I know.
Jason E. Liebowitz

I would like to dedicate this book to my parents, Hae Ja Yoon, MD, and Kyung Hwa Seo, MD. All that I have become I owe to them.
Philip Seo

We would like to dedicate this book to all the clinicians who have touched our lives, helped us to become the physicians we are today, and continue to foster our growth.
Marcy B. Bolster, Jason E. Liebowitz, and Philip Seo

Contents

Foreword

Medicine changes your brain. Most of us, I suspect, come to think about this for the first time in medical school, and sometimes we're thrilled, and sometimes we're disoriented, or even disturbed: "my perspective is being warped; my familiar way of perceiving the world is being altered by this rigorous and sometimes disconcerting set of new experiences and disciplines."

What is really changing, whether you know it or not, is your relationship to the stories all around you. You start diagnosing yourself—or other people—before you really know what it means to diagnose. You feel new kinds of responsibility and new kinds of terror. (I can remember sitting on an airplane, as a first-year medical student, thinking: "oh no, they're calling for a doctor—but I don't know anything—but shouldn't I be doing something to help?") You watch a movie or a TV show, and your brain gets stuck on some aspect of the medical plot, even while the actors go on playing out the drama.

And, after all, you do want to become a physician. That's why you're in medical school in the first place, and, in many ways, maybe you welcome the new perspective, as part of your eagerness to identify as a member of your chosen profession: "I'm starting to think like a doctor, react like a doctor, talk like a doctor." Ours is meant to be a transformative training, and, in fact, your way of understanding the stories of the world is changing. And so is your way of participating in those stories, and so is your way of telling those stories.

Masterclass in Medicine: Lessons from the Experts offers a chance to listen in as experienced and dedicated physicians reflect on so many different aspects of the job, from the personal relationships with patients to the cognitive, scientific, ethical, and even political challenges that arise out of taking care of people. These are writers of vast professional experience taking the time to do what we often do not do in our busy medical lives—to reflect on practice and to examine the lessons learned. In medicine, we are all regularly grateful for the presence of the experts around us and among us, our exemplars, our teachers, our colleagues. And yet we all know, from personal experience, that we are in a profession in which even the experts we most admire continue to wrestle with uncertainty.

That wasn't how I thought it was going to be, back at the beginning, when I truly knew nothing and therefore aspired to confidence and certainty, which I was sure were waiting just ahead. I remember being positive, as a fourth-year medical student on the wards, constantly struggling with a sense of my own overwhelming ignorance and with that fear that I might somehow do some damage, that the senior residents knew absolutely what they were doing. I don't think it would even have occurred to me as a distant possibility that the attendings were ever visited by self-doubt or regret. (Nowadays I sit on the airplane, thinking: "oh no, they're calling for a doctor—but surely they don't need a general pediatrician—but shouldn't I be doing something to help?") And in fact, airplane emergencies aside, one of the glories of the job we do is that more experience and more knowledge teach us over and over not only about victories and miracles but also about uncertainties and tragedies.

Probably any profession changes your brain, if you devote your life to it. That's part of what we've learned about the brain, after all, maybe most especially in my own field of pediatrics. Starting in early childhood (and before), your life experiences build your brain, so that the brain you take through life (that is, the brain that takes you through life) is shaped and changed by your experiences and by your learning. But what you'll read about in this book are the different—and special—kinds of experiences and learning required of us and granted to us as a consequence of our own strange and remarkable profession.

I still find myself getting stuck on the medical stories—I look at an illustration of a child with a crutch, and I want to know what happened (Congenital disability? Polio?), and that leads me into the medical literature where people argue why Tiny Tim was tiny, and why he needed that one crutch. I teach a class where undergraduates read Camus's novel, *The Plague*, about an outbreak of bubonic plague in North Africa in the 1940s, and I can't stop worrying about why there are no sulfa drugs in the book. Medicine has changed my brain, and it's changed the way I hear and tell stories. I loved getting to listen to the voices in *Masterclass in Medicine* and hearing the authors' thoughts on the jobs they do.

Medicine is a storytelling profession but not always a reflective profession. It's a profession of great privilege—yes, the privilege of continuing to learn, but most of all, the honor and privilege of caring for people, being allowed into the rooms and lives and stories of other people. I think you will hear that sense of privilege reflected over and over in these essays, articulated in so many different ways by physicians who know so much and who are taking that opportunity now to reflect: lifelong students of medicine who are thinking about what they have been taught by their practices and their patients and lifelong teachers reflecting on what they have learned.

Perri Klass, MD
Professor of Journalism and Pediatrics
New York University

Preface

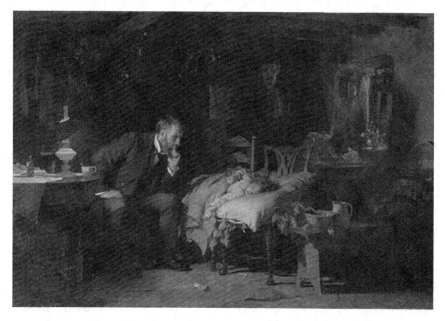

"The Doctor" by Luke Fildes (1891). Reproduced with permission of the Tate Gallery, London.

In 1891, Luke Fildes completed his painting *The Doctor*, a work that is considered to be one of the most significant depictions of the practice of medicine in the annals of art history. In this painting, a young girl appears pale and listless as she lies with one arm draped over the side of her bed, her eyes closed and her body still as she languishes from illness. In the background, her parents despair—the mother sits with her head buried deep in her arms, hands clasped together in a sign of prayer; her father stands with his palm on his wife's shoulder while he looks expectantly toward his daughter and the man sitting next to her. The seated man is a physician. He leans toward the girl with hand on chin, wearing a look on his face that is a mixture of intense contemplation and consternation. The artist has illuminated the figures of both the girl and the doctor, clearly drawing the viewer's attention to these two individuals and making them appear almost celestial.

The painting is frequently shown to medical students, and one would be forgiven for thinking that it was based on real-life events in which a brilliant doctor is able to solve his patient's medical mystery and provide a cure. However, the true story is much more complex and surprising. Fildes's was inspired by his own family's tragedy in which his one-year-old son Philip died of typhoid fever on Christmas morning in 1877. The son had been visited by a doctor as he lay dying, and, although the physician could not save Philip's life, Fildes was moved by the compassion and worry that the doctor displayed on behalf of the young boy.

As you will read in the chapters of this book, medicine is not always about finding the right answer or providing a specific treatment that resolves a medical condition. Instead, the practice of medicine is so often about the development of a deep and meaningful relationship between two individuals, a bond that is multifaceted and frequently evolves over time. Doctors often meet patients and their families in times of great need and, through the combination of empathy, cooperation, and a willingness to truly listen, they seek to provide the emotional and spiritual support that is as much a part of a person's health and well-being as is their response to a particular medication.

Our goal for this book is to allow for physicians widely considered by colleagues to be master clinicians to share their stories and reflections on what has allowed them to achieve this level of clinical excellence. When we approached these doctors with invitations to pen a chapter, each one protested in calling themselves an "expert" or "master clinician." The academic achievements and reputations of these authors clearly demonstrate that they are indeed among the best and brightest of physicians. However, their chapter contributions reveal a quality that they all possess and that, as you will see in reading this book, is essential to good doctoring: humility. Indeed, as these incredible physicians write eloquently on such wide-ranging topics as dealing with uncertainty, communicating and collaborating with patients, respect, and more, you will see that their most profound lessons routinely come from unexpected sources, including their own mistakes or personal tragedies. With introspection, humor, creativity, and a refreshing openness, these physicians describe in rich detail what it means to develop one's own skills as a lifelong learner, mentor, and role model while providing truly outstanding and humanistic care for patients.

The contributing authors, whose work we share with you, represent a diverse array of physicians across many specialties, ages, geographic locations, and backgrounds. Although each author is a medical doctor, the lessons contained in this text are widely applicable to any health professional providing care to patients. We also strongly believe that, for anyone who has already or will one day interact with the health care system—which describes all of us—the stories contained in this book are relevant, timely, and highly worthy of your attention.

These authors teach by example and demonstrate the value of humility in both the clinical setting and through their writing. We consider it a tremendous privilege to have been able to communicate with and review the prose of each of these masters of medicine, and we hope readers experience satisfaction and joy in their reading of this book.

Marcy B. Bolster, MD

Jason E. Liebowitz, MD

Philip Seo, MD, MHS

Editor Biographies

Marcy B. Bolster, MD is a rheumatologist and Director of the Rheumatology Fellowship Training Program at the Massachusetts General Hospital, Boston, MA. She is Professor of Medicine at Harvard Medical School. She has a strong interest in medical education across the spectrum of learners, and she has helped train more than 70 rheumatology fellows. Her commitment to medical education focuses on curriculum design, assessment, mentorship, and professionalism. She is the recipient of the 2019 American College of Rheumatology Distinguished Program Director Award, the 2019 Partners (now Mass General Brigham) Outstanding Program Director Award, and the 2021 Arthritis Foundation Marian Ropes Lifetime Achievement Award.

Jason E. Liebowitz, MD is Assistant Professor of Medicine at Columbia University Vagelos College of Physicians and Surgeons. His research and writings have been published in *The New England Journal of Medicine, JAMA, JAMA Internal Medicine, Arthritis Care and Research,* and *The Journal of Graduate Medical Education.* He is a co-editor of the textbook *Clinical Innovation in Rheumatology: Past, Present, and Future* and a co-editor of the textbook series *Interdisciplinary Rheumatology.* He has a strong interest in medical education and serves as the co-director of the Rheumatology and Clinical Immunology medical student course at Columbia University.

Philip Seo, MD, MHS is Associate Professor of Medicine at Johns Hopkins University and the Rheumatology Physician Editor for UpToDate. He was Director of the Johns Hopkins Vasculitis Center and Director of the Johns Hopkins Rheumatology Fellowship Training Program for 11 years, and recently completed his tenure as Physician Editor for *The Rheumatologist,* a publication of the American College of Rheumatology. In 2021, he received the American College of Rheumatology's Distinguished Clinician Scholar Award, which is awarded annually to a rheumatologist who makes outstanding contributions in clinical medicine, clinical scholarship, or education.

Contributors

Nancy B. Allen, MD
Professor Emerita of Medicine
Rheumatology and Immunology
Duke University School of Medicine
Durham, NC

Ronald J. Anderson, MD
Distinguished Clinician Teacher,
    Department of Medicine
Director Emeritus, Rheumatology
    Fellowship Program
Brigham and Women's Hospital
Boston, MA

Katrina A. Armstrong, MD
Executive Vice President for Health
    and Biomedical Sciences
Dean of the Faculties of Health
    Sciences and the Vagelos College
    of Physicians and Surgeons
Chief Executive Officer of Columbia
    University Irving Medical Center
Harold and Margaret Hatch Professor
    in the Faculty of Medicine
Columbia University Vagelos College
    of Physicians and Surgeons
New York, NY

Michele Barry, MD, FACP, FASTMH
Drs. Ben and Jess Shenson Professor
    of Medicine and Tropical Diseases
Senior Associate Dean for Global Health
Director of the Center for Innovation
    in Global Health
Founder, WomenLift Health
Stanford University School of Medicine
Palo Alto, CA

**Arabella S. Begin, MD, PhD, MMSc,
    MRCPCH**
Audrey and Lewis Cannell Fellow
    and Director of Studies in Clinical
    Medicine
Lincoln College, University of Oxford
Oxford, England, UK

Rita Charon, MD, PhD
Professor of Medicine
Chair, Department of Medical
    Humanities and Ethics
Executive Director of Columbia
    Narrative Medicine
Columbia University Vagelos College
    of Physicians and Surgeons
New York, NY

**John Patrick T. Co, MD, MPH,
    MBA, FAAP**
Vice President, Graduate Medical
    Education, Mass General Brigham
Associate Professor of Pediatrics,
    Harvard Medical School
Massachusetts General Hospital
Boston, MA

Mark R. Cullen, MD
Professor of Medicine, Epidemiology
    and Biomedical Data Science (retired)
Founding Director, Stanford Center
    for Population Health Sciences
Stanford University
Palo Alto, CA

Marcela G. del Carmen, MD, MPH
President, Massachusetts General
    Hospital
President, Massachusetts General
    Physicians Organization
Professor of Obstetrics Gynecology, and
    Reproductive Biology
Harvard Medical School
Massachusetts General Hospital
Boston, MA

David B. Hellmann, MD, MACP
Aliki Perroti Professor of Medicine
Director, Johns Hopkins Center for
    Innovative Medicine
Johns Hopkins University School
    of Medicine
Baltimore, MD

Ralph I. Horwitz, MD, MACP
Professor
Lewis Katz School of Medicine
Temple University
Philadelphia, PA

Vicki A. Jackson, MD, MPH
Blum Family Endowed Chair in
  Palliative Care
Chief, Division of Palliative Care and
  Geriatrics, Massachusetts General
  Hospital
Co-director, Harvard Medical School
  Center for Palliative Care
Professor of Medicine, Harvard Medical
  School
Boston, MA

**David H. Johnson, MD,
MACP, FASCO**
Chair Emeritus, Department
  of Internal Medicine
R. Ellwood Jones Distinguished
  Professor of Clinical Education
UT Southwestern School of Medicine
Dallas, TX

James Kahn, MD
Professor of Medicine, Emeritus
Stanford University School
  of Medicine
Palo Alto, CA

Jerome P. Kassirer, MD
Distinguished Professor, Tufts
  University School of Medicine
Editor-in-Chief Emeritus, *New England
  Journal of Medicine*
Boston, MA

Perri Klass, MD
Professor of Journalism
  and Pediatrics
Director, CAS Minor in Medical
  Humanities
New York University
New York, NY

Suzanne Koven, MD, MFA
Valerie Winchester Endowed Chair in
  Primary Care Medicine
Writer in Residence
Massachusetts General Hospital
Associate Professor of Medicine
Associate Professor of Global Health
  and Social Medicine
Harvard Medical School
Boston, MA

**Robert G. Lahita, MD, PhD, FACP,
MACR, FRCP**
Director of St. Joseph's Institute for
  Autoimmune and Rheumatic Diseases
Professor of Medicine, Hackensack
  Meridian School of Medicine
Clinical Professor of Medicine,
  Rutgers, New Jersey Medical School
Wayne, NJ

**Stephen A. Paget, MD, FACP, FACR,
MACR**
Stephen A. Paget Rheumatology Chair
Professor of Medicine, Weill Cornell
  Medicine
Physician-in-Chief Emeritus, Hospital
  for Special Surgery
Director, HSS Rheumatology Academy
  of Medical Educators
New York, NY

**Roy Phitayakorn, MD, MHPE,
MAMSE, FACS**
Vice Chair of Education, MGH
  Department of Surgery
Associate Professor of Surgery, Harvard
  Medical School
Boston, MA

David S. Pisetsky, MD, PhD
Professor of Medicine and Integrative
  Immunobiology
Associate Vice Chair of Academic
  Affairs, Department of Medicine
Duke University Medical Center
Staff Physician
Durham VA Medical Center
Durham, NC

Daniel Shalev, MD
Assistant Professor of Medicine and of
    Medicine-in-Psychiatry
Division of Geriatrics and Palliative
    Medicine
Weill Cornell Medicine
New York, NY

Richard M. Silver, MD, MACR
Distinguished University Professor
Division Director, Emeritus
Division of Rheumatology and
    Immunology
Department of Medicine
Medical University of South Carolina
Charleston, SC

Rache M. Simmons, MD, MS, MBA
Professor of Surgery
Weiskopf Professor of Surgical
    Oncology
Associate Dean, Diversity and Inclusion
Director, Office of Women
Co-director, Women Physicians of NYP
Weill Cornell Medicine
New York, NY

Sharon D. Solomon, MD
Katharine M. Graham Professor of
    Ophthalmology
Johns Hopkins University School of
    Medicine
Baltimore, MD

Theodore A. Stern, MD
Chief Emeritus, Avery D. Weisman
    Psychiatric Consultation Service
Director, Thomas P. Hackett Center
    for Scholarship in Psychosomatic
    Medicine
Massachusetts General Hospital
Ned H. Cassem Professor
    of Psychiatry in the Field of
    Psychosomatic Medicine/
    Consultation
Harvard Medical School
Boston, MA

**Dean L. Winslow, MD, MACP, FRCP,
    FIDSA, FPIDS**
Professor of Medicine
Division of Hospital Medicine
Division of Infectious Diseases and
    Geographic Medicine
Stanford University School of Medicine
Palo Alto, CA

Roy C. Ziegelstein, MD, MACP
Sarah Miller Coulson and Frank L.
    Coulson, Jr., Professor
    of Medicine
Mary Wallace Stanton Professor of
    Education
Vice Dean for Education, Johns Hopkins
    University School of Medicine
Baltimore, MD

1 The Good Doctor

David H. Johnson

How does one define a "good doctor"? It's a question I have asked myself many times since entering the medical profession over fifty years ago. Almost every physician I know tells me they can identify a "good doctor." Many can instantly recall "the best doctor I have ever seen," but, when I ask them to describe the characteristics of that person, there is almost invariably a pause, a moment of hesitation. The most common response is either "I know it when I see it" or some other variation of former Supreme Court Justice Potter Stewart's famous axiom, and maybe that is the best answer. In the past, according to Swenson and colleagues, "a stereotypical good doctor was independent and always available, had encyclopedic knowledge, and was a master of rescue care" [1]. Today, a good doctor must have "a solid fund of knowledge and sound decision-making skills but also must be emotionally intelligent, a team player, able to obtain information from colleagues and technological sources, embrace quality improvement as well as public reporting, and reliably deliver evidence-based care, using scientifically informed guidelines in a personal, compassionate, patient-centered manner" [1]. Those comments resonate with me, but how do you know a doctor possesses these qualities, and can a patient tell?

A few years before Swenson and his colleagues offered that perspective, I was invited to speak at a university-sponsored lecture series known as the "Out of the Lunchbox Lectures." The talks were intended for the general public with the goal of "sharing practical knowledge" and "improving community relations." A distinguished professor from the Philosophy Department was assigned the task of organizing the lectures, fielding requests for topics, and inviting speakers. One day, quite unexpectedly, the professor called me to ask if I would speak to the group on "How do you know if your doctor is any good?" Initially I thought, sure, I can do that. But very quickly I realized I had no idea how to tell the public whether a specific doctor is "any good." So my academic instincts kicked in, and I logged on to PubMed to "look it up." I found numerous articles describing the features of a "good doctor" but none that defined how to *tell* if a doctor is good. And by "good" I mean capable of doing their job in such a way as to ensure optimal health for an individual patient. So I did the next best thing. I sought the opinions of physician colleagues and family members. Although I received a myriad of opinions, including quite a few in the "what *not* to do" category, the effort proved mostly unhelpful. I identified no singular characteristic or cluster of attributes that could serve as a definitive "tell." Consequently, I had to "wing it." In the final few days leading up to the lecture, I will confess to being increasingly anxious and troubled. I was concerned I might mislead the audience and leave them with impressions that were not fact based. At length I called the professor to let him know I wasn't sure I could go through with the talk. I told him much of what I would say was "nonscientific" and "opinion-based." He responded, "That's not a problem. The last lecture was kind of like that." Turns out the lecture before mine was titled "Cannibalism: What's in It for You."

With that note of encouragement, I proceeded with the lecture.[1] I began my talk by providing a checklist of good doctor behaviors noting that they start all encounters by putting their patients at ease and attempting to alleviate anxiety. I suggested that good doctors are respectful, unbiased, humble, team players, and empathic and that they serve as patient advocates. I stated good doctors invariably are good

DOI: 10.1201/9781003409373-1

communicators. They listen well, can convey that listening has occurred, and that the heard content is accurate.[2] Above all, a good doctor must be *competent*! In choosing a doctor I shared some of my biases such as the lack of utility of "Best Doctor" lists and the uncertain value of "experience" in the nonsurgical specialties (i.e., gray hair is not necessarily a virtue). In fact, a doctor who has practiced for many years may be "out of date" and therefore less familiar with the latest treatment options. By contrast, I opined that board certification was a useful surrogate of quality although admittedly a weak one. In my view it remains so today.[3] I also suggested that doctors who participate in teaching activities involving medical students and residents are often more "up-to-date," my argument being that such interactions prompt older doctors to review and learn new material. This was pure speculation on my part, but it seemed a reasonable postulate. Finally, I suggested good doctors tell patients how their practice operates and will introduce their staff members including nurses, medical assistants, and personnel at the front desk and back office. Crude measures to be sure but readily available for assessment. If a doctor does these things, it is quite likely they are attentive to the details required to deliver optimal care of the patient. Think of the rock band Van Halen who demanded the removal of all brown M&Ms in their backstage snacks. They made this seemingly outlandish request to assess the thoroughness with which the concert sponsors paid attention to the details of their stage setup.[4]

After the lecture, a few audience members approached me to share their thoughts and perspectives. Most were complimentary of their doctor praising the physician's personal qualities, including their friendliness, empathy, and communication skills. Several proffered laudatory comments like "He's the best!" or "She's amazing!" High praise indeed. Interestingly, no one said anything specific about their doctor's competence.

In the years since I gave that lecture, I continued to ruminate on how one can tell whether a doctor is any good. I searched for the elusive feature that distinguishes the good doctor from the not so good doctor—the exceptional from the average doctor. I know about quality and performance metrics and how they are often used to assess the "goodness" of individual doctors. But these parameters do not invariably correlate with the delivery of high-quality care. Moreover, physicians who score well in the quality domain do not always do well in the patient evaluation area. I am also aware of patient surveys that characterize the "ideal physician" as someone who is "confident, empathetic, humane, personal, forthright, respectful and thorough" [2]. But those characteristics tell us how physicians are perceived, *not* that they are good at what they do. Interestingly, that may not matter since patient surveys also indicate that desirable personal qualities are more strongly valued than scientific proficiency and technical skills when it comes to choosing a doctor [3]. Indeed, long before these surveys were conducted, I was told, in medical school that the key to a successful medical practice is defined by "the three A's . . . accessibility, affability and ability . . . *in that order.*" Regardless, the aforementioned characteristics seem necessary, but are they sufficient?

> I remember the time Shipman gave to my Dad. He would come around at the drop of a hat. He was a marvellous [sic] GP apart from the fact that he killed my father.

This quote comes from Christopher Rudol whose father, Ernest, was one of many victims of Dr. Harold Shipman, a general practitioner from Manchester, England, who is said to have murdered more that 200 of his patients [4]. Apparently, Dr. Shipman possessed many of the sought-after personal attributes just listed—except most obviously humanism—but he was hardly "good"—even though his patients viewed him as a "good doctor." Instead, Dr. Shipman proved to be the quintessential "bad doctor," inter alia imbued with "bad intentions, undesirable values, suspect—occasionally evil—motives" [3]. Bad doctors possess "serious defects of moral agency, even though these may coexist with commendable aspects of medical practice" [3]. While bad doctors are rare, they are more common than we care to admit [4]. And they seemingly come in varying degrees. Recall, for example, the rapid emergence of the doctors who, for unfathomable reasons, repeatedly spouted misinformation during the Covid-19 pandemic [5].

> When a doctor goes wrong, he is the first of criminals. He has the nerve and he has the knowledge.
>
> —**Sherlock Holmes,** *The Adventure of the Speckled Band* **(1892)**

Somewhere between the good and bad doctor is the "poor doctor." A poor doctor is generally "credited with good intentions but inadequate knowledge or skills required for the job" [3]. Defined in this manner, a poor doctor may possess every desirable trait imaginable except, of course, competence. As noted, for the layperson, determining competence is a challenging and possibly impossible task but seems foundational to choosing a good doctor. In retrospect, perhaps identifying the "poor doctor" would have been the better goal of that earlier lecture.

In reality, most doctors fall into the "average" doctor category, what might be labeled the "good enough" doctor. Good enough doctors are capable of managing most day-to-day medical problems in their specialty and do so in a way generally consistent with accepted medical guidelines and in a manner satisfactory to their patients. Thus, from a patient's perspective, the doctor is good—maybe even exceptional—even though the doctor's overall performance is average. Atul Gawande described this phenomenon in a 2004 *New Yorker* article titled "The Bell Curve" [6]. In it, he chronicled the case of Annie, a young girl diagnosed with cystic fibrosis. Annie's parents were desperate to secure the best care possible. Luckily, they got an appointment at a nearby prestigious children's hospital where Annie was seen by expert physicians and assorted staff skilled in the management of cystic fibrosis. At the end of the visit, Annie's parents were given a care plan designed to give her the longest life possible. One can only imagine the gratitude the parents felt as they drove away from the facility with the knowledge they had seen the best. Except that they had not! The performance of the doctors and the center Annie had visited was at the lower end of the bell curve for sites managing cystic fibrosis even though the site was a Cystic Fibrosis Foundation center of excellence committed to following accepted guidelines. Another academic center, just a few hundred miles away, achieved life expectancies nearly twice that achieved by Annie's doctors. It seems the doctors at the second site were somehow able to "stay ahead of the pack," leading to superior outcomes. How?

A few months after Dr. Gawande's *New Yorker* article was published, I was headed home after a busy day at the office. As I exited the hospital into the adjacent parking deck, I spotted a man getting into his car some distance away. He appeared to have a large bundle under his arm that he hastily shoved into the back seat. As he drove in my direction I recognized him as Dr. B, a highly respected, older internist known for his clinical acumen and genteel demeanor. He was considered a physician's physician, much admired by his colleagues and greatly beloved by his patients. In other words, he was a true role model. Dr. B was also in solo practice, a rarity even at that time but certainly much more so today. As he drew alongside me, he slowed to a stop, rolled down the car window and said hello. In the back seat, I saw several medical charts, easily identifiable by their distinctive covers and colorful section tabs. I jokingly inquired, "Are you behind on your dictations," half expecting him to answer affirmatively with a note of shared resignation. "No, it's my homework" was his surprisingly cheerful response. "Homework? I didn't know you were taking classes," I retorted. "I'm not," he replied. He continued, "Every few weeks I take a few [patient] charts home to review." Gesturing to the seat behind him, he said, "These are all charts of patients with thyroid disease. I'll go through them to make sure I've done what I needed to do. It's also a great way to review a topic and I always learn something new." With that he drove off. For me it was an "aha" moment, an epiphany. To wit, while a doctor may know what to do in a given clinical scenario, how many doctors take the time to examine what *they* do in that situation? Not that many, it turns out, and yet here was a solo practitioner assessing his performance for no reason other than a desire to know he was doing the right thing for his patients. The encounter immediately brought to mind Gawande's article in which he noted, statistically speaking, most physicians are "average." One might argue that is not a bad thing since physicians are comprised of highly intelligent men and women with the bell curve skewed to the right. But even among such an elite crowd, the majority are "average." Reflecting on this truth, Gawande asks a hard question: for anyone who takes responsibility for what they do, what if they turn out to be average? Gawande contends there is no shame in being average but notes, "What troubles people isn't so much *being* average as *settling* for it." Clearly, *not* settling for average was Dr. B's quest. It was not a vain effort to outperform his peers. Rather it was Dr. B's attempt to be the best *he* could be. To some, Dr. B's willingness to honestly self-assess might seem inconsequential—a little thing—but to me it was emblematic of Dr. B's dedication to his profession and to his patients.

The same year Gawande's "Bell Curve" article was published I had the privilege of serving as president of the American Society of Clinical Oncology, better known as ASCO. Typically, ASCO presidents have a "theme" for their term, and mine was "Cancer Survivorship," chosen to highlight the good work of the National Coalition for Cancer Survivorship, an organization founded by Dr. Fitzhugh Mullan and led by Ellen Stovall, both cancer survivors. I, too, am a cancer survivor, the first to serve as ASCO president in its more than 40-year history. Ironically, my successor, Dr. Sandra Horning, also is a cancer survivor. The fact that ASCO had never had a cancer survivor serve as its president and now had two in a row struck *New York Times* reporter Lawrence Altman (also a physician) as interesting and newsworthy. He wrote an article about Dr. Horning and me, using the opportunity to delve into the then relatively new field of cancer survivorship.[5] In turn, his article prompted Terry Gross, host of NPR's "Fresh Air" program, to interview Dr. Horning and me in a segment titled "A Personal Stake in Beating Cancer."[6] In a wide-ranging conversation, Mrs. Gross queried us about our professional and personal experiences with cancer. I was as much a listener as I was a participant, and one response from Dr. Horning struck me as particularly revealing. At one point during the interview, she expressed considerable gratitude toward her surgeon for the promptness with which she had provided the pathology results of a lymph node dissection. The action of Dr. Horning's surgeon was highly commendable and should be the norm, but alas it is not. However, when it does happen, it is telling, and I believe indicative of a really good doctor. It was a small point—a little thing—but Mrs. Gross immediately picked up on the significance of providing timely test results and noted how consequential it is to patients and their family members. I too had endured the wait for a biopsy result and can attest to the heightened anxiety one feels during the interregnum between procedure and outcome, so her comments resonated with me. In a similar vein, I recently had cataract surgery. On the first postoperative day my long-time internist called to ask how I was doing. To be clear, that meant he had made a mental note of my surgery date, remembered that date, and then took the time to call even though he had nothing to do with the procedure. No one prompted him to do that! It was a small but highly personal and meaningful gesture—a little thing.

Back in 1972, while reviewing the records of a newly admitted patient, a co-resident of mine suddenly remarked to no one in particular, "Good doctors leave good tracks!" In an era before electronic medical records, paper charts were the norm. Paper charts typically stayed with the office or hospital where they were generated. If a patient was transferred from one facility to another, you were lucky to get a photocopy of some portion of the chart, sometimes consisting of the odd pages or the even pages but usually not both. If outside records were provided, they were often thrown together in a non-chronological fashion with copious extraneous, often useless data included. It took perseverance to work one's way through such records. Rare was the circumstance when a carefully prepared medical summary accompanied the patient. That day in 1972 happened to be one of those rare circumstances for my co-resident. With a curt "Look at this!" he handed me a sheet of paper. It was the referring physician's handwritten summary of the patient's hospital course. It was clear and concise with all the pertinent details—a little thing but a godsend on a busy admit day. As I looked up from reading the summary, my co-resident declared, "A 10-point buck made those tracks," which was his folksy, roundabout way of saying, a good doctor wrote the summary. Even as a non-hunter, I had to agree.

Are these three physicians examples of "good doctors"? Possibly the answer can be gleaned from the life of William Osler, considered to be the greatest clinician of the 20th century, whose influence on the practice of medicine reverberates to this day. Contemporaries spoke glowingly of Osler's medical skills, his joie de vivre, his creativity, and his humanity. He was enormously productive, writing hundreds of scientific articles and singlehandedly authoring the first comprehensive textbook of medicine. He was by all accounts a good doctor. What set him apart? What special skill or talents did he possess? Michael Bliss, one of Osler's biographers, proclaimed [7]:

Osler was committed to excellence in the practice of medicine in a way that dazzled both his students and his colleagues. He never cut corners, never avoided confronting his mistakes, never became set in his ways. Most of the students and colleagues who observed Osler with patients thought he was the best they had ever seen. Most of the patients thought so too.

The essence of Osler's greatness is perhaps best captured in this observation written in 1927 by his colleague James C. Wilson [8]:

He had a trait that so many of us lack—greatness in little things—method, system, punctuality, order, the economic use of time. These have been the handmaidens to his greater gifts. These have enabled him to widen his usefulness to lands beyond the seas.

—Seest thou a man diligent in his business? He shall stand before kings.

So how does one define a "good doctor," and how can you tell? To be sure, the good doctor possesses all of the characteristics desired by patients, but, more than that, good doctors strive to be the best they can be, not for personal glory or public approbation but because the profession demands it and it's what patients expect.[7] Good doctors simply do not settle for being "average." It's their "greatness at little things"—a willingness to self-assess, a timely phone call, a well-crafted summary, all done quietly without fanfare or publicity—that sets them apart. These supposed little things—done out of habit—are indicative of a commitment to excellence. "Excellence, then, is not an act, but a habit" [9]. In short,

Good doctors are defined by what they do when no one is looking.

That is why it is so difficult to define the good doctor. Hopefully, you'll know it when you see it.

NOTES

1 In case you're wondering, I was told my lecture was *almost* as engaging and informative as the cannibalism lecture.
2 "The single biggest problem in communication is the illusion that it has taken place."—George Bernard Shaw
3 Full disclosure: I am a former member of the American Board of Internal Medicine (ABIM) Board of Directors.
4 www.npr.org/sections/therecord/2012/02/14/146880432/the-truth-about-van-halen-and-those-brown-m-ms
5 www.nytimes.com/2005/05/24/health/policy/at-the-helm-oncologists-with-cancer.html
6 https://freshairarchive.org/segments/personal-stake-beating-cancer
7 When was the last time you were at a dinner party and heard someone praise their doctor for being "really average"?

REFERENCES

1. Swensen SJ, Meyer GS, Nelson EC, Hunt Jr. GC, Pryor DB, Weissberg JI, Kaplan GS, Daley J, Yates GR, Chassin MR, James BC, Berwick DM. Cottage industry to postindustrial care—The revolution in health care delivery. *N Engl J Med* 2010;362(5):e12.
2. Bendapudi NM, Berry LL, Frey KA, Parish JT, Rayburn WL. Patients' perspectives on ideal physician behaviors. *Mayo Clin Proc* 2006;81(3):338–344.
3. Hurwitz B, Vass A. What's a good doctor, and how can you make one? *BMJ.* 2002;325(7366):667–668.
4. Kaplan R. The clinicide phenomenon: An exploration of medical murder. *Australas Psychiatry* 2007;15(4):299–304.
5. Sun LH, Weber L, Godfrey H. Doctors who put lives at risk with COVID misinformation rarely punished. *The Washington Post*, 2023.
6. Gawande A. The bell curve. *New Yorker*. December 6, 2004.
7. Bliss M. *William Osler: A Life in Medicine*. New York, NY: Oxford University Press, 1999.
8. Wilson JC. Dr. Osler in Philadelphia, teacher and clinician. In Abbott ME, ed., *Appreciations & Reminiscences of Sir William Osler, Bart*. Toronto, ON: Murray Publishing Co., Limited, 1927: 245–248.
9. Durant W. *The Story of Philosophy*. Garden City, NY: Garden City Publishing Co., Inc, 1926.

2 Personomics

Roy C. Ziegelstein

I wasn't particularly fond of the first two years of medical school. We spent most of our days mainly in the classroom. What we learned was interesting; however, it was never connected to a particular patient or to a patient's story, at least not intentionally, and making a connection to any individual with any life experience was left up to us and our imagination. This frustrated me so much that I actually gave serious thought to dropping out of school, but I soldiered on, eventually making it to my first clinical rotation.

And then it was like magic!

I was introduced to patients. Sure, they had interesting medical conditions, some of which I had learned about during the first two years of medical school, and they required drugs or operations, some of which I had learned about during the first two years of medical school, but they also had lives! Stories! All the medicine I was learning was now connected to someone's life. It was somehow much easier to remember and far more interesting. I learned about diseases and treatments, and I felt fulfilled because I was able to care for other human beings.

Of course, the concept of Personomics [1]—which I coined 30 years later—was unknown to me at the time by that name, and yet I would say the value of knowing the patient as a person was clear even then. Or perhaps I should say one aspect of that value proposition was clear: it made me feel engaged, fulfilled, and rejuvenated. I think in retrospect I probably exhibited symptoms of burnout the first two years, although I don't recall anyone ever using that word, and I don't think I knew what it was. In fact, the term "burnout" had been described by Herbert Freudenberger less than ten years earlier [2]. In retrospect, it was from that experience and from the extraordinary feelings I developed from getting to know patients that the concept of Personomics began to take shape. Moreover, I suspect it was at that time that I began to recognize that Personomics could be an antidote for burnout, even though I didn't know either term.

What is Personomics? It describes the collective information needed to know the patient as a person. It is a term that should be reserved for health care, and so it is more specifically the information needed to know the patient as a person to provide individualized care—and often to optimally diagnose and treat a patient—in the context of the specific health care setting. It is not knowing that the patient was born in New Jersey or that they have a dog named Spike unless, of course, that information is relevant to the patient's care. It is information about the patient's psychological, social, cultural, behavioral, economic, and unique life circumstances that influences their predisposition to certain health conditions, how those conditions may manifest in a given patient, and how the patient may respond to treatment [1].

Actually, if I really think about it, the concept of Personomics was born more specifically in my first year of medical school on one particular day and in one specific setting. A group of us were sitting at a table in the library studying for an exam. The self-appointed leader of the study group announced it was time to take a break. Before the break, though, she asked us all a question:

If you had to choose, which would you rather be: a doctor who was technically skilled and knowledgeable or a doctor who knew the patient well as a human being?

DOI: 10.1201/9781003409373-2

One by one, the self-appointed group leader went around the table. One person chose "technically skilled and knowledgeable," and the next chose "knowing the patient," and so on. Then it came to me. I said the first thing that came to mind:

I don't think you have to choose.

In fact, I would say it differently now. It's not just that you can be technically skilled and knowledgeable and know the patient as a person at the same time; it's that you can't really practice medicine optimally and deliver great care without knowing the patient as a person.

Fast-forward to my internal medicine internship. One day in particular stands out. On that day, one of the true giants in medicine who made a discovery that changed how we understand human health was one of nine patients I admitted one evening on call. He was 92 years old and was still working in his office when he got up on a chair so he could reach a book on the top shelf of his bookcase. He stumbled and fell, striking his flank on a radiator heater. He went to the Emergency Department to see if he had done any serious damage and was found to have a couple of red blood cells per high power field on a urinalysis. He was admitted for a possible renal contusion and microscopic hematuria. Not surprisingly, he was my least sick patient that evening, and the other patients got far more of my attention. In fact, between all the admissions and cross-cover, I never really talked to him beyond asking the standard questions interns were supposed to ask to complete an admission note. His personal attending physician came the following morning and appropriately and understandably told me to complete his discharge paperwork, which, of course, I did with pleasure, since my service had swelled overnight.

There were many reasons to hospitalize a patient in those days, including microscopic hematuria, so it seems. However, keeping a patient in the hospital so the intern could get to know him as a person was not on the list, and so this patient was discharged without my having the opportunity to get to know him at all. I had no chance to ask him about his life or about his work. Not long after, I realized that I had admitted one of the most legendary figures in medicine and biomedical science, and I had wasted the opportunity to talk to him, let alone to get to learn about his life.

I was demoralized, emotionally exhausted, and burned out. I thought I was a terrible doctor.

So one of the values of Personomics is clearly that it makes medicine more enjoyable. More fulfilling. More rewarding. More engaging. It is—as I wrote earlier—an antidote to burnout. I think this value should be sufficient to make Personomics part of every clinician's practice and of every medical student's training. While the value to patients of being known as people seems intuitive, the potential value *to physicians* of having patients feel understood has also been emphasized. Knowing patients as people may engender more positive feelings to physicians that then make physicians feel better about their work [3]. Now two decades ago, Horowitz et al. [4] published findings from workshops with physicians in which they were asked about "a work-related experience that they found meaningful, defined as 'something that you found to be important and fulfilling or that reaffirmed your commitment to medicine.'" Among the findings about what doctors find meaningful in their work, the authors concluded that:

we were struck that nearly all the doctors, although given deliberately general and nondirective instructions, described a [sic] nontechnical, humanistic interactions with patients as experiences that fulfilled them and reaffirmed their commitment to medicine. Rather than recounting tales of diagnostic and therapeutic triumphs, they uniformly told stories about crossing from the world of biomedicine into their patient's world.

So Personomics can add meaning, fulfillment, and joy to the practice of medicine. However, there's something else.

Again, back to internship. I remember another day when I admitted two patients in the same two-bed hospital room. The person in the A bed was in his eighties. He had many medical problems and was taking a laundry list of medications. He was an immigrant from East Asia. He weighed only a little more than 100 pounds. The person in the B bed was in his early thirties. He was otherwise healthy and took no medications. He was from the local community, as was his family. He weighed more than 300 pounds. As I reviewed my admissions for the evening, I realized that these two patients had the same diagnosis and were being treated with the same medication at the same dose—even though they couldn't have been more different. It occurred to me that this seemed silly, even primitive. I thought about the day when we would be able to tailor medical care to the individual patient. I'm not going to say that I coined the term "precision medicine" that day; in fact, it is not my term at all. I will say, though, that I realized the need for precision medicine that day and that, when the concept was finally coined and popularized, I became a big fan and still am.

Now fast-forward quite a number of years to when I was a cardiologist attending in the clinic, precepting several fellows. One of the fellows saw two patients that day, both of whom had recently been discharged after sustaining a myocardial infarction. In each case, the fellow assessed the patient perfectly; reviewed the medication list to make sure it contained aspirin, a beta blocker, and a statin; and discussed a heart-healthy diet. The first patient was a fairly wealthy attorney who lived in the suburbs, just a short drive in her luxury car to the neighborhood gourmet food market. The second patient lived in a low-income part of the city, with no affordable or healthy fresh food anywhere nearby and no access to transportation to get to a store that sold healthy foods. Unfortunately, the fellow didn't know that because he didn't ask. His dietary recommendations to both patients were the same. Indeed, he didn't even know that, while the first patient had two refrigerators in her home, the second did not even have a working refrigerator in his apartment. The notion of treating these two patients the same and not tailoring treatment recommendations to each patient based on knowledge of the patient's unique life circumstances is as silly and as primitive as recommending the same medication at the same dose to individuals whose genomics, proteomics, pharmacogenomics, and metabolomics are as different as the neighborhoods, incomes, and access to transportation and healthy foods as the second pair of patients. It seems to me just as valuable to know whether a patient has a working refrigerator as it does to know if they have a gene affecting their response to a particular medication.

That's the second benefit of Personomics: the ability to provide sophisticated, precisely tailored diagnostic and treatment recommendations that make sense for individual patients based on knowledge of their social, psychological, economic, and other unique life circumstances.

Let me provide an example that illustrates how Personomics can assist in diagnosis. Some years ago, an older man was referred to me for evaluation of near-syncope. He had numerous cardiovascular risk factors, including diabetes and hypertension, and the referral indicated that the patient often felt like he would pass out when he exercised. That story alone suggested something bad. Exercise-induced syncope or near-syncope often suggests aortic stenosis, severe myocardial ischemia, or perhaps a dangerous ventricular arrhythmia. However, the patient had had an echocardiogram and cardiac stress test several years earlier, and they were both normal.

Something dangerous was certainly still possible, but what that something might be was a bit of a mystery.

I spoke to the patient and asked him to tell me about himself as a person. He was retired and lived with his wife in a modest home in the outskirts of the city. The home had two levels with a finished basement. In the basement was a television, a couch and lounge chair, a coffee table, and a treadmill. I asked the patient what he liked to do for fun. He and his wife were avid churchgoers, and they enjoyed going shopping and spending time together. His wife was in very good health. Wanting to keep up with her, he tried to better his own health and manage his cardiovascular risk factors. He and his wife both ate a healthy diet, and he exercised nearly every day. He and his wife walked outdoors when the weather was nice, and he never had any chest discomfort, shortness of breath, or lightheadedness on those occasions. The same was true when he walked up stairs or when he did yard work. However, it was a different story when he used the treadmill. On those occasions, he felt very lightheaded, and in fact on several occasions he almost passed out, having to ease himself down to the carpeted floor in his finished basement.

I asked him about the specific circumstances of treadmill use that made him feel this way. As I noted in the published description of this patient's presentation [5], he told me that he actually felt fine while on the treadmill, and only after stopping did he experience any sensation of lightheadedness. Wanting to understand the circumstances better and not having the opportunity to travel to his home with him to ask him to act out a typical episode, I asked him to imagine himself in his home on his treadmill and show me step-by-step what he did when he stopped exercising. He proceeded to walk in place as if on a treadmill, and he then "got off" the treadmill and stopped walking in place. He told me, "Now I check my pulse, and that's when I get really lightheaded." I asked him to act that out as well. He proceeded to press on his neck to check his carotid pulse, and he then started to stagger and had to be eased down in a chair. The diagnosis of carotid sinus hypersensitivity then became obvious. I asked our assistant in the clinic to connect him to an electrocardiography machine, and I prepared him for carotid sinus massage.

I would argue that, without getting to know these aspects of this patient's life circumstances around his near-syncopal events, many additional cardiac tests would have been arranged and performed. His care would have been more expensive, and it would have taken much more time, likely weeks or months for the tests to be arranged and resulted. In fact, those tests would almost certainly not have led to the correct diagnosis and might well have led to additional unnecessary diagnostic tests and treatments. This scenario illustrates how the process of getting to know the patient as a person—which some feel takes too long given the realities of modern medical practice—actually can make the process of care more accurate and also more efficient, so that the clinician gets to the right answer in less time.

So if Personomics is important, how can it be put into practice?

It may be daunting for the busy clinician to consider having to ask questions to get to know the patient as an individual. In addition to the perceived time sink, some clinicians may not be confident that they know the right questions to ask.

I would argue that the average clinician feels the same way about the "-omics" of precision medicine. In fact, I'm quite certain that the average clinician has more confidence asking questions to try to get to know the patient as a person than analyzing genetic information and communicating this information to the patient. And I suspect the average clinician also has more time for the former.

What questions should the clinician ask to get to know the patient as a person?

It depends on the context. It is not likely that a pediatrician caring for an eight-year-old needs to ask the same questions as the obstetrician caring for a pregnant patient or a colorectal surgeon evaluating a patient for a hemicolectomy. Perhaps the common thread is to ask a general question and then pause and listen. Tell me something about you. Tell me what you do in a normal day. Tell me what you think I need to know to provide you the best care.

Some years ago, we published a paper in which we asked physicians who had been recognized for their clinical excellence what questions or phrases they used to get to know patients as people [6]. We queried clinicians who had been inducted into the Miller Coulson Academy of Clinical Excellence at Johns Hopkins in part based on evaluation and feedback from patients. The physicians were from a range of specialties, including cardiology, critical care medicine, general internal medicine, geriatrics, nephrology, neurology, orthopedic surgery, and psychiatry. Some of the suggested questions included, "Tell me about yourself" and "What do you enjoy doing?" or "Tell me about your family and who is important in your life."

The mere fact that we had to research this question about how outstanding clinicians get to know their patients as people says something about the state of medicine today. Would we think of doing a research study in which we asked outstanding clinicians how they do anything else fundamental to good medicine? Would we ask how they auscultate the heart or palpate the liver? Would we ask how they interpret the basic metabolic panel or complete blood count? Would we expect that such a study would produce information considered novel or interesting enough to be published in a peer-reviewed journal? Of course not. The fact that this work was done and published tells us that most physicians today don't understand and appreciate the value of knowing their patient as a person or—if they do—they don't know how to find the information they need to do so.

So this would seem to beg the question: if today's physicians really don't know how to obtain this information or if they feel they don't have the time necessary to know the patient as a person, could this aspect of medical practice be performed by artificial intelligence (AI) or—better yet—*should* it be? I don't mean to ask here whether AI should *replace* a physician. Instead, I wonder whether AI could be added to the physician's tool kit to *assist* in this vital aspect of medical care. In the March 22, 1888, edition of the *Boston Medical Surgical Journal* (the predecessor of the *New England Journal of Medicine*), a "successful young physician in a prosperous country town" wrote an unsigned letter to the editor describing "the contents of my bag and buggy" [7]. It turns out that the contents of the "doctor's black bag" available to this anonymous country doctor have not really changed in the 135 years since. In a 2005 article entitled, "Revolutionizing the Doctor's Black Bag" [8], Hellmann et al. noted, "It is time to introduce modern tools into the black bag; in the process, what a physician can accomplish at the bedside can be transformed."

Think about how AI is used to perform complex, high-risk tasks that only humans were thought able to do in the past. Think about self-driving cars. Somehow AI determines which data are needed to operate a motor vehicle, even in traffic, and obtains that information through sensors and cameras, allowing it to then assist a person—or perhaps even to replace human decision making—by controlling steering, accelerating, and braking. AI uses machine learning algorithms and neural networks to collect, analyze, and act on data to perform many complex tasks where the cost of incorrect action may well be human life. AI can not only drive a car; it can also fly a plane. Martin Takáč, Associate Professor at Mohamed bin Zayed University of Artificial Intelligence in the United Arab Emirates, notes [9]:

An AI system can simulate millions of miles of flying involving thousands of scenarios—much more than a human pilot could ever do. Even with crises that will never arise, you can run through all these different variations. It's not doing X number of hours in flight school and you're ready to go. So in this sense, I think human pilots can be less safe than AI.

So could AI assist in the practice of Personomics? I actually think so. AI might help answer the question about what information each clinician needs to know about the patient in each circumstance. That information is likely to be very different in each setting and for each patient. Clinicians can add empathy, compassion, personal touch, and all the critical elements that are part of human–human connections, but the actual information may well be obtained by AI, perhaps even better than a human can do so and almost certainly with greater efficiency.

Recently, ChatGPT, a type of AI called a large language model, made headlines when an article [10] was published showing that it did a pretty good job with the United States Medical Licensing Examination (USMLE). In fact, *Business Insider* published an article [11] whose title screamed, "ChatGPT Is on Its Way to Becoming a Virtual Doctor, Lawyer, and Business Analyst." It is not hard to imagine that if AI can pass a test required to become a practicing physician, it just might be able to perform some of the functions of a practicing physician or at least assist in medical practice, especially in the realm of Personomics. This is not science fiction. This is reality.

It is reasonable to ask whether AI can develop an understanding of the components needed to know the patient as a person, especially if physicians cannot or will not. Perhaps AI can learn aspects about each individual that are of greatest relevance to that particular clinical encounter, obtaining these data from the patient, either through a written questionnaire or as a chatbot. The AI can then analyze the data to form a cohesive picture of the patient in order to tailor diagnostics and therapeutics to the individual, either alone or with the assistance of a human interface. In this way, AI could actually assist physicians with their work, much as a handheld ultrasound assists me in my work as a cardiologist, providing data that would not have previously been immediately available to me during the patient encounter and that I cannot determine through physical examination alone (for example, the patient's left ventricular ejection fraction or whether they have a pericardial effusion). Perhaps AI can help physicians be better diagnosticians and also add joy and fulfillment to their work. Perhaps AI can be the answer to both diagnostic errors and physician burnout.

In summary, medicine is the most wonderful career in the world, and getting to know the patient as a person is the most wonderful part of the practice of medicine. I think doctors today want three things, even if they are not optimistic about the possibility of achieving the trifecta. First, they want to be great doctors. Modern doctors. Doctors who diagnose and treat with a high degree of precision. And doctors who avoid mistakes. Second, they want to be happy. They seek joy. Fulfillment. They want to be engaged in their work. Third, they want to diagnose and treat in a way that is affordable and accessible to the patient and that is consistent with their obligation to be good stewards of society's resources.

It's understandable that doctors may feel pessimistic about achieving even one of these goals, let alone all three. The time clinicians can spend with patients is short. Practicing medicine with a high degree of precision is seen as requiring lots of tests and resources—some of which may not even be part of routine practice, like genetic testing—and all of which require a high degree of sophistication to interpret and communicate to the patient. Interpretation and communication take time for the clinician. Waiting for the results of tests takes time for the patient. Referral to other specialists who may be needed to perform and interpret these tests takes more time for both patient and clinician. And endless documentation in the electronic medical record—often charting things that seem irrelevant to patient care—eats into time with family and friends and sucks fulfillment and joy out of life like the Dementors in Harry Potter [12] consume someone's soul, feed on human happiness, and produce utter abject despair.

Personomics doesn't require a referral to another specialist. You don't need to wait for the results of a lab test. Personomics is never "pending." And yet it provides a high degree of precision, allowing the clinician to practice in a way that is relevant and meaningful to the patient, providing diagnostics and treatments tailored to the individual's unique life circumstances. At the same time, it restores fulfillment and joy in the practice of medicine. And it doesn't cost a dime. Personomics is the triple threat.

REFERENCES

1. Ziegelstein RC. Personomics. *JAMA Intern Med* 2015;175(6):888–889.
2. Heinemann LV, Heinemann T. Burnout research: Emergence and scientific investigation of a contested diagnosis. *SAGE Open* 2017; 7(1). https://doi.org/10.1177/2158244017697154
3. Dobler CC, West CP, Montori VM. Can shared decision making improve physician well-being and reduce burnout? *Cureus* 2017; 9(8):e1615.
4. Horowitz CR, Suchman AL, Branch WT Jr, Frankel RM. What do doctors find meaningful about their work? *Ann Intern Med* 2003;138(9):772–775.
5. Ziegelstein RC. Near-syncope after exercise. *JAMA* 2004;292(10):1221–1226.
6. Hanyok LA, Hellmann DB, Rand C, Ziegelstein RC. Practicing patient-centered care: the questions clinically excellent physicians use to get to know their patients as individuals. *Patient* 2012;5(3):141–145.
7. Anonymous. The country physician's armamentarium. *Boston Med Surg J* 1888; 118:306–307.
8. Hellmann DB, Whiting-O'Keefe Q, Ziegelstein RC, Martin LD, Shapiro E. Revolutionizing the doctor's black bag. A step to revitalizing primary care in medicine. *Pharos Alpha Omega Alpha Honor Med Soc* 2005;68(3):22–26.
9. Mohamed bin Zayed University of Artificial Intelligence. "Would you fly in a plane piloted solely by AI?" *Wired*. January 20, 2022. Available from: https://wired.me/technology/artificial-intelligence/would-you-fly-in-a-plane-piloted-solely-by-ai/
10. Kung TH, Cheatham M, Medenilla A, Sillos C, De Leon L, Elepaño C, et al. Performance of ChatGPT on USMLE: Potential for AI-assisted medical education using large language models. *PLoS Digit Health* 2023;2(2):e0000198. https://doi.org/10.1371/journal.pdig.0000198
11. Varanasi Lakshmi. ChatGPT is on its way to becoming a virtual doctor, lawyer, and business analyst. Here's a list of advanced exams the AI bot has passed so far. *BusinessInsider*. 2023. Available from: www.businessinsider.com/list-here-are-the-exams-chatgpt-has-passed-so-far-2023-1
12. Rowling JK. *Harry Potter and the Prisoner of Azkaban*. New York, NY: Arthur A. Levine Books, 1999.

3 Diagnosis

Jerome P. Kassirer

Expert diagnostic reasoning is an indispensable foundation of optimal medical care. It is the gateway to accurate prognosis, risk assessment, test selection, and especially appropriate therapy. Centuries of experience in making diagnoses, as well as recent advances in clinical problem solving, have yielded useful principles and a framework within which physicians assess information, identify illness, and offer advice. Striking recent advances in the medical application of artificial intelligence are already encroaching on the traditional diagnostic role of physicians, but the technology is evolving so rapidly that it is impossible to assess how much or how soon the role of doctors will be usurped by technology. Given the possibility that much of our cognitive approach might well be superseded by machine learning, it behooves us to understand the state of the art of diagnosis as currently practiced by humans.

Traditional admonitions to learn diagnostic reasoning by reading the first 100 or so pages of a prominent medical textbook were replaced in the mid-20th century by a proposal that Venn diagrams, namely overlapping circles containing symptoms or signs, would lead to diagnostic clues or even clarity, but the application of these intersecting circles in the real world of medicine faltered and was abandoned. Studies of clinicians actually engaged in clinical problem solving exposed a far more complex process consisting of elements that mirrored the scientific process itself [1]. Concepts such as hypothesis generation, context formulation, evolving hypotheses, accumulation and evaluation of new evidence, probabilistic reasoning, and validation of working hypotheses comprise the components of the diagnostic process and have opened these components to an examination of their accuracy and sources of potential errors. The rediscovery of Bayes theorem, an 18th-century, long neglected mathematical formulation for combining and interpreting data, including diagnostic hypotheses represented as probabilities, provided another basis for understanding, using, and teaching fundamental diagnostic approaches [2].

In this chapter, I cover, sometimes in broad brushstrokes and sometimes in detail, the basic tenets of the diagnostic process based on research and personal experience for more than six decades. I have interlaced personal and pragmatic approaches with mathematical methods and have liberally instantiated unfamiliar and sometimes arcane concepts with cogent examples.

HYPOTHESIS GENERATION

Diagnostic reasoning begins with the receipt of a cue or set of cues: often the cue is a patient's reason for seeking medical advice (known as the chief complaint), or a new test result, or a chance finding on a scan or X-ray. The cue may be simple (such as, "A 70-year-old man with pain in the chest") or detailed and complex (such as "A 70-year-old man with severe hypertension with sudden excruciating back and chest pain"). Studies show that expert clinicians rapidly formulate preliminary diagnostic hypotheses that generate a context for further data gathering, interpretation, and action. One preliminary hypothesis might be "heart disease"; another might be much more specific, such as "dissecting aortic aneurysm." Often the preliminary list is a large nonspecific group of disorders, all of which could explain a patient's initial clinical manifestations. These initial hypotheses are first approximations of a final diagnosis and are based on doctors' clinical experience, preliminary patient

DOI: 10.1201/9781003409373-3

data, and relevant background information. Sex and age occasionally are such clues; recent falls or exposure to toxins or new medications are others. The population that includes the patient can also be critically important: such demographic information often adds importantly to the specificity of the preliminary hypothesis. High fever in a patient who returned days ago from equatorial Africa, for example, generates far different diagnostic hypotheses than the same high temperature in a patient who recently ate raw pork in Milwaukee. Further testing and information gathering in such circumstances are critically dependent on such inferences.

HYPOTHESIS REFINEMENT

The next step in the diagnostic process, namely hypothesis refinement, involves gathering more data, reconsidering the initial diagnostic hypotheses, and iterating toward a final diagnosis. The data sources are exceptionally broad: new information can come from the patient's history, physical examination, or existing laboratory test results that might strengthen, weaken, solidify, or disprove the initial hypotheses. An assessment is made whether additional testing is warranted. The physician ponders, "What best test or tests, including blood tests and scans, might get us closer to a correct answer?" From the beginning of a diagnostic session to the end, the list of hypotheses evolve as new information is incorporated. What first may seem to be acute pericarditis may eventually turn out to be acute pancreatitis: although the initial symptoms and signs may have pointed to a cardiac event, the actual inflammation might instead be found many inches away when the patient's serum is found to be milky or when a markedly elevated serum lipase result is reported. Such surprises are the exceptions, not the rule; more often, the evolution of the set of diagnostic conditions (the so-called differential diagnosis) is gradual, and it often involves a cluster of possible items (such as pleuritis, pneumonia, myocardial infarction, pericarditis, and myocarditis), each of which might enter or leave the changing list of hypotheses as evidence accumulates. Often in retrospect, the final and correct diagnosis may not have been considered in the original differential.

The major processes that contribute to hypothesis refinement include causal (physiologic) reasoning, pattern recognition, probabilistic reasoning, and the use and interpretation of diagnostic tests.

Causal Reasoning: Until recently when probabilistic models were introduced, causal and physiologic reasoning were the principal bases for diagnostic inquiry. Causal reasoning is dependent exclusively on fundamental knowledge about physiologic function and dysfunction and the cause-and-effect relations among physiologic variables. As such, it is specific to disease entities and independent of the patient population [3]. Metabolic pathways of the endocrine systems are illustrative. In a patient who feels chilly and sluggish, an elevated thyroid stimulating hormone level would clinch a suspected diagnosis of myxedema, and a high concentration of sodium in the urine of a hyponatremic patient with lung cancer would confirm the presence of inappropriate secretion of antidiuretic hormone. Despite this high degree of specificity, causal reasoning must be applied carefully. Chains of causal connections can be strong or weak, and weak ones may not be reliable. The strength of a causal link can be assessed by checking whether a given change in response correlates closely with the change in stimulus, whether the time sequence between the stimulus and its response is appropriate, whether an examination of the entire causal chain is credible, and whether statistical relations between one event and another correlate closely. Still, there is no certainty in causal attributions or even in correlations that pass the test of statistical validity. A final test in assessing a causal hypothesis is testing it against alternative possible explanations. An apparent explanation by a given causal hypothesis of a set of findings does not necessarily prove that the proposed connection is correct: maybe some other mechanism explains the findings better.

Pattern Recognition: No consideration of the diagnostic process would be complete without a mention of pattern recognition as a diagnostic aid. Many recognizable patterns are derived originally from physiologic models; others are discovered during long experience by expert clinicians. A patient with clay-colored greasy stools and dark urine, for example, should be suspected of having obstruction of the bile and pancreatic duct, likely by an undiscovered pancreatic cancer. A weak patient with severe hypokalemia and a non-anion gap metabolic acidosis and an alkaline urine has type 1 renal tubular acidosis until proven otherwise, and a patient whose muscles are slowly atrophying and who, on close examination, demonstrates muscle fasciculations should be immediately suspected of having amyotrophic lateral sclerosis. Although these patterns are often correct and may give the impression, when invoked correctly, as having been a magical diagnostic "hit," they cannot be relied upon for everyday clinical use: they simply do not encompass the wide extent of disease entities.

Probabilistic Reasoning: After initial hypothesis generation, probabilistic reasoning often dominates the diagnostic process. The principles of Bayes theorem are the basis for probabilistic thinking and for the clinically useful language that has evolved with it. In a Bayesian analysis, one assembles a set of diagnostic possibilities that could explain the clinical and laboratory findings. This step is critical, simply because neglecting one diagnosis might result in omitting the correct one. Then each relevant possible diagnosis is defined by a "pretest" probability, one that denotes how likely it alone could explain all of a patient's findings. The array of individual pretest probabilities (the initial differential diagnosis) adds up to 1.0, reflecting the assumption that all possible diagnostic alternatives have been included. Independently, an assessment is made of a series of "conditional probabilities." A conditional probability is the likelihood that a given item of data (a symptom, a physical sign, or a test result) is found in each of the diseases in the differential diagnosis. The ratio of the probability of the finding in one disease versus another is known as the "likelihood ratio." If one is trying to distinguish between acute pancreatitis and acute cholecystitis, for example, a disproportionately high serum amylase in one disorder versus the other (the likelihood ratio) strongly favors pancreatitis.

Once all conditional probabilities are assessed, a calculation is made that includes both the prior probabilities and the conditional probabilities, yielding a set of "posterior probabilities" that reflect the likelihood of each relevant diagnostic consideration given the data item. Details of the calculations of Bayes theorem are readily found elsewhere [3, 4]. Referring again to the distinction between pancreatitis and cholecystitis, a markedly elevated serum amylase, even with a low to moderate prior probability of pancreatitis would still yield a high posterior probability of pancreatitis. Contrarily, a normal serum amylase and lipase would cast doubt; that is, it would lower the posterior probability of pancreatitis even if its prior probability had been quite high. Making actual calculations can give some precision to these relationships. Given time constraints and other factors, Bayesian calculations are not often made, and both the prior probabilities and the conditional probabilities are combined intuitively.

Testing Principles: Diagnostic testing can be viewed in terms similar to the probabilistic principles described under hypothesis refinement [3, 4]. The data a lung scan generates can be interpreted similarly to the results of a series of blood tests. Similarly, a chest CT scan provides data on heart size, lung parenchyma, pericardial or pleural fluid, and thoracic bony integrity; a serum immunoelectrophoresis yields data on serum albumin as well as a variety of serum globulins and globulin fragments. No matter where we are in the diagnostic process, we might iterate toward a final diagnosis by ordering a diagnostic test. Before doing so, however, it is worth asking whether the test result has any chance of altering subsequent decision making. If not, why order the test? Similarly, if ordering further diagnostic tests to ramp up a diagnostic likelihood to near certainty is likely to have no additional therapeutic benefit, the fruitless tests should be discarded, especially given their added costs and risks. Decisions to test should be based on test accuracy, the risk of performing the test, and, most importantly, the test's potential usefulness in therapeutic decision making.

When considering which test or tests to order, we begin with a physician's diagnostic hypothesis, a prior probability that may have been modified already by all information collected up to this point, as just described. Key in deciding which test to order is the performance of the test itself. The performance of each individual test in each individual disease is defined in terms of the test's sensitivity and specificity. Sensitivity is the probability of a positive test result in patients known by some criterion to have a certain disease (the true positive rate); specificity is the probability of a negative test result in people known to be free of the disease (the true negative rate). Both of these rates are based on actual data derived from high-quality clinical studies. High-sensitivity tests yield a small number of false negative results; thus, when such a test is negative, a suspected diagnosis can effectively be excluded. High specificity tests yield a small number of false positive results; thus, when such a test is positive, the disease under suspicion becomes highly likely. Of course, tests are imprecise because test values in normal individuals and those with disease overlap. Positive tests may be falsely positive, and negative tests may be falsely negative. Adding to the challenge are diseases such as seronegative rheumatoid arthritis, in which a test for the disease is consistently negative.

With these considerations in mind, the results of a positive or negative test can be incorporated with the pretest probability to obtain a post-test probability in a formal calculation using Bayes theorem. Alternatively, testing judgments can be made by using a simple likelihood ratio nomogram. One starts with a pretest probability of disease, lines it up with a known likelihood ratio (for example, the probability of a true positive test in patients with a particular disease divided by the probability of a false positive test in patients without the disease), and thus identifies the post-test disease probability. Many specific likelihood ratios are well-known, but if one is not available, it can be identified from existing clinical data. Ordering the right test for the right condition is invaluable diagnostically, and, despite a given test's cost, using it may avoid risks of invasive procedures and save patients days of hospitalization.

HYPOTHESIS VERIFICATION

As hypothesis refinement proceeds and more information (test results, physical findings) accumulates, probability assessments are repeated sequentially. Some diagnoses under initial consideration become untenable as their posterior probabilities drop to vanishingly low values; some rise to the top. There exists no magic probability of disease (for example, 0.95) at which a diagnosis can be considered definitive. In the final analysis, intermediate or even final diagnoses are a measure of a physician's confidence in the accuracy of a diagnostic assertion. Even with the use of the most sophisticated testing (genetics, special histologic stains), every diagnosis, according to these precepts, must be considered somewhat tentative or incomplete. Nonetheless, at some point when the evidence points to an increasingly likely diagnosis, final diagnostic verification should be carried out. A test of diagnostic adequacy checks whether the final diagnosis accounts for all of the patient's findings, both positive and negative. A test of diagnostic coherency checks whether the patient's findings are consistent with the altered pathophysiology of the proposed disease state. A final, or working, diagnosis is one that has survived the refinement process, is unambiguous, highly likely, and has passed the adequacy and coherency criteria. The working diagnosis can reasonably be used for prognostication, risk assessment, further test selection when necessary, and treatment selection. The mechanisms of how a working diagnosis interacts with the risks of harms and benefits of therapeutic decision making are described next.

TESTING AND TREATMENT THRESHOLDS

The connection between uncertainty in diagnosis and the risks and benefits of tests and treatments is rarely made explicit, yet it is critical to optimal therapy. Diagnostic probabilities, test accuracy, and therapeutic risks and benefits merge under the concept of testing and treatment thresholds [5]. Because of inherent diagnostic uncertainty, some patients with a given disease may not receive treatment, and some people who do not have the disease will inappropriately receive treatment. In either case, harm can result. Calculating or estimating a diagnostic threshold provides guidance as to what level of uncertainty treatment should be appropriate. Consider the case of suspected appendicitis with rupture. When the probability of appendicitis is very low, laparotomy is rejected; when the probability is near certainty, surgery is mandatory. Yet clinical medicine is full of pitfalls: abdominal symptoms may be atypical, abdominal tenderness may not be precisely where it is anticipated, and even an abdominal CT scan may be somewhat ambiguous. This diagnostic uncertainty puts the surgeon in a quandary: what is the likelihood of the condition and how likely does it have to be before the benefits of surgery outweigh the risks? The probability below which surgery should be avoided and above which surgery should be carried out is the therapeutic threshold.

When a treatment for a suspected disease is highly effective and minimally risky and a physician, based on prior testing, believes that the likelihood of the disease is quite high, the optimal choice is to treat and not to employ any additional tests. When a treatment is less effective or is associated with substantial risk, confidence in the accuracy of diagnosis, namely a high probability of disease, would justify using the treatment. Explaining these relationships calls for two additional examples: prescribing statins and prescribing chemotherapy. Take the case of statin use for vascular disease. Statins are highly effective in improving lipid profiles and lowering the risk of myocardial infarction and stroke. At the same time, the risks of statins are low and rarely serious. For these reasons, the probability of vascular disease events (and the confidence of the physician in the diagnosis) would need to be low to prescribe the drug. By contrast, most chemotherapeutic drugs for cancer have limited efficacy in terms of long-term survival, and they risk serious multisystem side effects. For these reasons, the probability of cancer or lymphoma must be nearly certain (the physician must be highly confident in the diagnosis) to prescribe the drug. The demand for a clear histological or genetic diagnosis before treating cancer is the embodiment of this concept.

The treatment threshold concept entails the possibility of adding a diagnostic test in therapeutic decision making [6]. Within the divergent choices of no treatment on the one hand and treatment with a specific agent on the other, there is a single therapeutic threshold, as just described. But suppose that, to further increase or decrease the disease probability, a diagnostic test is also available. In that case, there might be two thresholds: a no-treatment/testing threshold and a testing/treatment threshold. In this case, the test is used to decide between treating or not. Below the no-treatment/testing threshold, treatment is withheld because the test would not raise the probability sufficiently to cross the threshold. Above the testing/treatment threshold, treatment is given because a test result would not lower the probability enough to cross the threshold. Between the two thresholds, the test is carried out. If negative, the chance of disease is lessened and treatment is not preferred; if positive, the probability of disease increases and the benefit and risks of treatment become more favorable. Whether or not these thresholds are calculated or estimated, the cognitive principles connecting diagnosis and treatment clarify previously unrecognized relationships between diagnostic confidence and treatment characteristics.

PRAGMATIC ACKNOWLEDGMENTS ON DIAGNOSTIC TESTS

Modern enhancements in diagnostic testing deserve special mention. Diagnosis has been revolutionized over the past 50 years by vast improvements in diagnostic testing: so much so that the cognitive aspects of assembling diagnoses are often eclipsed by new noninvasive scanning methods that shortcut the diagnostic process and permit safer invasive testing when requested [7]. Furthermore, new serological and genetic tests have sliced existing diagnostic categories thinner and thinner, creating opportunities to narrow down treatment selection based on known therapeutic responses. Often, especially in emergency departments, relevant scans are ordered even after only minimal clinical information is at hand: merely a hint that even a young person who just returned from a 12-hour plane trip has sharp chest pain would, appropriately, merit a CT scan today or even a more invasive vascular scan. Though it is true that scans in particular—CTs, ultrasounds, MRIs, PETs—have made many kinds of diagnoses faster, more accurate, and safer, they are no panacea: they must be ordered at the right time and for appropriate indications. Scanning is expensive and, as for nearly all diagnostic tools, imperfect. For all these reasons, diagnostic testing requires expert cognitive assessment. Issues include when to use a scan; whether the likelihood of a certain disease influences the need for a scan; which of many scans is most likely to yield a result for a given body area; when scans are in short supply, which patients should jump the waiting line; and which criteria should be used in making these judgments. A particularly knotty problem is the so-called incidentaloma: an abnormal and unexpected scan finding occasionally identified when no such finding had been anticipated.

Despite technical improvements, some invasive diagnostic tests still entail risk. Harms may include bleeding, viscus perforation, and kidney damage, among others. Fortunately, tests such as organ biopsies and sample collections from body cavities that previously were accompanied by serious complications have become safer over the years. These procedures are no longer hit-or-miss operations, in part because they are often performed with guidance by imaging. Moreover, advances in sampling by perfecting biopsy equipment, as well as histologic and bacteriologic sample assessment, have made testing less invasive and more precise. Despite these advances, any procedure-related risk must be incorporated into diagnostic decision making when the possible benefits of a test are being contemplated.

THE ESSENTIAL NATURE OF CLINICAL DATA

It stands to reason that the validity of the data employed in diagnostic reasoning is a crucial factor in getting the correct answer. Massive efforts have been expended since the end of the 20th century to get clinicians to search the medical literature for reliable clinical data for use in medical decision making. Experts have opined on the relative value of various kinds of medical data derived, at one extreme, from unreliable anecdotal and personal opinions to the highly reliable double-blind controlled trials or systematic reviews of diagnostic test performance. Websites of the National Institutes of Health and other prominent medical institutions also contain vast amounts of scientifically valid information. Compiled clinical data sources based on expert opinion, now widely available online, have become more and more useful as their content is reexamined regularly. Given the wide availability of solid data, there is scant excuse for not using valid information when assembling diagnoses.

Regrettably, rigorous attempts to ensure the inclusion of correct information can easily falter if the fundamental inputs, namely the patient's history and physical findings, are sloppily accumulated. The trite phrase, "garbage in, garbage out," applies notably here. It is never sufficient to be satisfied with a patient's complaint of weakness, for instance, without drilling down on what the symptom represents medically (lightheadedness? loss of consciousness? inability to brush their teeth or rise from a chair?). Neither should one be satisfied with a physical examination that omits the status of the neck veins in a breathless patient or fails to check the ankle reflexes in a sluggish patient because the patient is inconveniently bedridden. And it is essential to gather all relevant findings, including tests and diagnoses, from recent doctor visits or hospitalizations. The aim is simple: get all the data; use the best data.

COGNITIVE DIAGNOSTIC ERRORS

We all use shortcuts or rules of thumb in making judgments. These so-called heuristics are generally accurate, yet sometimes they can be misleading. In laboratory experiments, using young normal individuals as test subjects, cognitive researchers have identified several of the common heuristics that lead to errors in assessments of probabilities and numerical calculations. One error occurs when assessing the likelihood of an event based on its close resemblance to another well-defined event. Another occurs when assessing the chance of some event based on readily recallable similar events. A third occurs when assessing an outcome based on a particular starting point. Careful examination of actual discussions during the diagnostic process has revealed the existence of these and other cognitive errors in medicine [8]. Improper interpretation of clinical cues can lead to defective hypothesis generation; overly specific expectations for a disease can lead to inappropriate exclusion of diagnoses; and overestimation of variation in disease manifestations can lead to erroneous diagnosis verification. In short, cognitive errors occur in all stages of the diagnostic process. Though some errors have trivial or no consequences and are often identified and corrected subsequently during diagnostic inquiry, some have serious consequences, including delay of treatment, inappropriate treatment, and unnecessary testing. Avoiding these errors involves understanding that they happen, identifying them, and providing instant feedback when possible. Sharing diagnostic decision making with others probably reduces the chance that such errors will occur. Unfortunately, general, nonspecific debiasing approaches are mostly untested. It is imperative to appreciate that errors in diagnosis have as their etiology many other causes: inexpert interpretation of tests, failure of communication, incorrect sample identification, use of flawed or incomplete data, and many more. In this section, only those based on flawed cognition are considered.

TEACHING DIAGNOSTIC REASONING

Diagnosis is a cognitive task. It is a classic example of human problem solving under conditions of uncertainty. It is not dissimilar to the kind of iterative problem solving that mechanics employ when examining a clunky car engine or a wobbly airplane. Diseases are many and their manifestations enormous. From one patient to another, the same disease may have quite different manifestations, different responses to therapy, and different time courses. Given this exceptional variation, finding the kernel of truth in a morass of signs, symptoms, and test results can be difficult. Clinicians have invented a variety of aids to help themselves and others wander through this thicket, including diagnostic flowcharts, algorithms, lists of clinical characteristics, practice guidelines, and menus of findings that are added numerically until a final sum assures a diagnosis. Though all these aids are designed to simplify the process, in the final analysis human cognition is the only solution. Ideally, it would be helpful to have a universal inductive problem-solving method that could be imparted to students;

unfortunately, no such method exists. Diagnosis often requires a slog through myriad data, employing the squishiness or firmness of each data point.

Lacking a universal problem-solving algorithm to impart diagnostic expertise, what can we do? First, we can impart a language of hypotheses, iterative testing, sensitivity and specificity, thresholds, and the known elements of the diagnostic process. Second, we can avoid expecting students to solve clinical problems before they have accumulated substantial medical knowledge. Third, we can acknowledge the critical role of deep medical knowledge in clinical problem solving. Although the emphasis in this essay has been on unstructured problem solving, little has been said about the knowledge that underpins clinical cognition. In fact, rich detailed knowledge of diseases and their manifestations is a fundamental requirement of problem-solving expertise. Expertise of all kinds requires a rich knowledge base, amplified by substantial experience; studies show that some 10,000 hours of sustained intentional learning are required for an individual to develop expertise, and medicine is no exception. Diagnostic (and therapeutic) problem solving depends on a vast knowledge base to generate diagnostic hypotheses and to recognize when an existing hypothesis falls short of explaining a complex set of clinical findings.

Teaching by example, however, is a powerful tool, and illustrative cases can be used not only to impart medical knowledge but to exemplify and explain clinical problem solving, both expert and erroneous approaches. Using the case method effectively requires careful preparation [9]. The cases must be selected to illustrate specific aspects of the diagnostic process, such as hypothesis generation or hypothesis revision. Ideally, the cases should be actual patient narratives and not idealized instances that fail to reflect the messiness of actual problem solving (such as false positives, false negatives, and red herrings) that are regular occurrences in the real world. Instant feedback on suggestions is particularly valuable in spotting possible cognitive errors. A student, fresh from the hematology rotation who reflexively offers a diagnosis of lymphoma for every febrile patient can be corrected on the spot. Feedback on the actual clinical course of the described patient is essential. Experts in the disease and its pathophysiology should be present to explain causal connections and to critique suggestions about diagnostic approaches. The atmosphere must be a friendly give and take with respect for individual opinions. Such sessions can be valuable for a range of audiences, from medical students to seasoned clinicians.

REFERENCES

1. Kassirer JP, Gorry GA. Clinical problem solving: A behavioral analysis. *Ann Intern Med* 1978;89:245–255.
2. Fagan TJ. Nomogram for Bayes theorem. *N Engl J Med* 1975;293:257.
3. Kassirer JP, Wong JB, Kopelman RI. *Learning Clinical Reasoning*, 2nd edition. Philadelphia, PA: Wolters Klewer/Lippincott, 2009.
4. Sox HC, Higgins MC, Owens DK. Chapter 4: Understanding new information: Bayes Theorem. In *Medical Decision Making*, 3rd edition. Hoboken, NJ: Wiley-Blackwell, 2013.
5. Pauker SG, Kassirer JP. Therapeutic decision making: a cost-benefit analysis. *N Eng J Med* 1975;293:229.
6. Pauker SG, Kassirer JP. The threshold approach to clinical decision making. *N Engl J Med* 1980;302:1109–1117.
7. Kassirer JP. Imperatives, expediency, and the new diagnosis. *Diagnosis* 2014;1:11–12.
8. Kassirer JP, Kopelman RI. Cognitive errors in diagnosis: Instantiation, classification, and consequences. *Am J Med* 1989;86:433–441.
9. Kassirer JP. Teaching clinical reasoning. Case-based, coached. *Acad Med* 2010;85;1118–1124.

4 Fun Stuff

Suzanne Koven

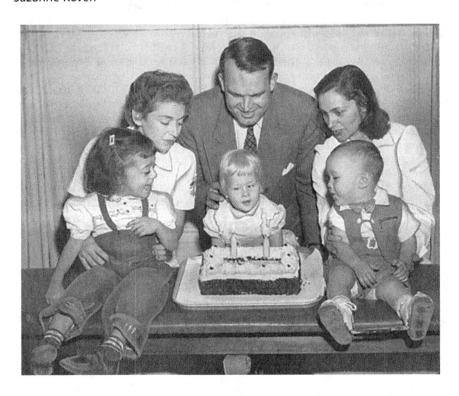

The older I get, the more I miss my parents. Sometimes I google them hoping for news. The same few items always pop up: a handful of real estate transactions, donations to defunct charities and forgotten political campaigns, their obituaries. But every now and then I come upon something I haven't seen before. Not long ago, during one of my digital séances, an unfamiliar black and white photo appeared. Published in 1952 in the *Brooklyn Eagle*, once America's largest circulation afternoon newspaper, it shows my father, then a young orthopedic surgeon, wearing a suit and tie, standing between two women dressed in starched white uniforms. They form a triangle with my father at its apex. Three small children in party clothes sitting in front make up the base. All eyes are fixed on a cake with two candles. A caption identifies the occasion as the second anniversary of the outpatient cerebral palsy clinic at the Jewish Sanitarium for Chronic Diseases in Brooklyn. The women are an occupational and a speech therapist. The children are patients. My father, the clinic's director, is beaming.

It strikes me that this image belongs to a lost world, a world before ubiquitous color photography, before the internet, before the women's movement, and the Americans with Disabilities Act. A world of starched white uniforms and neckties

DOI: 10.1201/9781003409373-4

and afternoon newspapers. The one nod to the future, which I find moving, is that the speech therapist, "Mrs. Betty Jones Hoffman," per the caption, uses her maiden name as her middle name, a bold statement for a woman then. I google her too. She wrote several books and articles about speech therapy for children, and her married name was actually spelled with two n's: Hoffmann.

I can't know if there are other errors in the old newspaper clipping, but one fact I insist upon: my father was as happy in his work as he seems in this photo. In addition to directing the cerebral palsy clinic, he performed surgery at the Brooklyn Jewish Hospital in which he, my mother, my brothers, and I were all born. Nearby he had a solo orthopedic practice, where he was king. His secretary and X-ray technician, both women (dressed in starched white) took turns making his lunch every day. He spent as long as he liked with each patient, often eliciting an entire life story over a broken arm or an arthritic hip. For most of his career, he set his own fees, and every Friday he stopped at the bank on his way home from work and personally deposited the cash and checks with which his patients paid him.

Surely being a doctor then was stressful, as it always has been. But I don't think I'm romanticizing to say that the stress that my father experienced as a physician in the 1950s through the mid-1980s wasn't existential; it didn't resemble the burnout so prevalent among doctors today. He worked long hours doing a difficult job: being responsible for other people's health and lives. I recently asked an older colleague whether doctors back then thought they had it better than doctors today think we do. An insightful and honest man who tends not to sugarcoat things, I expected him to remind me that *every* generation thinks they had it the hardest. He didn't. He said: "Yes. We were fully aware that we were lucky to be practicing in the golden era of medicine."

Doctors in mid-20th-century America had every reason to feel lucky. They were mostly married white men whose wives stayed home, as my mother did. Even if their wives had jobs, they still managed the household and the children, leaving husbands free to devote themselves to medicine (and golf) unambivalently. Respect for physicians, fueled by the development of vaccines to prevent infectious diseases such as polio, was at an all-time high, as was reverence for science in general, boosted by the space program. Medicare wasn't passed until 1965, and private insurance companies were new and relatively unintrusive. There were few malpractice suits and no computers. TV shows such as *Dr. Kildare, Ben Casey,* and, later, *Marcus Welby MD* portrayed doctors as compassionate, all-knowing, and heroic.

When I graduated from medical school in 1986, not long after my father retired, I expected to be the kind of doctor he had been: autonomous, esteemed, and happy. For many years I felt I *was* this kind of doctor. Early in my career as a primary care physician, my stresses weren't much different from those I imagined my father experienced: I worked long hours and bore responsibility for people's lives and health. Two pressures I faced that my father didn't face were balancing work with raising children and placating increasingly demanding and well-informed patients. I'm pretty sure my father never raced out of his office to be on time for school pickup, and I'm certain no patient ever waved a printout from WebMD at him. Headaches in the form of hospital politics, balky insurance companies, and frozen screens arose, but, as I often told people back then, when the exam room door closed, it was just me and my patient, and nothing else mattered.

A photograph from the *Boston Globe* in 1996 seems to verify my memory of my contentment. I'm leaning toward an elderly woman, my stethoscope slung around my neck. I'm smiling broadly, so is the patient, and so is the medical student who happened to be shadowing me that day. The photo was staged by a *Globe* reporter, an acquaintance for whom I'd agreed to pose as a favor. But my pleasure was real.

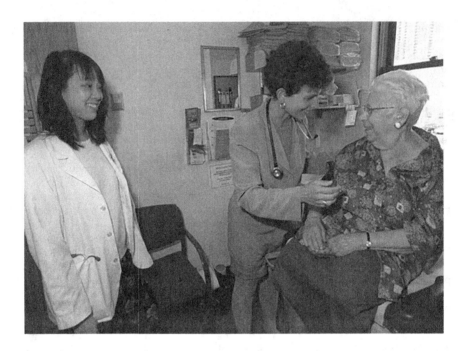

The elderly woman was one of my favorite patients. She lived alone in an apartment a couple of blocks from my office and often made appointments just to talk. I was delighted to see her that day as always, and delighted to show the medical student just how delighted I was. Still, the occasion for the photograph was less felicitous than the second anniversary of my father's clinic in 1952 had been. The headline of the *Globe* article that the photo accompanies reads: "Fees May Affect Doctor Care: Incentives on Pay Prompt Question about Whether Patients or Profit Come First."

In the past five or ten years, many articles have appeared claiming that physicians are unhappy in our work. Among these are "How Medicine Became the Most Miserable Profession" (*Atlantic* 2014), "Why Doctors Hate Their Computers" (*New Yorker*, 2018), and "The Moral Crisis of America's Doctors" (*New York Times Magazine*, 2023). In these and countless other publications in the lay and medical press, as well as in lectures and conferences geared toward medical professionals, the same depressing statistics are repeated about high rates of burnout, alcoholism and addiction, and suicide in physicians (especially women); about physicians discouraging their children and other young people from entering the profession; about increasing numbers of physicians (especially women) leaving the profession long before the usual retirement age. A Facebook group for doctors seeking nonclinical careers includes thousands of members, many of them quite young. A startling 2019 study revealed that 40% of female physicians start practicing part-time or leave clinical medicine altogether within six years of completing residency.

The Covid-19 pandemic both exposed and exacerbated doctors' woes. Especially early on, health care workers were at particular risk of contracting and dying of the virus. Many physicians chose to send their children away to live with relatives to avoid infecting them. Doctors in their twenties and thirties left copies of their wills taped to their refrigerators so that if they died at the hospital, the necessary postmortem paperwork would be readily accessible. Even physicians not on the front lines faced extraordinary stress. At work we struggled to provide patients with sound medical advice as our knowledge about the coronavirus evolved daily—and disinformation spread just as rapidly. At home we struggled to educate and entertain our children and contain our parents' anxiety. With sitters scarce and schools closed, female physicians, as ever, were more likely than male physicians to fill gaps in childcare, and so the pay inequity between men and women in medicine widened.

If, as some believe, joy in medicine is dead, its autopsy might read something like this: in the mid-1990s, corporatization and digitization eroded the satisfaction physicians find in relationships with patients. Endlessly meeting "metrics" and clicking through templates have made our work dreary and have cost us the respect and trust of our patients who feel, rightly, that we're rushed and distracted and that we aren't paying enough attention to them. A change in the portrayal of physicians on television has reflected this loss of respect. Beloved TV doctors of old have been replaced by an assortment of angry, sex-obsessed, or just plain weird characters in shows like *Grey's Anatomy*, *Scrubs*, and *House*. The added stresses of practicing medicine during the Covid-19 pandemic, along with the rise in distrust of medicine and science during the pandemic, delivered the sucker punch.

I know my own satisfaction must have waned gradually since that cheery photo in 1996, but I refused to acknowledge this, even to myself. I'd always been proud not only of my work but of the pleasure I found in my work, particularly when that work was the most challenging. I tried to take scheduling mishaps, late patients, rude consultants, and unexpected clinical complications not only in stride but with good humor. Until my very last day in practice, I privately referred to myself with a secret nickname, "Happy Warrior," a sobriquet coined by William Wordsworth in an 1806 poem and applied, in recent decades, to politicians such as Hubert Humphrey and Ronald Reagan who, under duress, maintained sunny dispositions. To be other than optimistic and cheerful, especially under duress, I believed, was a sign of weakness in a clinician. Maybe I feared that if I stopped smiling, I would feel too much: too much frustration about the demands placed on me, too much sadness at the suffering I witnessed every day. But one gray spring day in 2016 my resolve cracked. I started weeping uncontrollably during a meeting at my hospital. I'd teared up at work before when a patient died or told me a particularly moving story, but never anything like this.

The meeting during which I broke down was about, of all things, the new electronic medical record system my hospital had just installed. There had been much apprehension among my colleagues about the arrival of this system, which was rumored to be extremely burdensome, adding to the time clinicians spend staring at screens and clicking. Many of my older colleagues threatened to retire when it arrived, and many did. Several decamped to concierge practices that didn't use this system.

I'd been to a few of the requisite training sessions supervised by representatives from the company that created this medical record system. These sessions were held in sterile downtown office spaces filled with computer stations. The reps, whom we doctors treated with eye rolls and sarcasm as if they were substitute teachers and we were middle schoolers, guided us through the electronic charts of test patients with names like Santa X. Claus and Grizzvaldo Zyzzez. We were instructed to enter all medical information in problem lists. If a patient had anxiety-causing chest pain while quarreling with his spouse on the same day he was fired from his job, this unfortunate tale was to be disarticulated into a list: *chest pain, anxiety, marital discord, unemployment*. Though I ultimately became facile with this system, I never found it easy to decipher what had actually happened to a patient by perusing her problem list. The patient's information was all there, but her story was missing. At the training sessions, my mind wandered as I imagined how Cinderella might be retold in list format: *fatigue, cold exposure, soot inhalation, family conflict*.

At the end of the training period, each doctor was offered an opportunity to meet with a local "superuser," a colleague who'd mastered the system and was able to answer questions before we "went live." (I noticed during this period that corporate-speak replaced medical jargon at the hospital.) As I sat in a conference room with a superuser and a couple of trainee colleagues, I looked out the window and saw the flag proudly announcing my hospital's early 19th-century origins flapping in the cold early spring wind, its metal grommets clanking against the metal flagpole as if in ghostly protest. The superuser asked if we trainees wanted to take a turn "driving" the keyboard through a variety of hypothetical clinical scenarios. When my turn came, I declined. Instead, I started bawling.

"I'm in *mourning!*" I wailed, sounding to myself like a character in a Chekhov play. "In mourning for our profession! How has it come to . . . to . . . *this*?" All that was good and sacred in medicine would be lost, I cried, most importantly the doctor–patient relationship. Were we healers or data entry clerks? How could we truly listen to our patients with our eyes glued to the screen, pecking away at the keyboard, "populating" our lists?

The superuser made a sympathetic face as I ranted. I don't remember what my other colleagues did; I imagine they were embarrassed for me. But I wasn't embarrassed. Despite my sobs, I felt wonderful. I relished my righteous anger and enjoyed the release, however impotent, of a tension that had been long building.

A month after this incident, I went to Italy for a weeklong conference held at an inn set in a vineyard in the Umbrian hills. The trip was funded by my department. (Had they heard that I was on the verge of cracking up? This possibility just occurs to me.) I was sent there to learn, with a dozen other doctors from around the world, about Balint groups, gatherings at which doctors share morally, ethically, or psychologically challenging cases.

The food, the wine, the countryside dotted with olive trees and grapevines were perfect antidotes to the bland offices and endless screens that had upset me so. Most helpful of all were the daily Balint group meetings. Conceived in the 1950s by the British psychiatrist Michael Balint, the groups follow a strict protocol that helps create the space in which doctors can share and respond to stories freely: participants promise one another absolute confidentiality, and the person presenting a case remains silent while the case is discussed by his or her colleagues. I recall only one of the cases presented by someone else that week—a physician distressed by a beloved patient's request that she assist in his suicide—but I remember in detail the two stories I told. Both concerned patients about whom I had uncomfortable feelings. The first was a widow I'd cared for my entire career, from her sixties to her nineties. She always came to visits alone using a ride voucher provided to the elderly and always spoke glowingly and at length of her son's attentiveness. I saw little evidence of the son's devotion, though, since every time I called him, at my patient's request, to discuss an upcoming procedure or new condition, the son seemed annoyed at the inconvenience. The one time the son called me was when the patient, then age 97, was hospitalized. The son was enraged at me for doing whatever it was I must have done or not done that caused his mother to become so ill. The second was a retired physician who refused to wear a gown for his annual physical. He greeted me at each yearly visit with a hearty handshake from my exam room chair on which he sat, in the nude.

I vaguely recall the constructive reframing of these stories offered by my colleagues. Had I considered that the son might be dealing with his own problems or that he might be projecting his guilt about neglecting his mother onto me? That the retired doctor could possibly have subtle dementia causing disinhibition? Or that he was just lonely? But I remember viscerally my sense of relief at having told the stories. By the end of my week in Italy, I felt lighter, more alive. I took a selfie with my head wrapped in a scarf, sporting enormous sunglasses and smiling enigmatically with the Umbrian hills in the background. I look relaxed. More than relaxed, beatific.

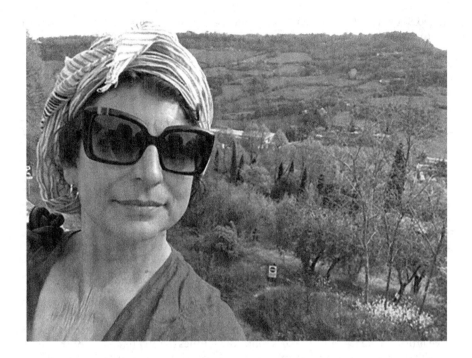

How could I bring this bliss home, though? The vineyards, the food, I knew these were not transportable. In the past I'd come home from vacations and, for a day or two, try in vain to reproduce their salutary effects, but in February the fresh-squeezed orange juice available for exorbitant prices in Massachusetts never tasted like it had in Florida the day before. There was one thing I could bring back, though. In fact, it was something I already had: opportunities to sit with my colleagues and talk openly and at leisure.

A few years earlier, I'd started leading a monthly literature discussion group for my colleagues. For the first few years, we met after work in a fluorescent-lit dining room across the hall from the main cafeteria in the basement of the hospital. The room, used for staff meetings such as ours, is called Garden East, though there is nothing garden-like about it except for the appearance, once, of a mouse. There, in Garden East, over tepid pizza and Diet Coke, amid steamy cafeteria smells, month after month, until we migrated to Zoom during the Covid-19 pandemic and, most recently, to "hybrid," my colleagues and I have discussed poems, short stories, essays, novels, memoirs, plays, and other literature related—sometimes tenuously—to health care. In this group, my love of medicine, strained by the demands of the computer screen and the pressure to see more patients in less time, was renewed. My colleagues—doctors, nurses, chaplains, therapists, administrators, and other hospital workers—have told me that our meetings have done the same for them.

I've often thought about why this low-tech, low-budget program has affected me and others so profoundly. One reason, I think, is that doctors, nurses, and others who work in health care tend to enjoy getting to know people, hear their stories. And yet the modern hospital and clinic are structured to keep us isolated: we mostly see patients one at a time and, because of privacy laws and the fast pace of our work, we can't share stories except in narratively arid rounds, conferences, and electronic medical records. Over the years, immersed daily in trauma, sadness, death—and sometimes even comedy—we build up a backlog of unexpressed emotion. In the monthly literature discussion group, talking about Tolstoy or Toni Morrison, we're invited to express that emotion. We feel less alone, more connected to one another and to the deepest meaning of our work—and also to its strangeness.

Yes, strangeness. I practiced medicine for over 30 years, and not a day went by when I wasn't struck by the strangeness of this activity. I've imagined explaining my job to a Martian. "You see," I tell the little green man, "I meet someone for the first time and ask them very personal questions. Then, a few minutes later, I tell them to take their clothes off." I touch their breasts and testicles, put my finger in every orifice. This odd interaction requires a frame, a willing suspension of disbelief, the temporary construction of an alternative world in which such interactions are normal.

Our profession has developed several tricks to help both the patient and the doctor ignore this strangeness including comfortingly familiar costumes—white coats and badges and even the hated hospital johnny—jargon, and bits of choreography that enforce a distance between what happens in the clinic and hospital from everyday life. Deviations from this choreography feel awkward. For example, while usually a medical assistant brings a patient into the exam room, I've sometimes brought the patient into the exam room myself—and then felt the urge to step out, close the door, and reenter after knocking. Just to start the scene over from the beginning.

This artifice, this suspension of disbelief, takes a toll. The narrow confines in which doctors and patients interact, not to mention the increasingly limited time in which these interactions occur, can make communication seem incomplete. Often both doctor and patient feel unheard or misunderstood, gaslighted. So much remains unsaid and unacknowledged; we're forced to pretend that love, lust, hate, anger, fear, and uncertainty, as well as politics and family and financial worries, have little or no place in that airless room. Sometimes the awareness of this pretense gathers so much pressure it erupts to the surface with shouts, tears, threats of lawsuits. Mostly it simply roils, often leaving both doctor and patient angry, ashamed, and unmoored. The patient feels she is not being healed. The doctor burns out. There have been many attempts to relieve this pressure: patient empowerment manifestos, physician wellness programs. For me, it has been literature.

When I returned from the conference in Italy, I reflected that perhaps I had not so much lost joy in medical practice but that my joy had been obscured by busy-ness and busywork, like the gleam of silver hidden beneath a layer of tarnish. My literature and medicine group seemed, at least monthly, to restore the shine—or, more accurately, my ability to see it—by reducing the isolation in which shame, anger, and emotional exhaustion thrive.

Here's an example of how this works: one evening we talked about Roz Chast's *Can't We Talk about Something More Pleasant?* In this funny and heartbreaking graphic memoir, Chast recounts how, in her sixties, she managed the declining cognitive and physical health of her nonagenarian parents, who'd made no preparations whatsoever for old age. At first the clinicians present spoke about older patients for whom we'd cared and about how challenging family dynamics can be at the end of life. Soon, though, the conversation turned more personal. Older participants voiced concerns about retaining their identities after retirement from medicine, and their younger colleagues expressed worry about dealing with their own aging parents. The divisions between clinicians and nonclinicians, between clinicians and patients, among hospital staff in various roles and at various stages of their lives and careers melted away. Chast's book had given us a means to share our vulnerability and our humanity with one another and, I have no doubt, increased our empathy with our patients, with our own families, and with ourselves.

Each month, a few days before our group meets, I send participants an email with the subject line "Fun Stuff." The email includes questions raised by the assigned texts plus links to video clips, interviews, and other material to supplement our reading. I borrowed the term "Fun Stuff" from literary critic James Wood, who used it as the title for an essay about legendary drummer Keith Moon of The Who. Moon, whom Wood idolized as a teenage drummer growing up in England, was known for inserting wild, unexpected excursions between beats, as if some internal rhythm, barely contained beneath the surface, were escaping in exuberant bursts. This seems to me a perfect description of what happens in our hospital reading group.

I've always resisted the idea that the group is recreational and blanch when some of the participants refer to it as a "book club." Similarly, I'm irked when programs similar to ours are offered at other hospitals as part of "wellness" initiatives. What we talk about in this group doesn't feel like an add-on, a perfunctory fix to what's gone wrong in medicine; it *is* medicine, the part that lives in the interstices, the subtleties, the silences. The part for which there no longer seems to be any time or space.

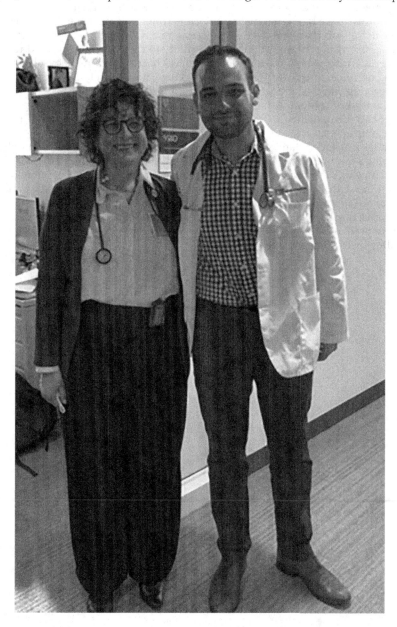

One more photo, from 2021. My son, then a first-year medical student, had stopped by my office to get a lift home for Thanksgiving, coming straight from his clinical skills course. I made him put on his white coat and stethoscope, which were in his backpack, and handed a colleague my phone to take our picture. I'm beaming. I'm not a physician who discouraged her children from entering the profession I still love, and I'm as thrilled to stand with my son, side by side with our stethoscopes, as I appear. I try not to be an overbearing doctor-mother, but it's hard for me to hide my glee in my son's choice of career. And I long to tell him what I wish I'd understood decades ago: that the way to find joy in medicine isn't, as many suggest, to maintain strict boundaries with patients. Rather, I've felt most joyful in the moments when I've let down my guard with my patients, opened my heart to them.

Administrative tasks that distance doctors from patients make these moments more elusive than they once were. Many doctors have chosen to cut back on clinical time, sacrificing income and the opportunity to do work they love and trained so long and arduously to do, in order to feel less harried and more joyful. By 2021, nearing retirement from my practice, I was seeing patients just two half days a week and devoting most of my professional life to writing, teaching, and facilitating workshops like the monthly literature discussion group. These last years in practice, when I had few patients, were among my most satisfying—part of why I look so happy in this photo.

But the current system in which doctors feel they can find satisfaction only by practicing a few hours a week or not at all isn't any more sustainable than the archaic system in which my father worked as a solo practitioner. Patients need more meaningful time with doctors, and doctors want more meaningful time with patients. I think my dad would applaud the efforts many are now making to reduce the number of tasks that keep doctors from fully engaging patients or to delegate these tasks to other professionals who are capable, sometimes more capable than doctors, of handling them. I imagine him smiling.

5 Mentorship in Medical Education and Training

Theodore A. Stern

OVERVIEW

Mentorship is a process in which an experienced person provides guidance to someone who is less experienced and facilitates academic success, promotes personal growth and emotional well-being, and encourages a gratifying work–life balance. Mentorship is more than traditional teaching (e.g., about clinical care and the conduct of research) [1]. Nevertheless, it is often difficult to define, and it leaves several who, what, where, when, why, and how questions unanswered (Table 5.1). Alternative terms for mentors include advisor, guide, counselor, consultant, coach, guru, overseer, protector, role model, sensei, and teacher. Yet these terms fail to capture the essence of mentorship or how a mentoring relationship can be formed, built, and sustained. Nevertheless, whichever synonym is used for mentorship, at its core, it relies on trust between mentee and mentor, as vulnerabilities and weaknesses need to be unearthed before they can be strengthened, thereby enabling growth and mastery [2].

Not surprisingly, when embarking upon a mentor–mentee relationship, it is important to consider whether the pairing should be initiated by the mentee or by the mentor or whether it should be assigned by a service chief, training director, or administrator. Many inexperienced mentees lack perspective on who their mentors could or should be, as they don't have institutional knowledge about whether a highly successful faculty member has been or would be an effective mentor for them (either because their expertise may not dovetail with the mentee's area of interest, or they have conflicting personality styles, or they have less than an optimal amount of time available for mentoring) (Table 5.2).

Given that mentees are often involved in a bevy of activities (e.g., patient care, research, lecturing, publishing, and teaching), it is no wonder mentees often seek out more than one mentor to ensure that they are being prepared to succeed and excel at most, if not all, of these activities. The goals of mentoring are to further the mentee's intellectual and emotional development and growth.

When establishing a mentor–mentee relationship, it is wise to establish clear expectations and goals (with short-term and long-term targets) for both the mentor and the mentee (Table 5.3). These might include writing and submitting an abstract, grant, or paper; presenting at grand rounds or at a national meeting/conference); being promoted.

WHAT MAKES A MENTOR–MENTEE RELATIONSHIP SUCCESSFUL OR UNSUCCESSFUL?

Successful mentor–mentee relationships rarely arise and develop without a modicum of trust and respect. Such trust allows for a safe place to express thoughts and feelings, confidence to be built, and confidentiality to be maintained. Successful mentorship is a "two-way street," with each half of the dyad feeling better (e.g., appreciated, gratified, and rewarded) and having grown.

Mentors should convey to their mentees that there is more to life than work. Mentees often need to be reminded that they should find joy and meaning in many spheres of their life (e.g., home, work, and community), while maintaining physical fitness and overall health.

DOI: 10.1201/9781003409373-5

Table 5.1 The Who, What, Where, When, Why, and How Questions Related to Mentorship

Who

Who needs a mentor?

Who should your mentor be?

Who needs more than one mentor?

What

What is mentorship (and how does if differ from supervising, coaching, providing opportunities/invitations, editing)?

What can facilitate the development and maintenance of a mentoring relationship?

What skills can mentorship offer? [e.g., writing/editing, public speaking (on Zoom, in person, in seminars/large venues), research opportunities, grant writing, enhancing emotional intelligence, understanding the politics of the workplace, learning how to collaborate]
as well as enhancing autognostic (self-knowledge) awareness, empathy, collaborations, and facilitating advocacy, minimizing burnout, serving as a sounding board for work–life decisions, debriefing mistakes, learning from peers, facilitating diversity

What goals could I establish for my mentorship? (e.g., preparing/submitting a poster/abstract/paper/chapter/grant/oral presentation/curriculum)

Where

Where should mentoring be conducted? [e.g., private setting, such as an office or at home, or in less than private settings (such as a cafeteria, at the bedside, or at national meetings)]

When

When should I contact a mentor/mentee (and should it be self-initiated or assigned)?

Why

Why is having a mentor valuable?

Why do some mentor–mentee relationships fail while others succeed?

How

How can I get the most out of my mentorship relationship/meetings? (e.g., planning with the help of an agenda, setting objective goals, preparing/reading/reflecting on what will be discussed, and creating an action plan with due dates based upon feedback received)

How often should mentors and mentees meet (and for how long)?

Table 5.2 Facilitating a Match between Mentor and Mentee

Decide what you need or want from a mentor.

Determine whether you will need one or more mentors.

Determine whether and how your potential mentor is likely to help you reach your goals.

Learn who the mentor has mentored and what the result of their mentorship has been.

Assess how much time you are willing to invest to make the mentorship effective.

Although mentors are endowed with a myriad of qualities that are highly valued by their mentees, it would be unlikely that your mentor(s) will possess each of these attributes (Table 5.4).

HOW CAN MENTORSHIP FACILITATE PROFESSIONAL DEVELOPMENT?

Mentorship is not a one-size-fits-all endeavor. In the clinical realm, mentorship might involve learner-centered experiential learning using an apprenticeship model that includes case presentations, observing interviews/physical examinations,

Table 5.3 Potential Goals of Mentorship

Enhancement of Professional Development:

by using a learner-centered experiential learning/apprenticeship model

by observing case presentations

by observing interviews/physical examinations

by observing how mentors formulate complex cases and lead teaching rounds

by receiving and delivering feedback

by reviewing articles

by communicating effectively

by submitting (and receiving feedback on) abstracts, manuscripts, workshops, symposia, grants to the best venues

Enhancement of Skills

by learning how to deliver better presentations

by learning how to write/publish scholarly manuscripts

by learning how to teach using a variety of methods

by learning how to get the most out of networking and participation in national organizations

by learning how to write grant proposals

by learning how to collaborate effectively

by learning how to be more efficient and productive

by learning when and how to say "no"

Table 5.4 Valued Qualities of Mentors

Responsive

Caring

Thoughtful (considers context and opportunities)

Connected to multiple networks/colleagues across the country

Respectful

Nonjudgmental

Organized/efficient

Supportive/confidence building

Inspiring

Generative

Creative

Savvy (attends to "the lyrics and the music")

Productive/prolific

formulating complex cases, running teaching rounds (often using the Socratic method of questioning), presenting didactics, delivering feedback, providing/ reviewing articles, communicating effectively with patients and colleagues, engaging in simulations, facilitating leadership opportunities and networking, all the while encouraging and maintaining a healthy work–life balance.

In addition, it helps to determine how you like to learn and learn best [e.g., by hearing, seeing, reading (before a meeting and then discussing what has been learned), doing (role-playing, simulations, demonstrations), reflecting]. Preparing for success with strategies that play to your strengths will facilitate learning and growth.

For example, when teaching a sport, such as golf, some instructors start by and focus on illustrating the mechanics of the swing and then having the student hit practice shots on a driving range, whereas some coaches play a round of golf with the student and then discuss their shot making and course management (i.e., where they were aiming to increase their odds of putting themselves into the best position for the next shot). These strategies often change depending on the experience level and skill of the student. However, in general, I prefer to look at the student's swing, analyze their mechanics, learn what other sports they have played (and had success at), and then shape the mechanics of their golf swing to maximize control and power. Then real-time adjustments can be made, swing by swing, while observing the results and by preparing one's body to enhance the swing.

In the academic realm, parallels to teaching the golf swing can be recreated (e.g., looking at written works or listening to presentations; analyzing their approach to and mechanics in creating a work product; discussing what they have achieved/done well before; and identifying components of their work output that maximize efficiency, productivity, and creativity), while shaping their approach to the tasks at hand. As with golf, thinking too much often increases tension, which alters (and shortens) the "swing mechanics" and decreases the likelihood of hitting your best shot. This allows for mentorship to be a creative and exhilarating process. Moreover, since negative thoughts typically inhibit performance, a wiser behavioral strategy is to "think positive" and "be confident." Practice as if each shot counts (to facilitate state-dependent learning), while improving your technique (rather than repeating the same error-filled efforts). The goal is not merely to hit the ball and see how far it goes; it is usually to have each shot's trajectory match the path that you want it to take, so that it hits its target. Focusing on the process rather than on the result requires thoughtful reflection and leads to enhanced understanding and satisfaction.

EXAMPLES FROM MY MENTORSHIP

Most mentorship relationships involve learning and developing skills (e.g., learning how to deliver better presentations, to write/publish scholarly manuscripts, to teach using a variety of methods, and to get the most out of networking and participation in national organizations) that are essential for academic and personal growth.

PUBLIC SPEAKING

For several decades, I have held an interactive seminar on public speaking, titled "How to Give a Talk" [attended by each of our psychiatry residents, our fellows in psychosomatic medicine, and members of other departments at the Massachusetts General Hospital (MGH)]. At these sessions, participants hear and see me talk about and demonstrate effective public speaking techniques; then they deliver a one-minute presentation to the attendees based upon a slide that I prepared.

I then provide them with feedback on their delivery, including volume and pace, eye contact, ability to shift their gaze from one audience member to the next by using a search-in-silence method, improvisation/ad libing, and effective use of body language. This goes hand in hand with suggesting alternative words suggested to strengthen the presentation, as well as feedback on how to make their slides more readable, organized, and memorable. Although these ultra-brief presentations evoke anxiety in trainees, they receive well-intentioned and immediate feedback that is specific, thoughtful, actionable, and timely (recalled by the mnemonic "STAT"). This serves as a reminder of, and as a template for, what can be done better and then practiced to improve performance and diminish anxiety.

In addition, before they deliver talks to large gatherings (e.g., grand rounds), we reserve time in the auditorium to practice the presentation and to desensitize them to the arena, its technology, and its acoustics. As they stand at the base of an impressive amphitheater and practice their presentation, I move from one area of the auditorium to another at different parts of their talk, so they can learn to shift their gaze among members of the audience, so everyone in the steeply banked auditorium feels as though they were being spoken to. I provide feedback of the same type that was offered in the public speaking seminar. We also review the clarity of their thinking/organization and their conveyed sense of mastery.

NETWORKING, COLLABORATING, AND GETTING THE MOST OUT OF PARTICIPATION AT NATIONAL MEETINGS

To help my mentees get the most out of going to national meetings, I meet with them in advance of their attendance at an organization's annual meeting (e.g., the Academy of Consultation–Liaison Psychiatry). We discuss what they hope to gain from their attendance at the meeting and whom they would like to meet (e.g., to facilitate a job interview, to meet key "players" in the field). Through thinking ahead, we can create a workable plan that will fit their schedule and mine.

Typically, my mentees want to meet the organization's leaders, those from other institutions who are likely to be posting job opportunities, those who are working in areas of shared interest, and those with whom collaborations would be welcomed. To facilitate this, we walk around together at the opening day poster session and look at and critique the posters. We meet scores of people who are standing beside their posters, as well as those who are reviewing the posters and seeking to reconnect with friends and colleagues. As we walk, I introduce my mentee (or mentees) to the poster presenter and/or their mentor so they can learn more about my mentee(s) and establish whether there are overlapping interests. By doing so, my mentees get to meet and "press the flesh" with senior members of the organization whom I have known for many years from my involvement in the organization and my attendance at annual meetings.

A similar tactic is applied at the meeting's opening night reception, where food and drink replace the posters. These more social gatherings help to develop relationships, collaborations, and committee appointments, as well as to brainstorm and create workshops/symposia at subsequent meetings. Given that there are numerous breakfasts, lunches, and dinners, as well as coffee/refreshment breaks, there are ample opportunities to converse with upwards of 100 people during the conference.

SCHOLARLY WRITING

In addition to leading a yearlong (every two week) seminar on scholarly writing for members of the MGH Psychiatry Department (which I have done for the past 35 years), I have delivered shorter seminars (lasting from one to four sessions) for those in other departments at the hospital. These seminars provide practical demonstrations of how to determine what to write about (and for whom), as well as how to outline and write a paper about something they have seen and that intrigues them. These sessions have led to numerous published reports [3, 4].

In the yearlong seminar, 5–15 residents, fellows, and junior staff each year learn the basics of scholarly writing. At the outset, we review what the writers want to write about, for whom (and why), the structure of papers, the information for the author's section of the journals to which they are likely to submit (so that writers will be able to decide on the proper target audience and journal for their articles).

For example, attendees at the seminar are asked whether they have been interested in any cases over the past two years and what was interesting about the cases. Then we clarify who the target audience could and should be and which journals would offer the best fit for the manuscript.

Next, an attendee presents a brief synopsis of the case/problem. This is followed by my asking a series of who, what, where, when, why, and how questions. These frame the discussion of the case. Detailed notes are taken in real time, so the crucial connections between the thoughts we have expressed and discussed are not over-looked. Then parameters for answering the questions are provided (e.g., answering each question with up to two pages of double-spaced text with up to 5 references/citations per question). After the text is then emailed to me, I provide track change edits, so the attendees can see why certain edits were made. Once the edits are reviewed, discussed, and accepted, the manuscript is submitted to a journal for publication.

Use of dictation, speech recognition technology, and the closed-caption function available on conference calls, enables thoughts to be "put down on paper" rapidly, without having to reconstruct the discussion. Moreover, this enables a draft to be created during the one-hour seminar.

Participants are uniformly surprised by how rapidly a working draft of a manuscript can be produced and by how the division of labor ("a divide and conquer" strategy) can reduce the time commitment of each collaborator. Most clinically oriented manuscripts can be completed with less than 15 hours of work by each person (including the time spent conducting a literature review needed to provide accurate and timely details and to make revisions). Scores of papers have been published using this method.

DISCUSSION OF CAREER OPPORTUNITIES/JOB PROSPECTS

My mentees and colleagues at my home institution and at institutions across the country often contact me when they consider making a career move. They are aware that their career changes will affect them, their families, and faculty and trainees at their home institution and at their new location. Changes in their position will impact their clinical work, research, teaching, administrative roles, leadership responsibilities, scholarly activities, career advancement/promotion, and salary.

For example, when a faculty member whom I had known for nearly two decades was thinking about moving to an academic center in another part of the country, he asked for a consultation. He had been remarkably successful as a clinician, teacher, investigator, and administrator/service chief; however, opportunities for advancement where he was working were limited. Now he was offered the chance to run a larger clinical service elsewhere, and he was weighing how this would affect his career and his family life given that he had school-age children. Our multifaceted discussion (which paid attention to his affect) addressed each of these issues as well as his salary support, the cost of living/housing, and his working relationships with others at the new institution. He trusted me to guide him through the complicated matters he was facing. Over the next decade, we have continued to discuss his career and his family.

COLLABORATION ON ARTICLES/CHAPTERS/BOOKS
WITH MEDICAL STUDENTS

I have always been an obligate teacher—whether it is in the hospital or on athletic fields.

In the medical arena, I have taught and coached Harvard Medical School (HMS) students in multiple venues. I have led sections of the first-year course "The Practice of Medicine" on interviewing, in which, along with other preceptors, students are coached on how to develop the components of the clinical assessment (e.g., the chief concern/complaint, the history of the present illness, the past medical history, the social history, the family history, the mental status examination) and how to practice compassionate care, among other topics. This places us in contact with students who are filled with potential but who are often short on life experiences as they encounter patients at the bedside for the first time.

In addition, I have led sections of The Developing Physician (TDP) for first-year and second-year HMS students, helping to guide them through the transition from being an undergraduate student to a medical professional. Several students have had their interest sparked by these sessions and have wished to develop their skills by learning more and by writing scholarly publications. They have used their patient encounters and clinical case conferences as a foundation for publishing articles for primary care physicians with an interest in psychiatric issues [5, 6]. As our collaborations have continued, our discussions have broadened and encompass readings, sports, educational opportunities/applications/recommendations for additional postgraduate degree programs, as well as career choice and development. Our mentor–mentee relationships have grown out of mutual respect and a willingness to share experiences that span health, well-being, and much more.

GENERATIVITY AND CAREER DEVELOPMENT OF FACULTY

While working as the Director of the MGH Office for Clinical Careers for a decade, I had the good fortune to oversee scores of seminars for clinical faculty throughout the MGH on the bedrock principles of academic success at HMS, the academic institution that provides promotions for its affiliated teaching hospitals (e.g., MGH, the Brigham and Women's Hospital, McLean Hospital). These seminars provided interactive discussions to facilitate skill building and the knowledge necessary for building an academic profile with seminars on how to deliver feedback, how to get the most out of national meetings, how to prepare your HMS curriculum vitae (CV) and your narrative, how to network, how to give a talk, how to write a book, how to advance academically, and how to write scholarly publications. These seminars were attended by several thousand faculty members over the years. In addition, I conducted one-on-one meetings with faculty members to discuss their academic and clinical interests; these meetings focused on myriad topics, which included helping them understand the criteria and process for academic promotion at HMS, helping them reformat their CV to the HMS style, assisting them in determining where they might focus their energy and effort in their academic endeavors (e.g., clinical care, research, teaching, administration) and discussing their lives outside the hospital. These individual meetings, which typically lasted 1–1.5 hours, were held with more than 1,000 faculty members over the years. Many of the meetings involved several sessions, and some spanned several years and involved more than 25 hours. Over and above these seminars/meetings, several of these coaching sessions developed into collaborations (e.g., helping mentees learn how to build curricula, enhance their reputation, and write/edit books in their field of interest and expertise). I walked them through the process of determining what they were interested in and whom they wanted to educate; we developed outlines for each book, created a list of potential collaborators/chapter authors, corresponded with the chapter authors and the publisher, edited each chapter, and engaged in marketing and fundraising efforts to disseminate the work product. These books strengthened their profile and facilitated their academic promotion [7–14].

There are others who have had less experience publishing peer-reviewed articles. They had significantly less exposure to writing and had little knowledge of people with whom they could collaborate. The process of outlining, writing, and publishing academically useful, peer-reviewed works led to more than a dozen publications.

In addition, I have collaborated with trainees at other institutions, often at the request of faculty at the other institution [15, 16]. These relationships built the mentee's confidence and provided them with templates for academic success; they learned how to write, edit, publish, delegate, cooperate, and proof their work.

Further, large multi-authored textbooks (where trainees, junior faculty, and senior members of our department collaborated) provided opportunities for becoming involved and developing expertise in a clinical area [17, 18]; by so doing, they "learn the ropes" and pay it forward, mentoring others in the future. Mentorship also facilitates the missions of gender and racial equity and diversity by preparing trainees and faculty to achieve their goals [19].

CONCLUSION

Some wonder how and why I do what I do. Although mentoring is time-consuming, it is a joy, not a chore. I love being generative and coaching others (as I coached baseball, soccer, and basketball for more than a decade in community organizations). Being involved, connected, and helping to shape the careers of others is not merely altruistic—it is gratifying.

As we have learned from the longitudinal study of Harvard undergraduates (lasting longer than 50 years) [20], our connections fill us with happiness. I recommend becoming involved as a mentor and paying it forward.

REFERENCES

1. Amonoo HL, Barreto EA, Stern TA, Donelan K. Residents' experience with mentorship in academic medicine. *Acad Psychiatry* 2019;43:71–75.
2. Gerken AT, Beckmann DL, Stern TA. Fostering careers in medical education. *Psychiatr Clin N Am* 2021;44(2):283–294.
3. Vaduganathan M, McCullough SA, Fraser TN, Stern TA. Death from Munchausen syndrome: A case of idiopathic recurrent right ventricular failure and a review of the literature. *Psychosomatics* 2014;55(6):668–672. https://doi.org/10.1016/j.psym.2014.05.013
4. Frank RC, Islam YFK, Johnson SW, Lander BS, Sharma S, Wallwork RS, Stern TA. Rules imposed by providers on medical and surgical inpatients with substance use disorders: Arbitrary or appropriate? *Prim Care Companion CNS Disord* 2018;20:18f02341. https://doi.org/10.3088/PCC.18f02341
5. Chipidza FE, Wallwork RS, Stern TA. Impact of the doctor-patient relationship. *Prim Care Companion CNS Disord* 2015;17(5). https://doi.org/10.4088/PCC.15f01840
6. Petriceks AH, Stern TA. Mild cognitive impairment, dementia, and the evaluation of patients who present with a concern about cognitive decline. *Prim Care Companion CNS Disord* 2021;23(5).
7. Wexler DJ, Celano CM, Stern TA, editors. *Facing Diabetes: A Guide for Patients and Their Families*. Boston, MA: MGH Psychiatry Academy, 2018.
8. Stanford FC, Stevens JR, Stern TA, editors. *Facing Overweight and Obesity: A Complete Guide for Children and Adults*. Boston, MA: MGH Psychiatry Academy, 2018.
9. Bolster MB, Stern TA, editors. *Facing Lupus: A Guide for Patients and Their Families*. Boston, MA: MGH Psychiatry Academy, 2020.
10. Kourosh AS, Stern TA, editors. *Facing Psoriasis: A Guide for Patients and Their Families*. Boston, MA: MGH Psychiatry Academy, 2020.
11. Reynolds KL, Cohen JV, Zubiri L, Stern TA, editors. *Facing Immunotherapy: A Guide for Patients and Their Families*. Boston, MA: MGH Psychiatry Academy, 2020.

12. De EJB, Stern TA, editors. *Facing Pelvic Pain: A Guide for Patients and Their Families*. Boston, MA: MGH Psychiatry Academy, 2021.
13. Chemali Z, Stern TA, editors. *Facing Memory Loss and Dementia: A Guide for Patients and Their Families*. Boston, MA: MGH Psychiatry Academy, 2021.
14. Williams WW, Ivkovic A, Stern TA, editors. *Facing Chronic Kidney Disease: A Guide for Patients and Their Families*. Boston, MA: MGH Psychiatry Academy, 2022.
15. Rustad JK, Stern TA, Prabhakar M, Musselman D. Risk factors for alcohol relapse following orthotopic liver transplantation: A systematic review. *Psychosomatics* 2015;56(1):21–35. https://doi.org/10.1016/j.psym.2014.09.006
16. Jiang S, Czuma R, Cohen-Oram A, Hartney K, Stern TA. Guanfacine for hyperactive delirium: A case series. J Acad Consult Liaison *Psychiatry* 2021;62(1):83–88.
17. Stern TA, Fava M, Wilens TE, Rosenbaum JF, editors. *Massachusetts General Hospital Comprehensive Clinical Psychiatry*, 2nd ed. Philadelphia, PA: Elsevier, 2016.
18. Stern TA, Freudenreich O, Smith FA, Fricchione GL, Rosenbaum JR, editors. *Massachusetts General Hospital Handbook of General Hospital Psychiatry*, 7th ed. Philadelphia, PA: Saunders/Elsevier, 2018.
19. Yeung AS, Trinh NT, Chen JA, Chang TE, Stern TA. Cultural humility for consultation-liaison psychiatrists. *Psychosomatics* 2018. https://doi.org/10.1016/j.psym.2018.06.004
20. Waldinger R, Schulz M. *The Good Life: Lessons from the World's Longest Scientific Study of Happiness*. New York, NY: Simon & Schuster, 2023.

6 Empathy

James Kahn

I've learned that people will forget what you said, people will forget what you did, but people will never forget how you made them feel.

—Maya Angelou

INTRODUCTION

Empathy is a central element in a master clinician's toolbox, and demonstrating empathy helps to sustain and elevate the clinician–patient relationship. Empathy is used in many clinical and teaching situations, and yet empathy is more than a contrivance applied in such settings; it is also a frame of mind. Master clinicians routinely practice it in everyday situations, seeking to expand their empathetic skill set. Master clinicians know that fostering relationships based on empathy—empathetic connections—often leads to greater understanding of the human condition. Developing these connections may help them experience protection, even shelter them from feelings of being separated or possibly discarded. In the clinical situation, empathy is among the most powerful feelings that sustain patients. Master clinicians initiate these empathetic connections and are keenly aware that how they help patients feel cared for is often the critical element for patient trust, improves understanding of the clinical situation, and may hopefully lead to better patient outcomes. Master clinicians are frequently master teachers and become role models for their students and mentees, helping them develop empathy as a critical competency. Demonstrating empathy is an important way to model and build an empathetic connection for learners.

The master clinician applies empathy to improve their relationship with patients, but is empathy an intuitive part of the master clinician's makeup or is it a cultivated trait that can be taught, enhanced, and shared with others? In this chapter, empathy will be defined and differentiated from sympathy and compassion. Once defined, the development of empathetic connections will be described. Next we will discuss whether empathy is a teachable skill and how one might improve empathetic connections. We will explore how to repair connections if there is a rupture in the relationship and how master clinicians rely on empathy to help repair relationships. Finally, we will discuss the application of artificial intelligence (AI) and whether AI will enhance empathy or if empathy will be a casualty of AI.

DEFINITIONS OF TERMS

"Empathy," "sympathy," and "compassion" are related terms that are often used interchangeably; however, they are very different, and master clinicians apply each concept in different ways. *Empathy* is the ability to understand and share other people's feelings. It involves an emotional attunement in order to understand others' emotions [1]. Master clinicians are quite insightful regarding patients' emotional situations. They also improve and strengthen their empathetic connections through careful listening to their patients, awareness of verbal and nonverbal communication cues, and the ability to communicate in an authentic and caring way. The author Brene Brown wrote: "Empathy has no script. There is no right way or wrong way to do it. It's simply listening, holding space, withholding judgment, emotionally

 DOI: 10.1201/9781003409373-6

connecting, and communicating the incredibly healing message of 'you're not alone.'"

Sympathy is an emotional reaction toward the misfortune of another and usually does not involve understanding the misfortune. Sympathy may lead to a consoling response to a distressing situation, but sympathy does not help you see the situation or the problem from another's perspective. Empathy is our ability to understand how someone feels, while sympathy is our relief in not having the same problems. Sympathy often involves problem solving and includes ideas and judgments about what a person should do and how they may feel [2].

In clinical care, sympathy can lead to a data-driven and factual planning process, and, while helpful, it may inadvertently contribute to barriers between the clinician and patient since there is very little emotional connection. While sympathy can involve genuine care and concern for others, it may not always involve the same level of emotional connection and understanding as empathy or compassion.

Compassion occurs when one is confronted with another's suffering and is motivated to relieve that suffering. Compassion involves a genuine concern for the well-being of others and a willingness to take action to alleviate their suffering. Master clinicians demonstrate compassion but also recognize that compassion is insufficient to build trust and understanding with patients. Compassion does not require an understanding of the suffering, and thus, as a tool to help in caring for patients, compassion may not reflect the training and skill set of master clinicians. Compassion is important, and the concern that is communicated is critical; however, the lack of understanding, of seeing the situation through the patient's eyes, makes this tool less powerful than empathy.

The master clinician tends to demonstrate an empathetic approach to patient care and occasionally also demonstrates compassion while greatly limiting sympathy. A 59-year-old woman with a breast mass presents a useful model to exemplify these terms and a master clinician's responses. A biopsy reveals cancer and, upon further questioning, it is discovered that this patient has two teenage daughters living at home and that the patient's mother died of breast cancer at an early age. She is worried, and so are you. A master clinician might say, "This is scary, but you are not alone, and I am here to help you. We will work through this together." That is empathy. The clinician expressed concern through understanding, gentle words, and a thoughtful tone; with appropriate body language and perhaps with the safe and appropriate touching of the patient's arm displaying a connection to the patient as well as competence and kindness. The master clinician is looking through the patient's eyes and understanding her fears while pledging support. Sympathy would be, "I am so sorry for you." Expressing sympathy, a learned behavior, may not be what your patient needs and, worse still, may short circuit the empathic connection. Patients need to tap into their resilience and develop understanding for the challenges they will likely face. A master physician, through their empathic connection, facilitates the patient's strengths, tries to understand her weaknesses, and provides the insight and knowledge for a pathway that hopefully leads to the best possible care. Sympathy may have a role, but planning for this patient's consultations and developing a treatment plan without recognizing her emotional needs might create a schism between the clinician and patient. The patient might then feel disconnected from the clinician, expressing bewilderment that the physician cannot perceive her situation and her fears. A master clinician grasps the need to help the patient connect with her feelings; providing pity is not helpful and may cause resentment, as well as contribute to patient detachment from her clinician and despondency from the reality of her situation. Compassion might be, "I am worried for you and for your daughters. We can help you, but, just as importantly, we can test your daughters for the cancer gene." This compassion and insight would be appropriate but not at this time. A master clinician understands that to begin the complex process of developing a treatment plan, it is most likely to be successful once you have connected with the patient. Without the connection to a patient, a treatment program, even if it is appropriate and effective, will not be completely satisfactory for the patient or her family. Many master clinicians will listen attentively to the patient, connect with her, and develop an empathetic response to her condition before treatment planning begins.

LEARNING EMPATHY

Empathy is a complex skill, but it is one that can be learned and developed. There are many different ways to learn how to develop an empathetic connection with others. In this section, the development of empathy will be explored.

Master clinicians are attentive listeners. They try to understand how their patients feel by attentive listening. Listening initiates the empathetic response. I remember a dignified master clinician, Dr. Philip Tumulty from Johns Hopkins, who was the most attentive listener I ever witnessed. He would sit on the patient's bed. He would look closely at the patient, occasionally hold their hand, and his face would mirror their concerns. He rarely smiled or frowned. I asked him about that, and he said, "I am not a judge, but a doctor, and doctors do not judge." I was not sure what he meant, but I knew it was profound. At first, I thought he modeled dispassion, withholding his feelings as a way to preserve his objectivity or even to remove himself from the intimate conversation I was watching. Over time I realized that I was wrong.

Dr. Tumulty was modeling empathy by helping his patients (and me) reflect on their own situations, their words and tone, and their body language. Dr. Tumulty was modeling that you cannot look at the situation through your patients' eyes unless you are willing to hear what they have to say. That's why listening skills are a vital part of building empathy. He was modeling how to give patients time to process and understand and then to express their feelings. He would not anticipate a patient's words but would wait for the patient to think about his experience and his feelings. His interactions were longer than others, and he never rushed his patients. His empathetic connection building required time, and Dr. Tumulty was never in a hurry. His patients loved him for his patience, and, although we were rushing to complete our tasks, Dr. Tumulty demonstrated that master clinicians did not hurry through forming these patient connections. Empathy could not be rushed.

Later in life, I would realize that providing patients with time through attentive listening was necessary for a true empathetic connection. This is important with all the distractions in our lives that interfere with attentive listening. Multitasking is a common barrier to active listening. The master clinician will not answer phone calls, will infrequently write notes, and would never read their email while speaking with patients. Master clinicians ensure that patients have their undivided attention. I am grateful to Dr. Tumulty for these lessons.

STAY CONNECTED TO YOUR EMOTIONS

Master clinicians try to stay in touch with their own emotions. A recent encounter provided me with an all-too-close experience of the essential importance of understanding and staying connected to my emotions. My father fell down a staircase and was rushed unconscious to the emergency room of a local trauma center. He was on an anticoagulant for atrial fibrillation. I was immediately distraught. For years, I was his lead clinician (but not his primary care physician). His brain MRI revealed a massive intracranial hemorrhage. My family turned to me for advice, insight, and recommendations. I did not want this role. It was not the responsibility that worried me, it was that I was so emotionally connected to him. I wanted to be his loving son and not his physician. I needed to stay in touch with my feelings. I felt love, loss, worry, and a deep concern for my father and for others in my family. Staying in touch with my feelings helped me become more aware of my emotions and the emotions of my family members and the health care team. I tried to stay empathetic to everyone. I worried about the loss we were all going to experience, and I wept for our loss and tried to stay focused on what my father needed. Eventually, we all realized that my father would not recover from his trauma and that it was time to discontinue life support. The team prepared to disconnect my father from the ventilator. They said he might survive for hours; I knew it would be minutes. My family members drifted out of my father's room, and so did I. My wife turned to me. "Don't leave him alone—he would want you there," she said to me. I stayed with him. My emotions and my feelings were raw, but in that moment, I felt an empathetic connection with my father. I wanted to stay in contact with my feelings. I tried to recognize them all. I wanted to share these with my father, but he was intubated. We could not speak, but I could talk to him, and I did. He was extubated and died soon afterward. I held his hand and witnessed his final breath. His final heartbeat. My training, my empathy enabled me to stay focused on my father. It was the worst feeling of my life as a son, and yet it is one of my proudest moments as a clinician. It was empathy that helped me through this sorrowful event.

Master clinicians are open-minded. Many clinicians are most comfortable with people who are like them, their culture, their skin color, their gender, their sexual identity, and their family. Many master clinicians thrive when they care for people who are "different" from themselves; they understand that the empathetic connection will make a difference between people because everyone wants to be accepted as their true selves. Yes, care is the focus, but the empathy that connects master clinicians with their patients, especially patients different from the master clinician, has its own special rewards. Master clinicians recognize that differences can be celebrated and not feared, and they do not see differences as barriers to empathetic connections.

MODELING EMPATHY

Modeling empathy is an important tool to teach empathy. Mentees and students sometimes may not recognize when they receive important learning. A master clinician, Dr. Karen Friday, carries a little sign with her when she is working during cardiology rounds. When she explains the pathogenesis of heart failure or she describes an unusual murmur or when she uncovers a previously unrecognized key element in a patient's history, she will raise the sign. It reads, "Teaching." In this way, trainees pay special attention to this new gift from Dr. Friday. The other side of the sign reads "Feedback" since feedback, an important aspect of teaching, is usually unrecognized by the learner. I wonder if such a sign would be useful when trainees observe an empathetic connection with patients. Dr. Friday also shows great patience. Learning empathy takes time, and master clinicians need to stay positive and limit discouragement. We all will find patients feeling sad, angry, or scared. We may feel unappreciated and burned out. We will have other pressing and important matters that require our attention, but the master clinician recognizes the need to limit distractions and focus on the patient's perspective. They will listen attentively, and the listening provides their patient with a sense of importance and the grit they will need to find a pathway to improved health.

NONVERBAL COMMUNICATION

Master clinicians recognize verbal cues that also convey messages. I have never witnessed a master clinician sitting with her arms crossed and looking away from the patient. If I find myself in this type of posture, I rapidly reposition my arms so the patient will not construe my body language as a sign that I don't want to listen to them. I do not want the patient to feel like I am a barrier to their communication. This is often hard when I am tired or when I have other commitments, particularly when I am feeling like I am not making progress with a patient. But that is when I try to "double down" and think about how they feel, how vulnerable they are, how they want to be helped, and I try to understand what they need and how I need to be empathetic.

Body language is also important for establishing empathetic connections. I have noticed that some people, when they are nervous, may spin their hair with their fingers or toss it with their hands. I don't have much hair, but I am sure there are other fidgety things I do that interfere with communication. Master clinicians are mindful of their own distractions and, once they are recognized, try to eliminate them from interfering with communication with patients. If you want to encourage the person to engage with you, use positive cues, such as a gentle smile and consistent eye contact, to project warmth. Trainees observing these interactions may need to be informed when they observe "Teaching," hopefully understand this lesson, and apply it in subsequent encounters. One can learn empathy by carefully observing modeled behavior by a master clinician.

VULNERABILITY STRENGTHENS EMPATHY

Being empathetic requires you to display vulnerability. When you hide behind an air of indifference, you make it harder for other people to trust or understand you. You also hold yourself back from feeling and understanding the full range of other people's emotions. Here are some ways you can reveal your vulnerability to others and, at the same time, feel safe in revealing your vulnerability.

We all can reframe how we think about vulnerability. Many of us might have been taught or believed that vulnerability is a form of weakness. Master clinicians do not fear their vulnerability. They may not embrace their own vulnerability, but they understand that opening up to others—trusting them to listen and accept their flaws—requires courage. Master clinicians emphatically connect with others even when they reveal their vulnerabilities. I know a master clinician who suffered a terrible loss, the death of his infant son. He wept as the small white casket traveled down the church aisle. I remember his bravery and his tears. He revealed to us all that he was a man saddled with unimaginable grief, and his pain would be reduced when he shared it with his friends and colleagues. He was a role model of mine, and the bravery he demonstrated in the face of sadness was inspiring and allowed us all to empathetically connect. I doubt that his empathy sprang from grief, but his bravery in revealing his sadness provided another plank for building his empathetic nature. The prism he used to understand his patients and provide empathy was forever changed by this sad event; it enabled him to reach inside and provide even greater empathetic connections to others.

Master clinicians reflect on their own emotional state, and they practice being vulnerable and authentic with others. I find that master clinicians are prepared to accept and communicate honestly despite the intensity of the conversation. This applies when you communicate difficult information, and feedback is often a difficult conversation. Master clinicians provide effective, authentic feedback, and often use empathy as a tool for the feedback. Feedback is difficult to give and hear because it should often lead to change. You should not fear a low rating by the listener if you have to give difficult feedback. Instead, remain vulnerable, understand the challenges in providing the feedback, but be confident that you are helping the listener become a better clinician, scientist, or friend. Master clinicians treat feedback as a "gift." What the listener does with the gift is difficult to know. Some people "return" the gift without much consideration of the thoughtfulness of the feedback and how it was tailored and specific. Persons receiving feedback may become defensive or may not consider the feedback authentic and thus lose an opportunity to improve themselves. Others simply regift the feedback to another without considering if it is appropriate and helpful. This is another lost opportunity to reflect and improve oneself. We all know how hard it is to find people who will be honest and helpful with feedback. The more time that is taken to provide authentic and thoughtful feedback, the more comfortable you will become with these conversations, and the more valuable the conversations will be for the listener.

Master clinicians want to empathetically connect with others, but they do not dwell on their reputation or their accomplishments. I vividly remember my first encounter with one of the truly great master clinicians, Dr. Victor McKusick. I attended a party at his home in Baltimore. I had never met him. I rang the doorbell, and a tall, gangly man in a white dinner jacket, black bow tie, and neatly combed white hair opened the door. He asked me in a soft voice who I was and what I wanted. I told him I was invited to a party by Dr. McKusick. He smiled and asked if he could take my raincoat. Certainly, I said, and thanked him for this courtesy. I entered the stately home, received a glass of champagne, and walked around meeting the other guests. I had a lot of fun, but I was desperate to meet the famous Dr. McKusick. Finally, I asked someone if they could point out Dr. McKusick to me. He laughed and pointed to the tall, gangly man welcoming new guests and hanging up their coats. I was shocked that this humble man (who I thought was a member of the party staff) was one of the greatest master clinicians I would ever meet. A few years later, I repeated this story to him. He smiled and laughed out loud. He did not remember that interaction, but he did say, "Always treat everyone like they are important, because they are." It is not about how I perceive others or how other people perceive me, but it is about how we communicate and bond with one another. Master clinicians embrace their humility, humanity, and honesty and, when combined with empathy, connect with others.

TEACHING EMPATHY

Teaching empathy to physicians is a crucial aspect of medical education. To instill empathy in physicians, medical schools and training programs can incorporate several strategies. A curriculum should focus on the human side of medicine and emphasize the importance of understanding a patient's emotional needs alongside their physical ones. Medical students can engage in role-playing exercises, and clinical simulations would be an effective tool for modeling emotional connections to help students gain a better understanding of the patient's perspective. These experiences allow students to practice active listening and develop the ability to look at the situation from the patient's perspective. In addition to experiential learning, it's essential to foster self-awareness. Encouraging them to reflect on their own experiences, such as when they feel misunderstood or unheard, can help sensitize them to the importance and impact of empathy. Medical schools can provide opportunities for students to engage in group discussions and reflective writing, allowing them to explore their own emotions and biases and how these may influence their interactions with patients. Self-awareness can be a powerful catalyst for developing empathy as it helps physicians reflect on their experiences. Moreover, mentorship plays a pivotal role in cultivating empathy among physicians. Master clinicians can serve as role models by demonstrating empathy and helping trainees recognize its value. Empathy is often observed and absorbed when master clinicians are vulnerable, and so practicing authentic responses that reveal vulnerability by a master clinician makes a powerful impact on students and trainees. Encouraging regular debriefing sessions and providing feedback can help trainees develop coping strategies that will likely reinforce the importance of empathy. By weaving these elements into medical education, we can ensure that future physicians not only possess the technical skills required for patient care but also develop the compassionate and empathetic approach necessary to optimally address the needs of their patients.

EMPATHY CAN HELP REPAIR RUPTURED RELATIONSHIPS

I have witnessed an empathetic break with a patient. Even worse, I think I precipitated it. It involved a patient in the intensive care unit (ICU) with significant heart failure and hypotension. He was hanging onto life by his fingertips. His faithful wife was his permanent bedside companion. There was a fragile balance between his heart failure as measured by his blood pressure and his multiple organ failure, represented by low urinary output and rising serum creatinine. He was making some progress on a daily basis, and I felt we enjoyed an empathetic connection. After morning rounds, I tried to present a factual and humane outlook on his health status and what the future might look like. I said, "This past Christmas was probably your last family celebration." They were shocked, and they were livid. They were right too. What was I thinking? I was trying to help them focus on the challenges they would face in the not too distant future. Yet our past conversations had focused on their hour-to-hour care and on the reality they faced and not on the longer-term challenges they would encounter. Suddenly because of my shifting focus on their future and away from their present, they lost confidence in me, and we suffered an empathetic break. I tried to apologize, but it was useless.

I excused myself and told them I would return in an hour and went to the team room. I reviewed his clinical situation with the team, as well as what I said and what I should have said. How would I reconnect with my patient and his wife? I needed to understand the situation from their perspective, look at it from their point of view. We needed to reestablish trust. I needed to be empathetic in a way that I had not been during the morning. I went to his bedside, and his wife was there. I was ready to give my best apology. Before I could begin my apology, they apologized for their outburst! I was shocked, yet I still tried to look at the situation from their perspective. They needed me to be their advocate. They needed me to be their interpreter of his health data. They needed me to be hopeful. They were just barely holding on, and I had tried to make them face their future instead of staying focused on their daily struggle. Indeed, they were trying to establish an empathetic connection with me.

For the first time, I realized that empathy could flow not only from me to my patients; it also could flow from my patients to me. They helped heal our breach. They needed me to be hopeful as well as empathetic. I never deceived them, and I did not focus on their future; they did not ask me what the future might bring. I understood what they needed, and they accepted me. I realized that sometimes empathy was not sufficient. Sometimes hope was just as important. I also came to understand the power of two-way empathy and to not fear that patients could also establish and even sustain empathy with me. Becoming vulnerable and open to this new realization has made the difference in my relationships with many patients. I am grateful to them for what they showed me and how they helped us heal our rupture and restore our empathetic connection. I learned the value of hope.

EMPATHY AND MAKING MISTAKES

Despite empathetic care, master clinicians make mistakes and learn from their mistakes. On the day of planned discharge from the hospital, a patient of mine suddenly became critically ill. He was rushed to the ICU, and, upon reflection and careful review, we deduced that he had received a high dose of medication. We had ordered it incorrectly. I reviewed all this with the team; the ordering intern was despondent, and the resident was forlorn. I was sad and told them it was not their error, but mine since I was the supervising physician. Every day my focus is how to help the trainees understand medicine, gain clinical insight, and model professionalism. We discussed the error, and we deliberated about how to improve his care. There was one more task for me to do. I asked the resident to walk with me, and we went to the patient's bedside. I told our patient that he was in the ICU because he received an overdose of one of his medications. I apologized for this mistake. I told him it was my error. He shocked us both by saying, "Doc, it's okay. You were just trying to do your best. This happens, and I appreciate your telling me." We were both surprised by his grace. I believe that because of our empathetic connection and our honesty, our patient provided us with understanding and forgiveness. At the end of the month when I provided feedback, I reviewed the lessons we learned during the past month including disease pathogenesis and disease management, but the most important lesson was how to deal with a mistake. I said we all would make mistakes, yet we had to learn from them and commit to not making the mistake again. Everyone looked around and nodded their heads. A few shed a tear, including me. Master clinicians reflect on their mistakes.

ARTIFICIAL INTELLIGENCE AND EMPATHY

AI has the potential to influence physician empathy especially if AI reduces the administrative burden and associated burnout induced through repetitive tasks. If AI reduces taxing repetitive work that may not add to patient care, then it may create the needed extra time for physicians to spend with patients. This time, if dedicated to actively listening, understanding patient concerns, and building trust, will hopefully improve patient–physician relationships and lead to greater empathetic connections. The added time may reduce burnout among clinicians. Burnout is the enemy of empathy. It is difficult to be empathetic if you do not have time to listen attentively to patients or to consider their specific needs. Burnout feeds on itself too. If you know you are not meeting your own standards of patient care or living up to the standards set by master clinicians, the feelings of burnout may accelerate. If AI provides more time for clinician–patient interactions, it will improve connections, thus promoting empathetic opportunities.

Another way AI may influence physician empathy is through personalized patient care. AI technologies can analyze large amounts of patient data and help to develop personalized treatment plans, thereby providing more tailored care. The aggregated data help the team address the unique needs of each patient and may lead to greater empathetic connections. This level of personalization can enhance patient experience and build physician empathy.

CONCLUSION

Developing, applying, and teaching empathy are lifelong practices, and master clinicians have learned the importance of empathy for patient care and for their everyday lives. They are purposeful with their preparation and achieve an authentic empathic connection that improves patient care. No doubt they have a "head start" because of their intuitive nature, but what distinguishes master clinicians is their determined focus on empathy, how they listen attentively to others, and how they truthfully communicate and provide hope. Master clinicians evaluate these emerging traits in their mentees and students. They support and, if necessary, provide feedback to improve the efforts of their trainees. Master clinicians modeling empathy enrich the education of their mentees and students. Their focus allows mentees and students to learn about and to practice developing this tool under a watchful eye.

We all have witnessed the growth of clinicians from students to trainees to colleagues. At the beginning of their careers, every clinician has nascent empathy, and, in retrospect, master clinicians do not begin their careers with more or less empathy than their colleagues. What seems to distinguish master clinicians from their peers is their commitment to strengthen and deepen their attentive listening. They learn to stay in contact with their emotions and become courageous enough to reveal their vulnerabilities. How do they gain these skills? Fundamentally, master clinicians reflect on their experiences, their feelings, and their own emotional development. They have a growing awareness of how empathetic connections improve patient care. They learn that empathy is important beyond patient care and that empathetic connections are crucial in their private and public life too. Master clinicians also learn from their mistakes. I know I have.

REFERENCES

1. Sinclair S, Beamer K, Hack TF, McClement S, Raffin Bouchal S, Chochinov HM, Hagen NA. Sympathy, empathy, and compassion: A grounded theory study of palliative care patients' understandings, experiences, and preferences. *Palliat Med* 2017;31(5):437–447.

2. Available from: www.psychmc.com/blogs/empathy-vs-sympathy#:~:text=The% 20Differences%20Between%20Empathy%20and%20Sympathy,Now%20that%20 we&text=Empathy%20is%20shown%20in%20how,not%20having%20the%20 same%20problems.

7 Clinical Reasoning and Judgment

Stephen A. Paget

Optimal medical care is critically dependent on the clinicians' skills to make the right diagnosis and to recommend the most appropriate therapy, and acquiring such reasoning skills is a key requirement at every level of medical education. Reasoning is the method by which this occurs, and judgment is the final decision.

Medical judgment refers to the process by which health care professionals, such as doctors and nurses, make decisions about a patient's care based on their training, experience, and the available information. It involves assessing a patient's condition, considering potential diagnoses and treatment options, and making informed choices to provide the best possible care. Medical judgment is a critical aspect of health care, as it influences patient outcomes and safety. It often involves weighing risks and benefits and adapting to individual patient needs.

The World Health Organization (WHO) has prioritized patient safety areas and included diagnostic errors as a high-priority problem [1]. In addition, a 2015 report from the National Academy of Medicine in the US, *Improving Diagnosis in Health Care*, concluded that most people will likely experience a diagnostic error in their lifetime [2]. A diagnostic error occurs when a patient's diagnosis is missed altogether, inappropriately delayed, and/or wrong, as judged by the eventual appreciation of definitive information, but these categories of missed, delayed, and wrong diagnoses overlap extensively. Cognitive failures, related to inadequate clinical reasoning—such as failure to synthesize all the available information correctly or failure to use the physical exam findings or test results appropriately—have been found to contribute to the majority of diagnostic errors. Regarding cognitive bias in decision making, the diagnostic failure rate in internal medicine is estimated to be about 10–15%, and diagnostic errors are mostly cognitive errors [3].

On the subject of cognitive errors, the human brain manages and processes information in two ways: intuitively and analytically. In the intuitive manner, there is little reasoning and the thinking is reflexive and fast. Many biases may serve as the main causes of cognitive failure, and this process, which is commonly used in everyday life, provides good odds of the right outcome but is not perfect. The analytic manner is a conscious process, is more reliable than intuitive thinking, and is rational and resource intensive. Cognitive failure avoidance demands critical thinking, debiasing, and purposeful self-regulatory judgment. Potential cognitive failures may include:

Anchoring: Fixing on a specific cause or likely diagnosis and having blinders on for other less likely but possible and more important alternatives

Search Satisficing: This is a portmanteau of satisfy and suffice, a decision-making strategy that attempts to meet an acceptability threshold. It is not the best option.

Framing: A cognitive bias in which people react differently to a particular choice depending on whether it is presented as a gain or a loss. One of the dangers of framing effects is that people are often provided with options within the context of only one of the two frames, such as the positive frame (i.e., if you take this medicine, you will live) or the negative frame (i.e., if you don't take this medicine, you will die).

DOI: 10.1201/9781003409373-7

Momentum: This is the carrying-through of an initial diagnosis or concept, hampering new thinking.

Bias/Branding: Holding on to a preconceived notion can close off broader and potentially more important possible diagnoses.

Avoidance of cognitive errors relies at least in part on metacognition, which is a method of introspection in which one is supposed to contemplate or reflect on one's own thinking because many cognitive errors are the consequence of inappropriate triggering of the intuitive component of cognition. Cognitive errors are susceptible to correction by analytic reasoning; however, some signal must be perceived in order to activate this checking process. There is little doubt that individuals can be forced to rethink their instinctive responses, and, when they do so, they seem to make fewer errors. Nonetheless, how much reassessing and revisiting intuitive responses occur in the real world is not known. In theory, there would be great value if individuals could use critical thinking skills such as emotional attachment that involves beliefs, perspective switching, and assessment of current context, but how to do so is difficult.

In the teaching setting of case discussions, the information is fresh, and the time is ideal for a retrospective analysis and immediate feedback, including a discussion of all kinds of errors if there were any. This approach has been used effectively in many facets of society and allows for an after-action review of events. If cognitive errors were made, this case wrap-up presents an opportunity to dissect and expose them. If the learners have been actively engaged in the problem-solving session, they will be personally invested in understanding how errors occurred. In wrapping up a case, a coach can also ask whether the diagnosis satisfies criteria of adequacy (were all findings explained?), coherence (did physiological linkages make sense?), whether there is a parsimonious explanation of the findings, what the major clues were that led to the correct diagnosis, whether and how a diagnosis could have been arrived at earlier or more efficiently, and whether the therapeutic approaches selected were rational or not. However, this discussion is devoted only to cognitive diagnostic errors, *not* to those involving system-level dysfunctions.

COMPONENTS OF CLINICAL REASONING

Several important components to clinical reasoning apply across many specialties in the world of medicine:

Data Acquisition: The initial step in clinical reasoning is obtaining a comprehensive and accurate patient history, which includes the nature, duration, and progression of symptoms, as well as associated factors such as age, gender, occupation, and family history. Physical examination, laboratory investigations, and imaging studies also provide valuable data that inform the diagnostic process.

Pattern Recognition: Pattern recognition involves the identification of clinical patterns based on common presentations, symptom clusters, and characteristic findings. Familiarity with these patterns assists in generating appropriate differential diagnoses.

Hypothesis Generation: Hypothesis generation involves formulating a list of potential diagnoses based on the identified patterns and clinical data. Clinicians should consider both common and rare diseases, keeping in mind the prevalence and epidemiology of various conditions.

Diagnostic Testing: Diagnostic testing plays a crucial role in confirming or excluding hypotheses. Clinicians routinely utilize a variety of investigations, including blood tests, imaging studies, and diagnostic procedures. Selecting the most appropriate tests based on clinical suspicion and evidence-based guidelines is essential.

Interpretation and Refinement: Interpreting the results of diagnostic tests in the context of clinical findings is essential to refine diagnostic hypotheses. It may involve reviewing patterns, ruling out certain conditions, or considering additional investigations. Clinicians should be aware of the limitations and pitfalls of tests to avoid misinterpretation.

Clinical Decision Making: After synthesizing all available data, clinicians must make informed decisions regarding treatment and management. This includes selecting appropriate pharmacological and nonpharmacological interventions, establishing follow-up plans, and considering patient preferences and comorbidities.

Clinical reasoning faces several challenges, which may include overlapping symptoms, variability of disease presentations, limitations in existing diagnostic markers, and overreliance on diagnostic tests. To surmount these obstacles, several strategies exist to enhance the process of clinical reasoning:

Continued Medical Education: Staying up-to-date with the latest research and evidence-based guidelines is essential for enhancing clinical reasoning in medicine. Clinicians should actively engage in continued medical education by attending conferences, participating in journal clubs, and utilizing online resources to stay abreast of advances in the field.

Case-Based Learning: Activities such as clinical case discussions and grand rounds provide opportunities for clinicians to apply their clinical reasoning skills to real-life scenarios. Sharing and discussing cases with colleagues can foster collaborative learning, encourage critical thinking, and expose clinicians to diverse perspectives.

Clinical Decision Support Tools: The use of these tools, such as diagnostic algorithms and smartphone apps, can aid clinicians in the clinical reasoning process. These tools provide structured frameworks for differential diagnosis and treatment recommendations grounded in evidence-based guidelines.

Multidisciplinary Collaboration: Discussions with other health care professionals, such as radiologists, pathologists, and other specialists, can enhance clinical reasoning. Seeking input from clinicians with different perspectives and expertise can help validate diagnostic hypotheses, assist with interpretation of complex test results, and optimize patient management. Face-to-face meetings among experts often will help sort out complicated scenarios.

Reflective Practice: Engaging in reflective practice, including regular self-assessment and critical reflection on clinical encounters, can promote continuous improvement in clinical reasoning skills. Clinicians should review challenging cases, analyze their decision-making processes, and identify areas for improvement or further learning. Once a diagnosis and treatment plan are formulated, nothing is more important than close follow-up and communication with the patient to assure that your initial diagnosis and treatment are correct and that things are moving in the proper direction for the patient. A personal favorite approach in the setting of the institution of a medication, such as corticosteroid treatment, might be carried out through electronic or telephone contact using the following language:

I have decided to treat you in the following manner. Each day I want you to contact me to grade your progress. 10 is the worst you could be, such as your current state, and 0 is back to normal. Each day, I want you to give me an overall grade that includes aspects of pain, fatigue, overall function, and any other prominent part of your illness. As soon as your grade is 0, I will begin to taper your medication. Or, if the therapy I chose is not helping, I need to rethink the diagnosis and treatment in order to achieve a better outcome.

THE CLINICIAN

Despite many revolutionary changes in the technology, concepts, and practice of medicine during the last century, there remains a single common title to distinguish doctors who treat sick people: clinicians. The word "clinician" comes from the Greek word meaning "bed," and the word "patient" is derived from the Latin *pati*, which means "to suffer." The clinician is the doctor at the sufferer's bedside, the doctor who accepts responsibility for the life entrusted to them by the patient. In caring for patients, clinicians constantly perform hypothesis testing. Although clinicians do not usually regard ordinary patient care as a form of experiment, every aspect of the clinical management can be designed, executed, and appraised with intellectual procedures identical to those used in any experimental situation. The important activities at the bedside and in the laboratory differ fundamentally, not just in their basic intellectual construction but also in their materials and mode of inception. The concept that a clinician performs various types of experiments in their routine therapeutic activities is entirely consistent with the definition offered by Claude Bernard, who is often regarded as a founder of experimental discipline in medicine. Bernard explained that the experimentalist is one who applies methods of investigation—be they simple or complex—in order to make natural phenomena vary or to alter them with some specific purpose. In the experiments of ordinary clinical treatment, however, the purpose is not to gain new knowledge, but instead to repeat a success of the past.

THE COMPLEXITY OF HUMAN DATA AND REASONING

A clinician observes at least three different types of data. The first type of data describes a disease in morphologic, chemical, microbiological, physiological, or other impersonal terms. The second type of data describes the host in whom the disease occurs. This description of the host's environmental background includes both the personal properties of the host before the disease began, such as age, gender, and education, as well as the properties of the host's external surroundings, such as geographic location, occupation, and financial and social status. A third type of data describes the illness that occurs in the interaction between the disease and the environmental host. The illness consists of clinical phenomena: the host's subjective sensations, which are called symptoms, and certain findings called signs, which are discussed objectively during the physical examination of the diseased host. When the diseased host seeks medical attention, they become a patient, and the clinician's work begins.

The clinician uses three types of data to make decisions about the present, past, and future of the patient. The decisions consist of determining a present diagnosis, which gives the disease a name and tells what is wrong; an etiology and pathogenesis, or how it got this way; and future prognosis and therapy, or what to do about it. Of these various decisions, only the choice of prognosis and therapy is distinctively clinical. The clinician must examine the patient to make effective decisions about treatment. Why did this happen to this patient at this time and in this place? The clinical symptoms and signs of the patient's illness, however, are discerned only by a doctor skilled in the clinical procedures of history taking and physical examination.

In using all these data for planning treatment, the clinician's reasoning can be broadly divided into two categories: therapeutic and environmental. The therapeutic decision deals with the mode of treatment, and the environmental decision deals with the management of the host—a choice of method of communication, accommodation, and human interchange that will best enable the sick host to bear the burdens of both ailment and treatment. The therapeutic decision answers the question: what is the best treatment for this particular ailment? In the reasoning of therapeutic decision making, the patient is a case, i.e., a representative instance of disease and illness for which treatment is chosen after comparison with results obtained in similar previous cases. In the reasoning of the environmental decision, the patient is a unique person for whom each aspect of management must be individualized.

A clinician's privilege and power in clinical therapy is her ability to make both the therapeutic and the environmental decisions concomitantly. The process of observation and reasoning used for these decisions is as diverse as the intricacies of human thought and is performed differently by each clinician. The process is usually regarded as an art-like, sometimes mystical, often intuitive procedure that seldom merits and rarely fulfills the intellectual demands of scientific thought. When a clinician makes decisions in the experiments of therapy, we generally assume that the procedure is too complex for scientific documentation. The clinician is usually permitted to justify her work on the basis of hunch or intuition or as nebulously defined by previous clinical experience. Her decisions are allowed a rationale that need not be overly rational and reasons that need not be particularly reasonable. If the clinician seems knowledgeable and authoritative and if her reputation and results seem good, she can be pardoned for most flagrant imprecisions, vagueness, and inconsistency in the conduct of therapy. The clinician does not even use a scientific name for her method of designing, executing, and appraising therapeutic experiments. She calls it clinical judgment.

To a clinician, the idea of treatment is not merely important; it is paramount. The care of the patient is the ultimate, specific act that characterizes a clinician. It differentiates her from all other medical doctors, biologists, and students of human illness. Its obligation is transmitted as the heritage of her profession. Its performance is their unique contribution to the multifarious services exchanged by humankind to sustain civilization and life. If treatment is an unimportant endeavor, the clinician has no useful purpose for her medical existence. Nevertheless, the basic intellectual problems of treatment receive comparatively little attention in contemporary clinical research. The clinicians of modern academic medical centers have become increasingly concerned with laboratory investigation of the pathogenesis of the disease or mechanisms of cellular biology. The problems of therapy are often dismissed as a mere application of the basic science studied in the investigator's laboratory. Behind this dismissal is the traditional belief that the therapeutic aspects of medicine can never be "science" and that clinical judgment can never be "scientific." Clinical judgment has a distinctive methodology for dealing with the tangible data of human illness, and clinical judgment in the present day has both the obligation and the opportunity to be accomplished with scientific taste, discretion, and quality. Never before have clinicians had to make decisions about therapeutic agents capable of such spectacular benefits and such potentially devastating harm. Never before have clinicians had available the intellectual assistance of new mathematical and computational systems to help manage the complex data assessed in their therapeutic decisions.

The scientific method is an intellectual concept. It refers to the quality with which an experiment is designed, executed, and appraised. Almost anyone can make some plans, carry them out, and see what happens. The scientific quality of the activity depends on the methods used for making the plans and for observing and interpreting what happens. In every aspect of experimental construction by the scientific method, the performance of clinical therapy is identical to a laboratory investigation. The differences between the clinical treatment and the laboratory work are not in the rational aspects of the scientific method but in the procedures and methodology used for the design, execution, and appraisal of the hypothesis testing. These procedures include the techniques used for preparation of material, selection of maneuver, and observation of response.

The clinical design is the preparation of the evaluation by examining a patient, arriving at a diagnostic classification, estimating a prognosis, and choosing a mode of treatment. In clinical therapy, the ultimate maneuver is the administration of treatment, or the clinician may elect to give no treatment specifically, allowing nature to take its course. In terms of results, the patient's response to clinical treatment and subsequent reactions constitute the outcome of interest.

Clinical and personal data are the responsibility of the clinician. She is the principal apparatus that observes and interprets the data as variables of human illness. The scientific function of this human apparatus is gravely impaired when the clinician's observations are imprecise and unstandardized and when her interpretations are made without appropriate criteria and without vigorous attempts to achieve uniformity and consistency. Clinicians usually accept these methodological deficits complacently, attributing them to the frailty of human capacities and concluding that, since the flaws are traditional, they must also be inevitable. Yet these human sensory organs give a clinician the power to make many observations of which no inanimate instrument is capable, and the human mind enables the clinician to make constant scientific improvements in the way she performs her observations and interpretations. The clinician cannot begin to improve these functions, however, until she recognizes herself as a unique and powerful piece of scientific equipment. She can then contemplate and, if necessary, revise the fundamental aspects of what she does and how she thinks when she collects the human data for which she is the main and often the only perceptual apparatus. The clinician who wants to contemplate the scientific performance of her bedside procedures soon finds her paths of thought blocked by a series of obstacles. The obstacles are a group of hallowed beliefs, transmitted as intellectual legacies by teacher to student and from one medical generation to the next. Each of these beliefs is like an axiom and established principle that, though not necessarily true, is universally accepted:

Motivation: The clinician believes that the main incentive for scientific research is to discover the cause of natural phenomena and that phenomena whose causes are unknown cannot be properly managed.

Reasoning: The clinician believes that her intellectual organization of clinical observations is rationally amorphous and that her thinking has too many intricate and unquantified elements to be expressed in the mathematical structure used for other types of scientific analysis.

Observation: The clinician believes that her description of the signs and symptoms cannot be scientifically precise because they often contain nouns, adjectives, verbs, and adverbs rather than the numerical dimensions of measurement.

Correlation: The clinician believes she finds a constant association between abnormal structures and abnormal functions that occur in human illness.

Classification: The clinician believes that she adequately identifies human illness by categorizing sick people with diagnostic names that represent the morphologic and laboratory abnormalities of disease.

Centrally important in the ultimate clinical equation is shared decision making with the patient. Their participation in their own care is as important in the final therapeutic decisions as the doctor. It is incumbent upon the physician to educate the patient and their family about the illness and the pros and cons of the various therapeutic options.

DETAILED STEPS IN THE CLINICAL REASONING PROCESS

First one needs to obtain and filter information that may be obtained primarily through reading, visual imagery, and listening. Other sensory inputs such as tactile and olfactory may be obtained. The next step is to formulate an initial small set of hypotheses in the context of identified questions and problems in a current case, as well as a knowledge base of prior cases, using schemas and pattern recognition. Experts quickly develop a small set of hypotheses with minimal clinical data to represent the problem to be solved. Experts will generally have the final diagnosis in this set within five minutes of starting. Novice and intermediate learners will take longer to develop a set of hypotheses. This is followed by obtaining additional information as directed by the initial hypotheses. The initial small set of hypotheses forms a framework for additional focused information gathering. This process is repeated and refined. One then uses a reasoning strategy (deductive versus inductive) to process the information in the clinical context of the case.

Deductive reasoning works from general to specific, in a "top-down logic." We develop hypotheses to explain the case problem and apply collected information to test the hypotheses in order to try to confirm or exclude them. In our hypothesis-deductive process, a classic rank-ordered list of differential diagnosis is generated: the process goes if-then-but-therefore (yes, no). If we have certain information, then certain hypotheses may be true, but we test against further information, and therefore it is true or not. This is akin to the scientific principle in which one tries to prove a hypothesis. Deductive reasoning offers the strongest support: the premises ensure the conclusion, meaning that it is impossible for the conclusion to be false if all the premises are true. Such an argument is called a valid argument.

Inductive reasoning works from specific to general, in a "bottom-up logic." One starts with information from the observations matched to an established pattern (algorithm) to come to a hypothesis. The hypothesis is then matched for fit to the problem in the case. Induction yields discoveries that are probable but not proven. Inductive reasoning becomes powerful when an expert-derived algorithm is followed. The algorithms have been derived with statistical relevance to real cases.

Abductive reasoning is a form of logical inference that seeks the simplest and most likely conclusion from a set of observations. Abductive reasoning, unlike deductive reasoning, yields a plausible conclusion but does not definitively verify it. Abductive conclusions do not eliminate uncertainty or doubt, which is expressed in the retreat terms such as "best available" or "most likely." This type of reasoning is commonly used in medicine.

The human body is very complex, and we cannot obtain all the information we want; thus, regardless of the reasoning process utilized, we can never absolutely prove or disprove most hypotheses. We arrive at the most likely diagnosis, but we may need to eventually consider others if more information becomes available or the outcome is different than expected.

Performance of an analysis of hypothesis by probabilistic and cause–effect means can be utilized in either deductive or inductive reasoning processes. Hypotheses are refined by Bayesian inference, which occurs when evidence or observations are used to determine the probability that a hypothesis may be correct. If tests are performed, such as laboratory tests, calculated results for test sensitivity, specificity, positive predictive value, and negative predictive value are useful in analysis. Hypotheses are refined by cause–effect analysis to apply principles of pathophysiology, such as biomedical knowledge, and determine whether a hypothesis is based on a sound scientific basis. Evidence-based medicine is another description of this process.

Next, we can employ abstract ideas and concepts that are interpreted and used effectively. In this situation, we avoid concrete thinking (childlike, literal interpretation, lack of generalizability) and avoid linear thinking (singular, unbranched series of cause-and-effect relationships).

We then formulate a final diagnosis and test the final diagnosis against positive and negative findings and standard criteria for the description of a disease process. The working diagnosis for a patient and prognostic or therapeutic recommendations are finalized only after they are assessed for their adequacy in explaining all positive, negative, and normal clinical findings. The pathophysiologic reliability of the diagnosis is a check on the reasonableness of the causal links between clinical events, ascertained from the use of biomedical knowledge. Does the diagnosis fit with cause and effect? Is the diagnosis consistent with pathophysiological principles? We must always consider other potential diagnoses to diminish the possibility of premature closure. We must evaluate the process and then stop, think, act, review, and ultimately communicate the diagnosis. Follow-up is key because clinical reasoning is improved when errors in information, judgment, and reasoning are discovered and discussed when reviewing the case. The quicker this happens, the greater the improvement will be. Experts apply pattern recognition with nonanalytic cognitive processing during the initial phases of considering a novel clinical case and then apply analytic processing in hypothesis testing. Novices may work the other way around. However, these two forms of reasoning can be interactive and not sequential; they are complementary contributors to the overall accuracy of the clinical reasoning process, each one influencing the other.

SHERLOCK HOLMES CONUNDRUM: THE DIFFERENCE BETWEEN DEDUCTIVE AND INDUCTIVE REASONING

Sherlock Holmes has always been lauded for his quote "science of deduction." Picture Sherlock snooping around a crime scene, collecting his information. He observes countless details about the scene and the victim and then, from that information, arrives at a conclusion that is not necessarily true but is probable based on the information available. Deductive reasoning begins with an accepted premise and seeks to prove another statement based on previously "known" information. An example of this might be found in how Sherlock walks into a dank bedroom with the premise that there have been a rash of murders in the area, so the woman on the floor is likely another victim of that same predator. He then gathers information and narrows the scope of that available information until his premise is the only logical conclusion remaining. This is the kind of logic that, in fact, many police investigators use. They have a suspect in mind based on previously available information that is not necessarily related to the case, and they then seek out evidence to prove the guilt of that suspect. Inductive reasoning, however, allows Sherlock to extrapolate from the information observed in order to arrive at conclusions about events that have not been observed. Here, we see the detective walking into the scene in a blank state— he has no presupposed ideas about what might have taken place. Then he gathers facts until he arrives at a conclusion.

TEACHING CLINICAL REASONING

Various clinical reasoning methods exist that can be applied to diagnostic problems by diagnosticians. Yet this does not imply that we cannot teach beyond repeated practice on a similar range of problems or observing others engaged in the process. If clinical reasoning cannot be taught either as a pure process or directly as a skill, teaching it in a case-based format might be a proper middle ground. What further features may an effective case-based approach require? First, it is important to take the term "reasoning" seriously. The teacher or supervisor should avoid overemphasizing the outcome (i.e., the "correct" diagnosis), for this may reinforce undesirable behavior, such as guessing or jumping to conclusions. In addition, teaching should consist of small steps, and teachers should not hesitate to frequently ask hypothetical questions or questions that probe a possible explanation of findings. What if . . . ? Can you think of other possibilities? Can you explain this? It should also be clear to both teachers and students that a differential diagnosis is a legitimate end point of the process, particularly if different diagnostic or therapeutic actions are associated with each alternative in the differential diagnosis.

There is limited evidence that the modeled schema characterizing disease into eight groups (congenital, traumatic, immunologic, neoplastic, metabolic, infectious, toxic, and vascular) can be helpful, but any other approach, as long as it is systematic, may also be used by early-stage learners. Moreover, to be effective, objectives and expectations must be clearly communicated before a clinical reasoning session begins. The best format appears to be small group sessions guided by a clinical tutor. In advanced groups, students can be asked to prepare and present the case. During sessions, students should be encouraged to actively participate and take notes. To avoid the "retrospective bias," that is, teaching problem solving as if one is working toward a solution known in advance, the method works best when the teacher is not familiar with the case but has access to exactly the same information as the students. Teaching clinical reasoning in a step-by-step fashion, with an emphasis on formulating a correct and comprehensive differential diagnosis, will be the best way to start clinical training. Expert clinicians store and recall knowledge as diseases, conditions, or syndromes—i.e., illness scripts—which are connected to problem representations. These representations trigger clinical memory, permitting the related knowledge to become accessible for reasoning. Knowledge recalled as in illness script form has a predictable structure: the predisposing conditions, the pathophysiological insult, and the clinical consequences.

One could argue that teaching clinical reasoning in the age of computer-aided diagnostic tools, artificial intelligence/ChatGPT/Bard, electronic medical records, and massive clinical electronic databases is superfluous. In actuality, it is more needed than ever. None of these digital modalities can yet substitute for an expert, experienced, empathic, and detail-oriented clinician.

REFERENCES

1. Cresswell KM, Panesar SS, Salvilla SA, Carson-Stevens A, Larizgoitia I, Donaldson LJ, Bates D, Sheikh A; World Health Organization's (WHO) Safer Primary Care Expert Working Group. Global research priorities to better understand the burden of iatrogenic harm in primary care: an international Delphi exercise. *PLoS Med* 2013 Nov;10(11):e1001554. https://doi.org/10.1371/journal.pmed.1001554

2. Committee on Diagnostic Error in Health Care; Board on Health Care Services; Institute of Medicine; The National Academies of Sciences, Engineering, and Medicine. Summary. In Balogh EP, Miller BT, Ball JR, eds, *Improving Diagnosis in Health Care*. Washington, DC: National Academies Press; 2015. Available from: https://www.ncbi.nlm.nih.gov/books/NBK338596/

3. Graber ML, Franklin N, Gordon R. Diagnostic error in internal medicine. *Arch Intern Med*. 2005 Jul 11;165(13):1493–9. doi: 10.1001/archinte.165.13.1493. PMID: 16009864.

8 Practicing Principled Medicine

Jerome P. Kassirer

Those fortunate enough to practice medicine should need no refresher on the fundamental principles of our profession, yet the vicissitudes of day-to-day patient care sometimes fail to remind us of why we eagerly return to the bedside. I have accepted this memory-jogging task, not, I admit, without reservations. I have no training in medical ethics, and I do not consider myself an ethicist. What I do bring to the discussion, however, is an exceptionally variegated career of more than 60 years during which I practiced, observed, and wrote about the profession I love. After making an astonishing diagnosis as an intern, I was propelled into academic medicine in Boston, where I practiced nephrology, took major administrative jobs, participated in research, was appointed editor of a highly prized journal, and ended up teaching and consulting at three more major academic institutions. My medical writings, aside from those related to the kidney and electrolytes, have covered diagnosis, clinical reasoning, physician accountability, joint physician–patient decision making, privacy, the use of scarce resources, overtreatment in fee-for-service reimbursement, undertreatment under capitation, physician–patient relationships, medical errors, conflict of interest, preserving the heritage of the profession, and many other topics. Time and experience did give me a lot to ponder and a lot to say.

THE CRITICAL ROLE OF TRUST

Trust holds society together. Our economy, our banking system, and our international relations are but a few aspects of society that depend on trust. Intimate personal relationships depend on trust; interpersonal trust in turn relies on the integrity of individuals. In medicine at large, patients must believe that the medical care system will act in their best interest, and in the one-on-one relationship between patients and their own physicians, trust allows individuals to safely experience interpersonal commitments that include an expectation that the doctor will maintain strict confidentiality and will always "do the right thing." Gaining trust reduces vulnerability, allowing people to depend on one another. Elements of trust include competence, caring, commitment, clarity, and consistency. Trust encompasses admitting when a medical error has been made and explaining how and why it happened. Without trust, relationships do not last. Trust is generally difficult to gain, yet easy to lose.

THE PHYSICIAN–PATIENT RELATIONSHIP

Starting from a fundamental basis of trust, the nature of the physician–patient relationship is the next essential ingredient of principled medicine. It has been traditional to refer to the sage comments of Dr. Francis Peabody nearly a century ago [1]. In his lecture to Harvard Medical School students, he referred to the highly personal experience of illness and the doctor's role. He urged his audience to understand that it was necessary to appreciate their patients' personal experiences of illness, and he observed that "the secret of the care of the patient is in caring for the patient." This empathic concept remains critical because patients are at their most vulnerable when they are threatened with illness. Few other circumstances require an individual to disrobe and bare the most intimate details of their lives. Given this vulnerability, it behooves us to appreciate small gestures that might remove the anxious

DOI: 10.1201/9781003409373-8

edge of a patient encounter. Just chatting about the patient's family and pastime preferences reduces tension. Refreshing any previous history before the encounter, sitting quietly and listening intently without interrupting and without typing on a keyboard, and identifying any emotional cues are important starters. My personal benchmark of genuine concern for patients was Sheldon Wolff, my boss (and friend) for 13 years. All patients referred to him, rich or poor, were treated to the same extent: Shelly personally arranged their tests and treatments at the patients' convenience; when the test or treatment was being administered, he showed up to ensure that the patient was well treated; he visited his hospitalized patients regularly and kept an eye on their clinical course even when others were the physicians in charge. He cared. My colleague Faith Fitzgerald's take on the centrality of the patient is also worth recounting [2]. She wrote:

If medicine is distracted by the business model of health care, or the wellness model of health care, or the management model of health care, we will erode the science base of medical education. And if we do that, we will erode the physician's central unique value—taking care of sick people. Patients trust physicians to do what is best for them, not for the health system, but them as sick individuals. If we are consumed with management and policy and with systems, real patients will languish in their beds wondering where their doctors are.

In several widely admired publications, Stanford physician Abraham Verghese has championed another important slant on the unique role of the physician in the patient encounter [3]. Verghese, a staunch advocate of teaching medicine at the bedside, initiated the idea that the physical examination represents far more than an opportunity to provide diagnostically relevant information; it constitutes a ritual that bonds physician and patient and that provides comfort to suffering people. To a modern medical school graduating class he said:

You are also participating in a timeless ritual . . . when you get to examine a patient. You are in a ceremonial white gown. They are in a ceremonial paper gown. You stand there not as yourself, but as the doctor. As part of that ritual they will allow you the privilege of touching their body, something that in any other walk of life would be considered assault. The ritual properly performed earns you a bond with the patient . . . The ritual is timeless, and it matters.

Echoing Peabody, Verghese mentioned his favorite quote from the ancient physician Paracelsus, "This is my vow: to love the sick, each and all of them, more than if my own body were at stake." Circumstances are such that some of these gestures and rituals may not always be possible, but when they are, a rich and deep relationship can form between doctor and patient that may not only help the healing process but make the work of medicine especially satisfying.

PROVIDING CARE
A primary aspect of principled medical care is the actual provision of care. The elements of this critical step include gathering all the necessary patient data, assessing the patient's condition, determining what diagnostic and therapeutic choices are optimal, formulating trade-offs between choices when necessary, explaining both the evidence and the decision making to the patient and/or family, assuring that the choices are understood, answering all questions, and evaluating whether patients have independence in making judgments that affect them personally. This enormous and complex responsibility today replaces a long-held paternalistic approach in which the physician briefly summarized the problem and told the patient what

he (in fact, it was almost always a he) was planning to do about it; the patient was allowed little say. At the outset, it should be pointed out that there is nothing wrong about asking physicians what their best choice would be when neither one nor the other of the possible options seems the most beneficial.

Many of us who became deeply involved in the emerging field of medical decision making in the late decades of the 20th century assumed that physicians could learn to employ some combination of evidence evaluation and formal decision analysis to help in making difficult medical decisions under conditions of uncertainty. Indeed, in expert hands, assembling a full decision tree with its probabilities and utilities (values) of outcomes proved successful and useful [4]. Unfortunately, even when the necessary calculations were fully automated, decision analysis was deemed by most physicians too complex for routine use. For this reason, complex decisions between competing choices are still being made implicitly, rather than formally.

Given that physicians' intellects remain responsible for collecting and evaluating evidence and making judgments about optimal testing and therapy, it is worth elaborating to some extent on both. Evidence-based medicine intends to replace intuition and nonsystematic judgments with data based on rigorous human experimentation and, in the proper hands, succeeds in doing so. In practical terms, however, the limitations of evidence-based medicine inhibit its ideal use. An individual patient may not be represented in any rigorous clinical trial; a clinical trial carried out under strict conditions may not reflect the "real-life" conditions of a patient at hand; and despite the vast number of clinical trials performed, the information from an individual trial or summary of similar trials may not be readily available. Requiring payment to review published material online can be a substantial barrier. Summary data in the form of expert reviews, clinical practice guidelines, and compiled, regularly updated electronic sources often substitute for original data. Needless to say, the use of these sources requires a facile use of computer search methods and often a willingness to pay for data use. Even when information from these sources is available, extrapolating a patient's full clinical manifestations, including test and treatment risks of harm can miss the mark. Sizing up choices for consideration by the patient can also be vexed because the ingredients of each choice, as well as the likelihoods and values of potential outcomes must be assembled implicitly. An added complexity is that both sides of the physician–patient relationship have known deficiencies. Physicians are, like other humans, often not logical calculators of probabilities. And on the patient side, emotions and personal experiences can influence sober judgments in their most difficult health decisions. During the time I was actively helping patients make such choices, I often wondered out loud whether the need of a patient to house a precious canine companion in a kennel had more influence on his decision to come into the hospital for more tests than the risks of harm avoiding the tests entailed. In the final analysis, the critically important synthetic task of combining data and judging its impact remains the job of a doctor; it is an awesome responsibility. Making difficult judgments constitutes the remaining vestigial art of medicine.

Once the data are assembled and interpreted, and once clinical judgments about the optimal approach to further testing and treatment are considered, the principled physician has another essential role, namely to inform and educate the patient. Educating patients may involve simply explaining the implications of a laboratory test result, interpreting a scan report sent to them directly from a laboratory, or describing the meaning of an independent search of an internet site, or even responding to some medical idea that originated in a conversation with a friend. Telemedicine or email can expedite these interactions. When it comes to complex decisions about invasive or risky testing procedures or treatments that may produce harm, a one-on-one patient encounter is vastly better. To begin with, physicians should be frank with patients who have heard, probably repeatedly, the flawed aphorism "do no harm." Of course, a doctor should never intentionally cause harm. Yet virtually all medical tests and treatments designed to enhance diagnostic accuracy or treat a serious ailment have the potential for harm. Because there is often some uncertainty in diagnosis, some patients who do not have a disease will receive a potentially harmful treatment and some who have the disease will fail to receive proper treatment. Similarly, some patients who do not have a disease will be harmed by a test, and others with the disease will be misdiagnosed because the test was never ordered.

Physicians are recommenders, not the prime decision makers. If the choice between two courses of action, say a surgical versus a medical approach, favors one over the other, they should express their opinion, and if they weigh both sides and assess that the choice is a decisional toss-up, doctors should try as best they can to explain why they reached this conclusion. Nonetheless, when patients ask for advice about these difficult choices, they will welcome a frank reply. In all of these encounters, the physician will have to assess whether the patient fully understands the components of the decision, his or her capacity to make a choice, whether the choice is consistent with the individual's values, preferences, and beliefs, and the patient's independence in making it. Patients' preferences matter: I once wrote about several instances in which, for one reason or another, physicians had abrogated patients' choices [5]. The cases had many features in common. I explained:

In each instance the medical consequences of the available choices were not well known, but the probability that the choice favored by the patient would have a seriously adverse consequence was very small. In each instance the patient was willing to accept a small chance of an adverse consequence as a condition for an improved quality of life. In each instance the physician stood in jeopardy if the outcome of the patient's choice turned out to be adverse. In each instance the physician attempted to impose a decision on the patient, and in each instance the patient rejected the physician's advice despite a previously trusting relationship.

I personally intervened in each case, allowing the patient to be the decision maker.

Physicians have another responsibility, one that is not ordinarily considered in discussions of the ethics of medical practice, namely to provide a ready portal of communication between themselves and the patient. With all the modern communication devices and methods, many people still have difficulty in reaching their doctor when the need arises. The intercession of intermediates including medical "portals" or medical assistants seems to have notably exacerbated the problem. In my view, a doctor should be readily available by phone or email, and in turn, patients should be parsimonious in the use of this form of communication, using it for true emergencies only.

Finally, physicians owe their patients a chance at getting optimal care. If it is unavailable locally, the patient should be referred elsewhere. I have experienced such referrals in my own medical care more than once, and I believe others should have the same benefit. Few interactions with physicians engender more trust in the dedication of one's doctor to providing the best care than such an experience.

PARSING OUT RESPONSIBILITIES

Until recently, the cognitive medical tasks described here have remained largely in the domain of physicians because computer systems have been insufficient to deal with the complexities of health and disease. A rapidly evolving field of machine learning and artificial intelligence based on the use of trained databases has created medical computer applications that mimic human behavior so eerily that it makes it difficult to know whether a human or a machine is creating responses to questions or analyzing data. Though the current iterations of these so-called chatbots are not yet in clinical use, experiments with them show promise in performing many of the human tasks that I have described in this essay. Because of the rapid changes and the continuing evolution of these computer methods, it is impossible today to guess how effective or flawed these programs will be when applied to real patients, yet it is safe to predict, I believe, that a substantial fraction of what physicians do now will change. How these changes will alter the traditional roles I have described is uncertain, but I have no doubt that divvying up the responsibilities between doctors and machines will be neither easy nor painless.

THREATS TO PRINCIPLED PRACTICE

Doctors, because of their unique positions of trust, are held to an exceptionally high standard in society, yet they have roles that often compete. One role is to provide care to the best of their ability, and another is to make a reasonable living, given the huge investment of time and money required to become a practitioner. An anonymous quote in an 1847 issue of the *Boston Medical and Surgical Journal* (the predecessor of the *New England Journal of Medicine*) titled "Profits of Medical Practice" that I came across in the 1990s sums up the issue as follows [6]:

> The fact is simply this, that the practitioner of medicine has a stomach to be filled, a body to be clothed, and in most cases a family to maintain—and a variety of relations which he bears to the whole community, renders it positively necessary that he should conform to the usages of civilized society. To do so there must be an adequate income from some source to meet the expense of being part and parcel of the general population.

I begin with the premise that most physicians, just like individuals outside of medicine, are motivated by money and that fee-for-service systems create financial rewards for more testing and treating, and capitated systems create financial rewards for less testing and treating. I was fortunate never to practice in either system. From the beginning of my long career at Tufts Medicine (its current name), I was salaried. I never had a contract: I was told at the beginning of each year what my salary would be and what was expected of me. I could make a few extra dollars, if I wished, by giving a few lectures a year at designated community hospitals; during my decades-long years of active practice, no one ever urged me to pay attention to the hospital's budget. My salary was meager but could sustain a small family. Without financial pressure on my testing and treatment judgments, I simply did what I thought was best for the patient. Given the camaraderie in the institution, there was no incentive to sit back and let others do the work. The experience was satisfying; I once remarked to a trainee on rounds that it was amazing that I was being paid for what I did because it was so much fun.

In my later editorial role, I began to worry about the effect that reimbursement in capitated programs might have on the morality of the entire profession [7]. I was concerned that doctors might "find themselves conforming to the restrictions and deceiving themselves that what they are doing is best for their patients." At the time, measures of the quality of care were widely introduced to assess the quality of care in all systems and to deter both underuse and overuse. Some of these efforts were successful, but many practicing doctors and physician-led hospital groups were dissatisfied with the additional burden of paperwork, the diverse demands for measurement from many different organizations, and the perception that these measures had impugned their reputation.

But it was another earlier experience that increased my sensitivity to a different threat that involved money, namely financial conflict of interest. Here is how I first got wind of it. After about a decade on the staff at Tufts, I was asked by one of the giant pharmaceutical companies to join their panel of lecturers, based on my developing expertise on the uses and risks of diuretics. Given the promise that I would have total control over selection of topics and all spoken material as well as a generous honorarium, I agreed, and over the next few years, I gave several talks a year. Representatives of the company showed up from time to time, but never commented on my presentations nor asked me to modify them. After I had given these talks for a few years, the company's representative offered to send me to a firm on Madison Avenue in New York City to improve my speaking style; I did so, with the implication that I might be sent to larger and more important venues. Once I had finished the training, the representative explained that I was ready (for the big time, I assume) and that all required was that I mention just one time, in each lecture, the name of their highly effective diuretic product that had recently been approved by the FDA. It was, in fact, an excellent drug, a major advance over existing diuretics, but I did not see myself as a hawker for a drug company and said I'd take a pass on doing that. From that time forward, I was offered no speaking engagements by the company.

I perceived the threat of financial conflicts of interest more clearly when I had become the editor of the *New England Journal of Medicine* in the early 1990s. This essay is not the place for an extended discussion of all the ways conflicts of interest have influenced principled practice and professionalism, but a few concepts are worth pondering here [8]. A conflict of interest exists when an individual is in a position in which professional judgment concerning a primary interest tends to be unduly influenced by a secondary interest such as financial gain. It exists when one duty tends to lead to the disregard of another, interferes with proper exercise of judgment, and when making a personal choice over a professional one violates a code, a promise, or a responsibility. I make another assumption that even small gifts can influence behavior. I make the additional assumption that the method most employed in medicine to deal with financial conflicts of interest—namely disclosure—is no solution at all. Disclosure is a necessary but not a sufficient part of a solution. Eliminating the conflict is the only real solution. In my view, all of the discord about lack of disclosure simply misses the point. The lack of disclosure is not the problem. The conflict is the problem. Despite books on the subject (one, my own [8]) and pronouncements of professional societies, the problem of financial conflict of interest remains incompletely solved in medicine.

Lest the reader is left with this impression that money is the critical driver of professional activities of doctors, I hasten to add that physicians' morality is a powerful counterbalance. In countless encounters with trainees over decades, I have been impressed that the overwhelming number decided on medicine as a career largely because of a desire to help people. This sense of responsibility provides a strong deterrent, not only in the routine practice of medicine but in other situations in which financial incentives might conflict with responsibilities to patients.

THE PRODIGIOUS REWARDS

Although all clinicians have had disappointing experiences (i.e., diagnosing untreatable illnesses, standing by when a long-standing patient fails to rally from appropriate therapy to treat and cure a dangerous infective endocarditis), other experiences such as keeping a patient with diabetes from developing complications for decades by careful management, bringing a terminally ill patient back to life from extreme acidosis and hypokalemia, and rescuing a patient from acute rhabdomyolysis and kidney failure are just a few of the counterbalancing rewards of practicing medicine. Being directly involved in the scientific and practical trajectories of medicine has its own gratifications. As a young physician, the only antibiotics available to us were penicillin and streptomycin; the only diuretic was a toxic mercury compound that had to be injected; the only antihypertensive drug was so erratic that too little had no effect and too much caused blackouts on standing. There were no organ transplants, no monoclonal antibodies for autoimmune diseases, and virtually no effective chemotherapeutic agents. Diagnostic testing was primitive. Not a single scan had yet been invented. In fact, the structure of DNA had not been identified.

Yet the personal rewards of medical practice vastly exceed the occurrence of medical "miracles." It is the personal bonds with patients that add to the joy of medical practice. An anecdote from my own practice may serve to illustrate this point. For decades, I took care of a patient with a rare kidney disease that had progressed so slowly that she was only on the verge of requiring dialysis 30 years later when I gave up my nephrology practice to be a full-time editor. Days after the announcement of my departure, I received her note, "You were always the Hospital to me. Thought you'd be there forever. I'll miss you more than you know. Hope I can hear about you now and then. I saw you on Channel 5. Take care and God bless you. Barb Farrell. PS. So long buddy." Barbara Farrell died three weeks later in her sleep. Here is a small excerpt from my letter to her daughter, Mary. "In all those years we had, I thought, the ideal doctor and patient relationship. I told her all. I comforted, cajoled, and encouraged her, and in turn, she trusted me and turned to me for advice of all kinds. Our encounters (hundreds over the years) brimmed with mutual respect and love" [9].

Medicine is a unique profession, truly a way of life. Rolling out of bed in the middle of the night to visit a newly hospitalized patient and to sign off on their care may feel like a burden at the time, but the doctor won't regret it, and the patient will long remember it. Being a doctor involves making a difference in patients' lives. Even though a business relationship may exist, the principles of each encounter are based on trust, mutual respect, and empathy. A doctor in our time is rarely alone but is working in a collaborative environment with others who often share these honorable attributes. It is not too sappy, I think, to describe medicine not as a job but as a calling. If one of my grandchildren or great-grandchildren should opt for a career in medicine, I would support their goal with enthusiasm.

ROLE IN SOCIETY

A penultimate word about principled medicine. To the extent that physicians as individuals and physicians as a group retain some esteem from the public, they must continue to live up to existing standards of professionalism that are spelled out for them by professional societies. Maintaining appropriate professional decorum and teaching the next generation of physicians are two such mandates. Another is becoming an advocate for health in situations in which local or national policies can adversely affect the health of the public: firearm availability is one example. Preserving society's resources should be another physician responsibility; doing so requires that physicians generally appreciate the cost of emergency department visits, patients occupying a hospital bed for a day, new monoclonal antibodies, multiple consecutive scans, and exchange transfusions, to name a few. It requires that physicians consider each test's possible value before ordering it and consider with cancer patients whether the latest vastly expensive treatment is worth it, in terms not only of enhanced life expectancy and quality of life but of its cost.

The concepts of being a principled physician are easy to describe and elaborate; they are not always easy to keep as a template for practice. But as Marilynne

Robinson wrote, "[A] standard is not diminished or discredited by the fact that it is seldom or never realized" [10].

Let these old standards stand.

REFERENCES

1. Hurst JW. Dr. Francis Peabody, we need you. *Tex Heart Inst J* 2011;38:327–329.
2. Fitzgerald F. Medical education and clinical research in the 21st century. A Report on a Conference of the NY Academy of Sciences October 18–19, 1999. NY Academy of Sciences Special Report.
3. Verghese A, Brady E, Costanza-Kapur C, Horwitz R. The bedside evaluation: Ritual and reason. *Ann Intern Med* 2011;155:550–553.
4. Plante DA, Kassirer JP, Zarin DA, Pauker SG. A clinical decision consultation service. *Am J Med* 1986;80:1169.
5. Kassirer JP. Adding insult to injury. Usurping patients' prerogatives. *N Engl J Med*, 1983;308:898.
6. Anonymous. Profits of medical practice. *Boston Med Surg J* 1847:203.
7. Kassirer JP. Managed care and the morality of the marketplace. *N Engl J Med* 1995;333:50–52.
8. Kassirer JP. *On the Take: How Medicine's Complicity with Big Business Can Endanger your Health.* Oxford: Oxford Press, 2005.
9. Kassirer JP. An ideal relationship. *Boston Globe.* September 6, 1991.
10. Robinson M. *The Death of Adam. Essays on Modern Thought.* Boston, MA: Houghton Mifflin Company, 1998: 48.

9 Diversity

John Patrick T. Co

It is the Fall of 2019. Two decades had passed since I had arrived in Boston and Massachusetts General Hospital (Mass General). Since then, I had completed a fellowship, gotten married, had two daughters, moved three times within the area, and the Celtics, Bruins, Patriots, and Red Sox had all won championships. I was getting ready to present the annual report on graduate medical education (GME) to the institution's senior leaders (including members of the C-suite, vice presidents, and department chairs), something not new to me. As director of GME for Partners Health Care (now Mass General Brigham), I had been doing the same for the decade prior. Presenters are asked to wait in the foyer area in a small seating area before being led into the conference room about 10 to 15 minutes in advance of the presentation. After being called into the room, I walked through the wooden double doors and turned to the right to take my usual seat at the far end of the rectangular room, on the side opposite to the front of the room where I would be presenting, affording me the ability to view all the attendees.

I always found the opportunity to present the annual report simultaneously exhilarating and somewhat anxiety provoking. Much as on prior occasions, I looked around the room to see who was there, scanning for faces of supporters as well as those who would ask the potentially challenging questions. As usual, there was a mix of both. Mostly I was hoping that those present would be paying attention instead of looking at their smartphones. For whatever reason that day, though, what I saw in the room was the same as usual, but the thoughts they evoked were different. I noted that in the audience of 40 to 50 people, as well as the portraits of accomplished leaders in the history of the institution, nobody looked like me. It caused me to reflect on presentations in recent years to leadership groups at institutions locally and nationally, where the diversity of the leaders was not reflective of either the populations being served or the providers they represented. I was not sure how to reconcile this with the fact that I had come to Boston two decades prior in part to experience and learn from diverse perspectives. I considered these leaders and my peers overall as like-minded.

Why is diversity important? What was my view of diversity when I began my career in medicine, and how has it evolved since then? What do I hope those who are entering the profession can learn from my experiences?

"Of all the forms of inequality, injustice in health is the most shocking and inhumane."—Martin Luther King Jr.

In 2003, the seminal report *Unequal Treatment: Confronting Racial and Ethnic Disparities in Health Care* described the existence, extent of, and impact of health care disparities in the US, their root causes, and some strategies to address them [1]. Recent National Healthcare Quality and Disparities Reports demonstrate that health and health care disparities persist across race, ethnicity, and other socioeconomic characteristics [2]. The COVID pandemic further amplified these root causes, including social determinants of health, structural racism, as well as overt bias and discrimination in how care is structured and delivered [3]. Addressing these causes can help ensure that health care delivered is not just the same or equal across populations but, more importantly, equitable, i.e., designed so that the needs of disadvantaged groups

DOI: 10.1201/9781003409373-9

are met, and their health can be maximized as it is for other groups. Accordingly, diversity and inclusion must be essential components of organizational strategies to achieve health equity. Why do gaps in these areas exist in health care, how are they contributing to inequities, and how can they be addressed?

"Even an outsider can do a good job."

In 1999, 20 years prior to my presentation, I arrived in Boston, moving into Charles River Park Apartments, the place often recognized by a sign on Charles Street that reads, "If you lived here, you would be home now." I can still picture driving into the parking lot in the U-Haul truck that held most of my possessions from my prior eight years of medical training in California and Maryland. The parking garage that housed my Toyota Camry is long gone, replaced by a high-end apartment building and underground garage. The cellular phone that I had at the time was a state-of-the-art Nokia with a battery that could support a few hours of talking time.

Why did I leave sunny, idyllic California as well as the friendships and the social and professional supports I had built over the prior eight years during medical school and residency? Even though at a young age I knew I wanted to be a physician, specifically a pediatrician, I also believed that learning about diverse fields and ways of thinking would in the end make me a better physician and person. It is why I chose a liberal arts education for college and left the East Coast, where I grew up for almost my entire life, in order to experience another part of the country as a medical student and afterward as a pediatrics resident. Certainly, I missed being closer to my hometown in upstate New York (but not the weather!).

Mass General's reputation, both positive and negative, preceded itself. On the one hand, this was Mass General and Harvard Medical School. They were world-renowned institutions at the forefront of scientific discovery and clinical medicine. As a budding academic, I saw an opportunity to learn health services research from Jim Perrin, Don Goldmann, Charlie Homer, Tracy Lieu, and Jonathan Finkelstein, all giants in the field with distinct interests and approaches that could help me identify and shape my own niche. On the other hand, I had heard the murmurings that prestigious institutions like these were places in which only insiders—those that did their residency training there—were fully accepted and likely to succeed. In addition, I was told: "Boston is a racist city, you won't like it there. Get some training and be FROM there, but you should plan to leave after your fellowship. You will want to leave." I also experienced imposter syndrome. How could the child of immigrant parents who did his medical training elsewhere and was ordinary in his medical career be accepted and succeed there?

As I was completing my health services research fellowship, I was fortunate enough to be offered a position to spend some of my time as the Associate Program Director for MGH's Pediatric Residency Program and to continue research projects I had initiated during fellowship. Medical education and quality and safety were my two passions, and I felt so fortunate that the start of my academic career seemed to be beginning on the right track to further those interests. Over the following five years, I was able to meet and work with most leaders and faculty in our department, through clinical care as well as via academic and educational pursuits. I felt that I was being accepted as someone who was now part of the Mass General community while contributing my diverse experiences and perspectives from being trained elsewhere. With the encouragement and support of my mentors, I then accepted a position to work in the GME Office of our health system. At the department's end-of-the-year dinner, in an attempt to recognize my contributions and upcoming transitions, one of the department's leaders stated, "And we want to thank John Patrick T. Co, who showed that even an outsider can do a good job." There was much laughter in the room at the time. I wasn't sure how to receive the backhanded praise. Was I still an outsider, and, if so, why was I being perceived that way?

"Take nothing on its looks; take everything on evidence. There's no better rule."—Charles Dickens, *Great Expectations*

As a school-age child in upstate New York, I often was asked by my peers and teachers, "Where are you from?" In my mind, my response to the question, "The Bronx," was obvious. Yet it was often met with quizzical reactions; people seemingly expecting a different answer, likely because my appearance suggested an Asian heritage. People's reactions to my response were difficult for me to comprehend or accept and seemed to be influenced by preconceived notions of my ethnic background. Their assumption was that I was "Oriental" and that I would name a country such as China, Korea, or Japan, not realizing that I was born and spent almost my entire life in the US. My mother served in the US Army Reserve for the love of and commitment to service of our country, retiring as a full colonel and serving on active duty as a medical doctor. People's view of my personality, character, interests, aspirations, and role in society were undoubtedly shaped by images of Asians in the media, including as nerds, people that are passive with no athletic ability, running grocery stores, and being the "model minority" [4]. The origins, existence, and detrimental impact of bias and discrimination against Asian Americans is underrecognized and not commonly taught about in structured curricula, though that is changing [5]. Stereotypes like these that are perpetuated about people of color further their feelings of being outsiders and limit their opportunities. Why did "Linsanity" occur in the US [6]? It was because an individual who did not conform to their society's imagery and mental model of what a National Basketball Association (NBA) player looks like was having success at the highest level of the profession. Because of the color of people's skin and appearance, are they relegated to certain roles and perceived as perpetual outsiders in certain professions, communities, or our society as a whole?

Stereotypes and biases based on race, gender, or other characteristics, especially for those in marginalized groups such as racial and ethnic minoritized populations, occur in the health care setting and can negatively impact the experience and care received by patients. To address this, the importance and ways to think of diversity must be promoted and integrated into the training of the next generation of physicians so that they learn to approach care for patients based on substance and not make assumptions based on biases or what they see on the surface. Having diverse perspectives, in combination with inclusive environments that allow those perspectives to be genuinely considered, can lead to more equitable outcomes [7]. The Accreditation Council for Graduate Medical Education (ACGME), the organization that accredits most GME training programs in the US, recognizes this. As part of their Equity Matters™ Initiative, the ACGME utilizes a framework for diversity, equity, and inclusion that I have found helpful (*ACGME Equity Matters*™) [8]. They note that diversity should be considered, in a sense, broader than demographic characteristics. Without this broader view of diversity, the importance of achieving equity and inclusion can easily be lost. Certainly, race and gender are important aspects of diversity to consider. Others though, such as culture, religion, orientation, and socioeconomic status are equally important. As we recruit the next generation of physicians, each person's experiences (the "road traveled" during their life's journey) as well as their talents and abilities (as opposed to their limitations or disabilities) need to be considered. Given the prevalence of disability in our population, the medical profession needs to ensure that those with disability are given the opportunity to practice medicine, contribute to the workforce, and inform how we deliver care equitably to these populations [9].

DIVERSE PROVIDERS FOR A DIVERSE POPULATION WITH DIVERSE NEEDS

I had not realized the importance of diversity in medicine until I began to seriously consider it as a career for myself, which prompted me to evaluate and better understand my parents' journeys toward becoming physicians and practicing medicine in the US. Both my mother and father were born in the Philippines to parents of Chinese descent. Unlike their siblings, who grew up assuming they would take over their respective family businesses, my parents each decided that they wanted to become physicians. Through the support of my grandparents, they became the first in their families to attend medical school and residency training, both in the Philippines. They came to the US through the J-1 Visa Program administered through the Educational Commission for Foreign Medical Graduates (ECFMG), now a division of Intealth [10]. They completed internal medicine (mother) and general pediatric (father) residency training in the Bronx, where my sister and I were born, before returning to the Philippines to practice primary care in the community. Several years later, they returned to the US and, for the rest of their lives, practiced primary care medicine in underserved communities in metropolitan and upstate New York. The person who served as my pediatrician in Vestal, New York, where I was in school from 3rd to 12th grades, had a similar pathway after attending school in Korea. He, like my parents and many other physicians in the US, left their extended families in their home countries to fulfill their professional dreams. Some of my parents' closest friends from the Philippines, who also pursued their medical training there, followed a similar path and became our extended family here in the US, providing support for each other as they transitioned into their medical careers and assimilated into a new culture.

The story of my parents is not uncommon among physicians in the US. According to the Association of American Medical Colleges [11], approximately one in five active physicians in the US were born and attended medical school outside the US and Canada. Most of these physicians, known as non-US international medical graduates (IMGs), are sponsored by J-1 visas and train in primary care specialties—including over half in internal medicine and another 10% in pediatrics [12]—and work in communities of underserved populations. Like my parents, many IMG physicians complete GME training twice: once in their country of origin and then again in the US in order to be able to obtain a medical license and board certification. Non-US IMGs are already an essential component of the US physician workforce for meeting the primary care and overall health care needs of the population. Given the projections for an increasing shortage of primary care physicians in the US, the role of IMG physicians in meeting these needs must be considered more fully, balancing this with ensuring the US is doing its part in educating clinicians who provide care across the world. As the COVID pandemic so clearly demonstrated, the health of populations across the world has never been more connected as it is currently [13]. Diseases can spread around the globe rapidly, as can knowledge, aid, and approaches to treatment. IMG physicians will continue to play a valuable role in providing health care worldwide, including in helping to diversify the physician workforce and address inequities here in the US [14].

Moreover, the US population has become increasingly diverse. In 2022, the percentage of the US population that was white (non-Hispanic) was approximately 59%, an almost 5% decrease compared to 2010, the largest decrease of any group during that time [15]. In that same period, the percentage of the US population that was Hispanic/Latino increased to nearly 20% and the percentage of people who identify as two or more races accounts for most of the increase in diversity, more than tripling to just over 10% between 2010 and 2020 [16]. With a growing and aging population, one that is becoming more diverse, our country will not only need more physicians to provide care but will also need these doctors to be able to do so in a way that promotes equitable, safe, and high-quality care [17]. During my tenure as Mass General's inaugural Medical Director for Equity, expanding prior years' work led by Joe Betancourt, Elizabeth Mort, Aswita Tan-McGrory, and Andrea Tull, we devoted much of our efforts toward laying the foundation for identifying and addressing the root causes of disparities in access to and delivery of care across specialties [18]. It was readily apparent how important it was to have diverse providers engaged in this work to express diverse perspectives in formulating the approach to our work, including understanding root causes and redesigning care.

YOU CANNOT BE WHAT YOU CANNOT SEE

In November 2022, I attended the AAMC's Learn, Serve, Lead Conference in Nashville, Tennessee. At the Leadership Plenary, Kirk Calhoun (MD, Chair, AAMC Board of Directors and President, The University of Texas at Tyler) recounted an episode of health care from his childhood, one where he was receiving care from an allergist in Chicago for asthma that was severely impairing him [19]. What struck him was that this person was, like himself, black, something that he had not encountered before. "For the first time in my life, I saw a doctor who looked like me. You cannot be what you cannot see." He recalled the doctor stating, "I know what this is, and I know how to fix it," and he recognizes how pivotal that experience was in inspiring him to become a physician. Stories like this underscore the importance of role models in cultivating a diverse workforce in medicine and why medical schools, institutions, and GME training programs must play a significant role in doing so.

How diverse is the US physician workforce? The racial and gender diversity of physicians in the US does not represent that of its general population. A study from the Urban Institute noted that among non-Hispanic/Latinx adults, Black adults were less likely than other adults to report racial concordance with their usual health care providers [20]. Fortunately, data from the AAMC shows that the diversity among medical school applicants, matriculants, and graduates has continued to grow [21]. The number of female applicants now surpasses the number of male applicants. The gains, though, have not been symmetric across groups, with the increase in Blacks lagging that in other groups. Prior research around the impact of racial concordance between patient and provider has been mixed, including its impact on influencing a patient's decision to seek care from a clinician, the likelihood of visiting their clinician for preventive care, satisfaction with the care received, and health care outcomes [22–25]. One study showed that Black, Latino, and Asian patients are three or more times as likely to have a concordant clinician than expected based on the diversity of the population of physicians, suggesting a strong preference for clinicians of the same race or ethnicity [26]. In my own experience, while caring for children and families of Asian ethnicity, I often sensed their being reassured by my being Asian, which typically surpassed any disappointment they had when I could not speak their language. In contrast, the many Hispanic families I cared for seemed both shocked and comforted with my being able to speak some Spanish, which I learned in school and used regularly during residency as I cared for a predominantly Hispanic population in a community hospital in San Jose.

Once underrepresented in medicine (UIM) trainees enter GME programs, what is their experience? Studies of residents in two primary care specialties suggest that they can experience bias in the assessments from faculty, including bias based on gender and race [27–30]. Black trainees report bias and higher scrutiny during their training, leading to higher rates of leaving or being dismissed from their programs [31]. If this is pervasive across programs and specialties, this can have significant and negative impacts on the trainee's success, future professional development, and workforce diversity. GME programs should learn from others who have implemented strategies that have been successful in promoting diversity and inclusion.

"DIVERSITY: THE ART OF THINKING INDEPENDENTLY TOGETHER." —MALCOLM FORBES

Early in my career, I had the great fortune of having mentors and supervisors such as Debra Weinstein, Jim Perrin, Tim Ferris, Peter Greenspan, Gregg Meyer, Kevin Johnson, and Ted Sectish who espoused integrating diversity in thought in leading, managing, and innovating. To achieve this, they did several critical things:

Developed teams that include individuals with diverse perspectives.

Created psychologically safe environments in which diverse perspectives could be shared and discussed.

Communicated how decisions were arrived at to demonstrate transparency and inclusiveness.

The most successful teams of which I have been a part or witnessed have been ones that were led by intelligent, principled individuals with a strong moral compass. While confident in their abilities and "comfortable in their own skin," great leaders are inquisitive and good listeners, asking for each team member's opinion because of genuine interest in understanding perspectives and ideas that they had not or perhaps could not have formed on their own based on their own experiences or biases. In teams with highly accomplished and opinionated people who have varying perspectives, discussions and decision making around challenging issues can be uncomfortable and more prolonged than on teams where all members of the team have similar backgrounds and experiences or on teams led by autocratic leaders. What I've learned, including from my own GME group, is that teams that reach decisions more quickly (because its members think in a uniform way) don't necessarily arrive at better decisions or ones that are reflective of the diverse stakeholders that they will impact.

My experience has been that teams that are able to consider and incorporate diverse perspectives in their daily work and decision making can achieve better outcomes than those that are more homogeneous. Rock and Grant [32] provide a great framework that captures my own experience around the underlying reasons for this, including:

More Focus on Facts: Teams with members who have diverse perspectives may push each other to be more objective in what they say. The diversity of views and experiences can lead to greater scrutiny and reexamination of other team members' statements and actions, empowering participants, improving group engagement in discussions, and making team members more aware of their own biases and blind spots, ones that can lead to errors and poor decisions.

Processing the Facts More Carefully: Having a different perspective on the team can lead each person to more critically scrutinize how information is interpreted and analyzed. I have learned that considering counterfactuals can be valuable in analyzing situations and that having diverse perspectives on the team can help ensure the inclusion of "outside" or varying perspectives. This difference in processing information can lead to consideration of more options and ultimately better decisions. Different perspectives can help avert confirmation bias from the uniformity of perspectives affirming prior beliefs without fully considering others.

Capacity for Being More Innovative in Developing Solutions: Diversity in the ways team members think and look or in their experiences can create environments that encourage innovation because sameness is not what they see and/or hear in their deliberations. Being around people who do not look, talk, or think like you can help team members and teams avoid conformity, which both inhibits working across boundaries and discourages innovative thinking.

Incorporating these principles into leadership and decision making can create environments where diverse perspectives can be expressed, discussed, and valued. These principles can promote decision making that crosses boundaries and addresses biases that have been deeply, yet imperceptibly, embedded into our ways of thinking and prioritization [33].

THE PATH FORWARD

It is the fall of 2023. I'm preparing to present the annual report of GME for the past academic year to institutional leaders. Four years have passed since my presentation to the group that evoked my strong reflections on diversity. Since then, we, like other organizations in medicine and health care broadly, have taken steps to more highly prioritize and better integrate diversity, equity, and inclusion into the fabric of our mission and operations [34]. Have we seen improvements? Thankfully, yes. The importance of diversity and inclusion in achieving equity are more tangible in our priorities and policies and in the work that we are doing around them. Is there much more work to do? Undoubtedly, yes. What is the path forward?

Diversify Senior Leaders: For sustained improvements in diversity, inclusion, and equity among leaders and their teams, senior leaders need to be diverse in their backgrounds, experiences, and ways of thinking. Perceptions of what leaders and effective leadership look like need to change [35]. Currently, senior leaders of academic medical centers are not representative of the diversity of the US population or of physicians overall, including in gender and race. For example, while Asian Americans constitute approximately 20% of the physician workforce [36], they constitute a much lower percentage of medical school department chairs [37]. Diverse individuals progressing through their medical careers should not set limits or view the highest levels of leadership as being unattainable. Critical to achieving this is being able to identify role models who have attained such success. Diverse senior leaders can help promote diversity in the work force overall, which can help improve team diversity and the solutions they formulate.

Define Diversity Broadly: While continuing to improve diversity in areas such as gender and race, medicine needs to continue to examine and expand its efforts to diversify the profession in other aspects such as gender identity, sexual orientation, religion, abilities, and, most importantly, ways of thinking. The impact of the Supreme Court decision on affirmative action on diversity in the medical profession has yet to be seen [38]. This needs to be monitored closely, critically examined, and countered should its impact on diversity be negative.

Strengthen and Increase Pathways to Diversify the Physician Workforce: Our system of medical education, including medical schools and GME programs, have done much to increase diversity in its learners. These efforts must continue and be linked to programs that provide financial, academic, and social supports for success at each phase, as well as support progression and retention. Better understanding, mitigating, and eventually eliminating bias in the assessment of trainees as they go through medical training are critical aspects of the overall support that must be provided [39, 40].

Improve Inclusion in the Work and Learning Environment: Verna Myers [41], who has championed diversity and inclusion in both the public and private sectors, has said, "Diversity is being invited to the party. Inclusion is being asked to dance." Successes in attracting diverse candidates must be accompanied by efforts to increase inclusivity and address bias and discrimination in the workplace, including how we educate and support our trainees throughout the continuum of medical education. Whether it be due to race, gender, sexual orientation, religion, abilities, or other characteristics, many individuals for one reason or another feel like outsiders in our societies, including in our health care systems. Improving inclusion can help us reach our goals, including the development and implementation of systems and solutions that promote equity in our health care delivery system.

If we are successful in these areas, what can we achieve? Improving diversity and inclusion can lead to the delivery of health care and ultimately health that is equitable and just. We must be unrelenting in our pursuit of this goal.

DEDICATION
I dedicate this chapter to my wife, Sylvia, and children, Chelsy and Kaylee. Without their love and unwavering support, my inspiration and career would not be possible. Sylvia has helped me reflect on and continually reexamine my perspectives on diversity, including its impact on my family and work.

REFERENCES
1. Institute of Medicine. *Unequal Treatment: Confronting Racial and Ethnic Disparities in Health Care*. Washington, DC: The National Academies Press, 2003. https://doi.org/10.17226/12875
2. Ma S, Agrawal S, Salhi R. Distinguishing Health Equity and Health Care Equity: A Framework for Measurement. *NEJM Catalyst*. March 7, 2023.
3. Trends in racial and ethnic disparities in COVID-19 hospitalizations, by region—United States, March–December 2020. *MMWR*. Available from: cdc.gov
4. Jin CH. 6 charts that dismantle the trope of Asian Americans as a model minority. *NPR*, 2021. Available from: https://www.npr.org/2021/05/25/999874296/6-charts-that-dismantle-the-trope-of-asian-americans-as-a-model-minority
5. Josephine M. Kim. *Race, Ethnicity, and Culture: Contemporary Issues in Asian America*. Cambridge, MA: Harvard Graduate School of Education.
6. Jeremy Lin finally loves 'linsanity' just as much as you do. *The New York Times*. Available from: nytimes.com
7. Vela MB, Erondu AI, Smith NA, Peek ME, Woodruff JN, Chin MH. Eliminating explicit and implicit biases in health care: Evidence and research needs. *Annu Rev Public Health* 2022;43:477–501. https://doi.org/10.1146/annurev-publhealth-052620-103528
8. ACGME Equity Matters™. Available from: www.acgme.org/initiatives/diversity-equity-and-inclusion/ACGME-Equity-Matters
9. Okanlami F. Disabusing disability: Demonstrating that disability doesn't mean inability. *You Tube*.
10. About Us. *Intealth*, n.d. Available from: https://www.intealth.org/about-us/
11. Active physicians who are international medical graduates (IMGs) by specialty, 2019. *AAMC*. Available from: https://www.aamc.org/data-reports/workforce/data/active-physicians-international-medical-graduates-imgs-specialty-2021
12. EVSP—Specialties pursued by J-1 physicians, 2022 [230822]. Available from: intealth.org.
13. Singh S, McNab C, Olson RM, Bristol N, Nolan C, Bergstrøm E, Bartos M, Mabuchi S, Panjabi R, Karan A, Abdalla SM, Bonk M, Jamieson M, Werner GK, Nordström A, Legido-Quigley H, Phelan A. How an outbreak became a pandemic: A chronological analysis of crucial junctures and international obligations in the early months of the COVID-19 pandemic. *Lancet* 2021;398(10316):2109–2124. https://doi.org/10.1016/S0140-6736(21)01897-3

14. Zaidi, Z, Dewan, M, Norcini, J. International medical graduates: Promoting equity and belonging. Acad Med 2020;95(12S):S82-S87. https://doi.org/10.1097/ACM.0000000000003694

15. 2020 U.S. population more racially, ethnically diverse than in 2010. Available from: census.gov

16. US population by year, race, age, ethnicity, & more. *USAFacts*, 2024. Available from: https://usafacts.org/data/topics/people-society/population-and-demographics/our-changing-population/

17. *2022 National Healthcare Quality and Disparities Report.* Rockville, MD: Agency for Healthcare Research and Quality, 2022.

18. AREHQ Report 2021-FINAL-REV-072822.pdf. Available from: https://www.mghdisparitiessolutions.org/_files/ugd/d0de3a_3c1653bd5b9b4f3c82d31bdef185d04f.pdf

19. Calhoun KA. Overcoming the headwinds. *AAMC*.

20. Dulce Gonzalez, Genevieve M. Kenney, Marla McDaniel, Claire O'Brien. *2022 Racial, Ethnic, and Language Concordance between Patients and Their Usual Health Care Providers.* Washington, DC: Urban Institute, March 2022. Available from: https://www.urban.org/sites/default/files/2022-03/racial-ethnic-and-language-concordance-between-patients-and-providers.pdf

21. Diversity in medicine, facts and figures, 2019 download. Available from: aamc.org

22. The association of racial and ethnic concordance in primary care with patient satisfaction and experience of care. *PMC*. Available from: nih.gov

23. Cooper L, Beach MC, Johnson RL, Inui TS. Delving below the surface. *J Gen Int Med* 2006;21(1):21–27. https://doi.org/10.1111/j.1525-1497.2006.00305.x

24. Cooper L. A 41-year-old African American man with poorly controlled hypertension: Review of patient and physician factors related to hypertension treatment adherence. *JAMA* 2009;301(12):1260–1272. https://doi.org/10.1001/jama.2009.358

25. Jetty A, Jabbarpour Y, Pollack J, Huerto R, Woo S, Petterson S. Patient-physician racial concordance associated with improved healthcare use and lower healthcare expenditures in minority populations. *J Racial Ethn Health Disparities* 2022;9(1):68–81. https://doi.org/10.1007/s40615-020-00930-4

26. Ku L, Vichare A. The association of racial and ethnic concordance in primary care with patient satisfaction and experience of care. *J Gen Intern Med* 2023;38(3): 727–732. https://doi.org/10.1007/s11606-022-07695-y

27. Boatright D, Anderson N, Kim JG, et al. Racial and ethnic differences in internal medicine residency assessments. *JAMA Netw Open* 2022;5(12):e2247649. https://doi.org/10.1001/jamanetworkopen.2022.47649

28. Klein R, Ufere NN, Schaeffer S, Julian KA, Rao SR, Koch J, Volerman A, Snyder ED, Thompson V, Ganguli I, Burnett-Bowie SM, Palamara K. Association between resident race and ethnicity and clinical performance assessment scores in graduate medical education. *Acad Med* 2022;97(9):1351–1359. https://doi.org/10.1097/ACM.0000000000004743

29. Walters J, Paradise Black N, Yurttutan Engin N, Cohen DE, Ben Khallouq B, Chen JG. Race and gender differences in pediatric milestone levels: A multi-institutional study. *Clin Pediatr* 2023:99228231200985. https://doi.org/10.1177/00099228231200985

30. Klein R, Ufere NN, Schaeffer S, Julian KA, Rao SR, Koch J, Volerman A, Snyder ED, Thompson V, Ganguli I, Burnett-Bowie SM, Palamara K. Association between resident race and ethnicity and clinical performance assessment scores in graduate medical education. *Acad Med* 2022;97(9):1351–1359. https://doi.org/10.1097/ACM.0000000000004743

31. The 'death spiral' forcing Black physicians out of their residency programs. Available from: advisory.com
32. Why diverse teams are smarter. Available from: hbr.org
33. Chrobot-Mason D, Aramovich NP Boundary-spanning leadership: Strategies to create a more inclusive and effective network. In Ferdman BM, Prime J, Riggio RE, eds, *Inclusive Leadership: Transforming Diverse Lives, Workplaces, and Societies* (pp. 135–148). Routledge/Taylor & Francis Group, 2021. https://doi.org/10.4324/9780429449673-10
34. Bryant AS, Healey JA, Wilkie S, Carten C, Sequist TD, Taveras EM. A health system framework for addressing structural racism: Mass general Brigham's United against racism initiative. *Health Equity* 2023;7(1):533–542. https://doi.org/10.1089/heq.2023.0077
35. Lee TH, MD, Volpp KG, MD, Cheung VG, MD, Dzau VJ. Diversity and inclusiveness in health care leadership: Three key steps. *NEJM Catalyst*. June 7, 2021.
36. Figure 18. Percentage of all active physicians by race/ethnicity, 2018. *AAMC*. Available from: https://www.aamc.org/data-reports/workforce/data/figure-18-percentage-all-active-physicians-race/ethnicity-2018
37. Asian American doctors largely left out of leadership. *STAT*. Available from: statnews.com
38. Supreme Court of the United States. *Students for Fair Admissions, Inc. v. President and Fellows of Harvard College*, 600 U. S. 181 (2023). Available from: supremecourt.gov.
39. Ibrahim H, Miller Juve A, Amin A, Railey K, Andolsek KM. Expanding the study of bias in medical education assessment. *J Grad Med Educ* 2023;15(6):623–626. https://doi.org/10.4300/JGME-D-23-00027.1
40. Ellis J, Otugo O, Landry A, Landry A. Dismantling the overpolicing of Black residents. *N Engl J Med* 2023;389(14):1258–1261. https://doi.org/10.1056/NEJMp2304559
41. "Diversity is Being Invited to the Party: Inclusion is Being Asked to Dance." YouTube, uploaded by AppNexus. December 10, 2015. <https://www.youtube.com/watch?v=9gS2VPUkB3M>

10 Peer Learning

Roy Phitayakorn

Peer learning or peer-assisted/-supported learning is probably the oldest form of education. It is loosely defined as teaching and learning that occur between individuals from similar social groupings without the involvement of professional teachers. Therefore, peer learning is a fluid educational process that includes activities whereby the participants may exchange roles of teacher or learner or even occupy both roles simultaneously [1]. An important psychological construct that is featured prominently in peer learning is the concept of cognitive and social congruence [2]. In general, teachers with a knowledge base that is just slightly more advanced than their learners are more effective teachers for certain topics than expert teachers who have a large cognitive incongruence from their learners [3, 4]. Peer learning groups with similar or high levels of social congruence may be better at creating positive learning environments because the participants are more familiar with the stressors and ways to mitigate them. Peer learning activities may also be better at making the "hidden" curriculum more explicit while also role modeling healthy behaviors or coping mechanisms.

Many different forms of peer learning have been described in the K–12 education literature. These forms are typically differentiated by the educational distance between the learners. For example, near-peer learning typically occurs when the peer teacher is just a few years senior to the learners. On the other hand, inverse-peer learning is where the peer teacher is junior to the learners. Lastly, true peer learning is when the individuals are at the same educational level, and there is no designated instructor. Although the rest of this chapter will focus on peer learning in physician education, it is important to note that the principles are essentially the same in postdoctoral or allied health professional training as well. In general, the three most important forms of peer learning that have been described in the medical education literature include peer tutoring, peer observation, and collaborative learning.

PEER TUTORING

Peer tutoring is an educational interaction where one person is the tutor or instructor and one or more persons are the designated student(s). The peer tutor should have advanced knowledge or skills that they are specifically trying to impart to the student(s). The knowledge or skills to be taught typically come from the actual faculty instructor in a previously arranged session where the peer tutor has been both taught and assessed to ensure they understand the material and are familiar with the skills of an effective teacher including active lecturing/listening, answering questions, and delivering constructive feedback.

For medical students or resident physician trainees, peer tutoring is an important component of both the Association of American Medical Colleges and the Accreditation Council for Graduate Medical Education competency frameworks. Specifically, it is helpful to remind our students and trainees that physicians should be expected to teach and that the word "doctor" originates from the Latin word *docere*, which means "to teach." Drs. Bulte and others have defined the role of a teacher as consisting of six activity domains: information provider/instructor, role model/behavior demonstrator, facilitator, assessor/evaluator, planner/logistics

DOI: 10.1201/9781003409373-10

coordinator, and resource developer/writer [4]. Peer tutoring can offer both theoretical and practical experience within all these teaching domains.

In undergraduate and graduate medical education, there are many advantages to utilizing medical students and resident physicians as peer tutors. For example, student or trainee peer tutors can augment faculty teaching efforts especially since the number of medical students has increased while the direct financial support of faculty for teaching has decreased at many academic institutions around the world [5, 6]. These tutors can also be empowered to function as peer mentors and often have many insights into clinical decision making and patient care workflow details that faculty instructors would lack. In addition, peer tutoring helps the student and trainee tutors by consolidating their own knowledge and skills likely through a combination of retrieval practice, metacognition development, and reflective practice [7]. These peer tutors also have increased intrinsic motivation to master the subject material as they prepare to teach and deliver the instructional content. Previous studies have found that peer tutoring by medical students does not appear to compromise the quality of learning [8] and improves the confidence of participants in their teaching skills [9]. This confidence likely influences students' self-perception and future teacher identity formation.

The disadvantage of medical student or resident physician peer tutoring is that it can provoke significant anxiety and should not be mandatory for all students or trainees. Also, it can be difficult to centrally standardize how the knowledge and skills are taught or received from the peer tutors. Lastly, there is also a "hidden curriculum" concern that the learners may wonder why the faculty are not teaching them directly and feel that student or trainee peer tutors are being used because their education is not as important as the faculty's clinical or research activities.

At a faculty level, peer tutors can be used for expert teaching, mentorship, and coaching. In terms of expert teaching, faculty peer tutors are often invited to give grand rounds or conference teaching whereby faculty experts can share their knowledge with the rest of the institutional or local faculty. This format allows many faculty to receive instruction simultaneously especially when virtual or hybrid on-site/virtual teaching is pursued. However, it can be difficult to regulate the quality of the teaching on a regular basis. Also, the formats tend to favor passive teaching methods such as large group lecturing; it can be difficult to teach technical or procedural skills using this format. Best practices for faculty expert teaching would encourage clinical departments to enhance and regulate presentation and teaching skills of their faculty expert teachers and give constructive feedback after conference sessions so that their faculty teaching quality can continuously improve. Facilities should also be available for simulation-based workshop formats to impart new technical skills and ensure that the faculty are up-to-date as procedural and device technologies advance.

In addition, faculty peer mentors are widely utilized for both professional career mentorship as well as managing work–life integrations. It is important to note that faculty peer mentors do not typically receive specific training in how to be effective mentors and therefore tend to give suggestions/advice to their mentees based on the mentor's lived experiences. Therefore, faculty mentees should be encouraged to have a "panel" of mentors, when possible, to ensure a balanced range of mentorship advice. Similarly, senior faculty mentorship is also frequently overlooked in many academic departments and clinical practices. Topics such as transition to retirement and financial planning must be discussed with senior faculty, ideally by senior faculty mentors [10].

Lastly, faculty peer coaches are an important aspect of peer tutoring and typically focus on topics including wellness, nutrition, exercise, and executive management skills. The number of medical faculty peer coaches has significantly increased since the start of the Covid-19 pandemic. Unlike faculty peer mentors, coaching is typically focused on helping the coaches create their own solutions instead of giving advice. Clinical departments should consider having one or several of their faculty become certified coaches (ideally from a program that is accredited by the International Coaching Federation) who can then work with their faculty peers on a regular basis.

PEER OBSERVATION

For medical students and resident physician trainees, peer observation programs have been trialed often in conjunction with history or physical examination assessments such as objective structured clinical examinations. They are also sometimes invited to observe a fellow student/trainee teach a class and then provide constructive feedback [11]. Interestingly, student or trainee tutors often enjoy peer observation programs but are significantly less confident in their abilities to complete peer assessments or conduct educational planning compared to the experience of teaching only [4, 12]. Therefore, careful pre-training is necessary, and clear centralized goals and objectives for the peer observership should be created in advance of any programs utilizing students or trainee physicians [13].

On the other hand, faculty peer observership programs require careful central organizational planning, but the goals and objectives should come from the faculty directly. There are many variations of faculty peer observership programs in the literature, but common themes are encouraging a growth mindset among everyone involved and supporting as much flexibility as possible [14]. Some programs feature faculty who request to be observed by their peers around predetermined activities or procedures and then receive constructive feedback afterward. Other programs seek faculty who want to observe "expert" faculty performing a certain activity or procedure, and then the observers reflect and meet with the expert to debrief how the observers can improve their own practice. The expert then observes the observers to help with development and retention of that activity or procedure. Regardless of the type of peer observation program, all efforts should be made to use standardized observer forms, when possible, for later programmatic evaluation [15]. Participants (observed and observer) should also always uphold a culture of psychological safety [16, 17].

COLLABORATIVE LEARNING

The last format of peer learning is the concept of collaborative learning, which can be loosely defined as when two or more individuals attempt to learn more about a topic or skill together. This knowledge creation may take the form of setting goals or clearly defined outputs and milestones for future group work. Collaborative learning is different from the other forms of peer learning in that neither learner has more knowledge or skills on the topic than the other learner(s). Therefore, a facilitator (not an instructor) is needed to help the group focus, ensure all ideas are considered, and help the group move forward in subsequent sessions.

For medical students and trainees, early collaborative learning efforts centered around problem-based learning have both advantages and disadvantages. Collaborative learning in these groups of learners seems to enhance intrinsic motivation in some instances but also to discourage other learners who find this approach to be time-inefficient, especially with skills training. Faculty may also be frustrated with not just teaching the material to the students and instead facilitating group work/thinking, which is prone to conflict and unnecessary detours. These issues have led many institutions to incorporate collaborative learning processes into case-based or team-based learning activities [18].

For faculty, collaborative learning is often used to help a specific work unit (research team, clinical section, division, department) create or revise workflows or regulatory or clinical issues with the understanding that the problem is too complex for any one individual to solve. This technique is often reserved for strategic planning sessions since it requires resources to find a trained facilitator, release teams from clinical activities, and reserve meeting room spaces. Newer project management technologies may allow easier and more frequent collaborative learning opportunities for medical faculty to address system-level problems. Best practices include providing time for faculty to do any necessary reading/learning before the collaborative learning sessions and ensuring that skilled facilitators are available to focus faculty on finding workable solutions instead of reviewing all the current problems.

In summary, peer learning has important implications for the education of students, resident trainee physicians, and faculty. Future work should include standardization of student- or resident-as-teacher resources as well as the incorporation of education technologies as a more streamlined method to provide constructive feedback and repetitive practice. Although most of the published research on this topic has focused on students and trainees, I believe that peer learning may be most effective for faculty development by creating a learning environment where faculty can share stressors/frustrations and best practices to move forward. Several years ago, our surgical division launched a peer learning experiment where we could observe our partners operate and then debrief afterward. Although this sounds routine, surgeons of the same specialty in our group very seldom operated together, and it was a significant loss of clinical income to lose an operative day. To enhance the educational opportunities, we were encouraged to create learning goals for the observation sessions and share them with our partners, so they knew what we wanted to focus on during the operation and the debrief afterward. Interestingly, our evaluations of these observations noted that the most valuable aspects of the sessions were not on the technical aspects of the operations but rather on learning how we manage complex teamwork issues, communication clarity, and promoting efficient workflows. Obstacles to such peer learning do exist, including in the form of the need for central coordination and having an administration that recognizes the value of these activities for faculty development. Nevertheless, I am hopeful that peer learning will ultimately be widely appreciated as an important form of continuing medical education that can support improved educational outcomes and enhance the care of patients.

REFERENCES

1. Topping KJ. Trends in peer learning. *Educ Psychol* 2005;25(6):631–645. https://doi.org/10.1080/01443410500345172
2. Ten Cate O, Durning S. Dimensions and psychology of peer teaching in medical education. *Med Teach* 2007;29(6):546–552. https://doi.org/10.1080/01421590701583816
3. Lockspeiser TM, O'Sullivan P, Teherani A, Muller J. Understanding the experience of being taught by peers: The value of social and cognitive congruence. *Adv Health Sci Educ Theory Pract* 2008;13(3):361–372. https://doi.org/10.1007/s10459-006-9049-8
4. Bulte C, Betts A, Garner K, Durning S. Student teaching: Views of student near-peer teachers and learners. *Med Teach* 2007;29(6):583–590. https://doi.org/10.1080/01421590701583824
5. Ross MT, Cameron HS. Peer assisted learning: A planning and implementation framework: AMEE Guide no. 30. *Med Teach* 2007;29(6):527–545. https://doi.org/10.1080/01421590701665886

6. Soriano RP, Blatt B, Coplit L, CichoskiKelly E, Kosowicz L, Newman L, Pasquale SJ, Pretorius R, Rosen JM, Saks NS, Greenberg L. Teaching medical students how to teach: A national survey of students-as-teachers programs in U.S. medical schools. *Acad Med* 2010;85(11):1725–1731. https://doi.org/10.1097/ACM.0b013e3181f53273

7. Benè KL, Bergus G. When learners become teachers: A review of peer teaching in medical student education. *Fam Med* 2014;46(10):783–787.

8. Haist SA, Wilson JF, Fosson SE, Brigham NL. Are fourth-year medical students effective teachers of the physical examination to first-year medical students? *J Gen Intern Med* 1997;12(3):177–181. https://doi.org/10.1007/s11606-006-5026-4

9. Tolsgaard MG, Gustafsson A, Rasmussen MB, Høiby P, Müller CG, Ringsted C. Student teachers can be as good as associate professors in teaching clinical skills. *Med Teach* 2007;29(6):553–557. https://doi.org/10.1080/01421590701682550

10. Anteby R, Sinyard RD 3rd, Healy MG, Warshaw AL, Hodin R, Ellison EC, Phitayakorn R. Passing the scalpel: Lessons on retirement planning from retired academic surgeons. *Am J Surg* 2022;224(1 Pt A):166–171. https://doi.org/10.1016/j.amjsurg.2021.11.025

11. Burgess A, McGregor D. Peer teacher training for health professional students: A systematic review of formal programs. *BMC Med Educ* 2018;18(1):263. https://doi.org/10.1186/s12909-018-1356-2

12. Whittaker E, Pathak A, Piya S, Cary L, Harden J. Peer observation of student-led teaching. *Med Teach* 2023;45(11):1300–1303. https://doi.org/10.1080/0142159X.2023.2229506

13. Eastwood MJ, Davies BGJ, Rees EL. Students' experiences of peer observed teaching: A qualitative interview study. *Teach Learn Med* 2023;35(1):1–9. https://doi.org/10.1080/10401334.2021.2006665

14. Steinert Y, Mann K, Anderson B, Barnett BM, Centeno A, Naismith L, Prideaux D, Spencer J, Tullo E, Viggiano T, Ward H, Dolmans D. A systematic review of faculty development initiatives designed to enhance teaching effectiveness: A 10-year update: BEME Guide No. 40. *Med Teach* 2016;38(8):769–786. https://doi.org/10.1080/0142159X.2016.1181851

15. Pedram K, Marcelo C, Paletta-Hobbs L, Meadors E, Dow A. Twelve tips for creating and sustaining a peer assessment program of clinical faculty. *Med Teach* 2023:1–5. https://doi.org/10.1080/0142159X.2023.2252602

16. Sullivan PB, Buckle A, Nicky G, Atkinson SH. Peer observation of teaching as a faculty development tool. *BMC Med Educ* 2012;12:26. https://doi.org/10.1186/1472-6920-12-26

17. Nixon LJ, Gladding SP. Peer observation to promote a culture of teaching and learning. *J Hosp Med* 2023. https://doi.org/10.1002/jhm.13173

18. Fatmi M, Hartling L, Hillier T, Campbell S, Oswald AE. The effectiveness of team-based learning on learning outcomes in health professions education: BEME Guide No. 30. *Med Teach* 2013;35(12):e1608–e1624. https://doi.org/10.3109/0142159X.2013.849802

11 Establishing Rapport with Patients

Ronald J. Anderson

Any discussion of the process of establishing rapport with patients will be affected by the nature of one's experience. My career in medicine has essentially been spent in the practice and teaching of rheumatology and internal medicine in an academic medical center, the Brigham and Women's Hospital.

While many aspects in the care of patients transcend all specialties, some features in managing individuals with rheumatological disorders are unique. Most of the conditions are of unknown etiology, involve long-term care and follow a variable course over time. Spontaneous remissions, presumably related to the inflammatory process, are not unique. In addition, due to the systemic nature of many of the conditions, I frequently functioned as a *de facto* primary care physician for many of my patients.

My decision to completely retire from the direct care of patients in my late seventies was based on a desire to "quit while I was still doing a good job," rather than to gradually reduce my activities and availability to a point that would alter an essential mode of practice that I thoroughly enjoyed.

A little over a year into my retirement, I was offered a newly created position, Distinguished Clinician Teacher, by the Department of Medicine at the Brigham and Women's Hospital. This involved clinical teaching with the unique focus of observing and mentoring physicians in training while they were seeing patients. Although I had regularly served as a ward attending on the general medical teaching service and had spent close to four decades as the rheumatology training program director, my observations of and advice to trainees were predominantly based on decision making after the primary data had been acquired and the essential patient interactions had taken place.

Over the next several years, I observed over 300 physicians, predominantly medical residents, as they saw patients in the outpatient practices. The format employed was that I functioned as an observer with no responsibility for the care of the patients seen. I attempted to be "a fly on the wall" and not "an elephant in the room." At the end of the session, I sat down with the physician and discussed my observations of their patient interactions.

This experience led me to critically assess the process of establishing a rapport with patients and better defined my own past thinking on this topic and the advice that I was able to provide trainees. It reinforced my thoughts on the essentials of establishing and maintaining a productive and rewarding relationship with one's patients.

As a prelude to this topic, what are the barriers to the creation of such relationships?

Although most physicians choose medicine, at least in part, for humanistic reasons, these qualities are often not nurtured by the culture of medicine. Particularly, in the observational sessions just mentioned, I sensed that many trainees were reluctant or uncomfortable in expressing their own humanity. I believe that this served as a barrier in relating to their patients and altered both effective care and joy in the experience. Why should this be, and what can be done to correct this unfortunate situation?

DOI: 10.1201/9781003409373-11

Medicine has always been a hierarchal system, and the attitudes inherent in this structure continue to play a significant role. In 1889, Sir William Osler gave a farewell lecture, *Aequanimitas* [1], to the University of Pennsylvania as he left to assume responsibilities at Johns Hopkins, creating a new faculty and programs that for more than a century have been the model for academic medicine. The essence of this lecture was that "No quality takes rank with imperturbability. . . . The physician who has the misfortune to be without it, who (displays) indecision and worry, . . . loses rapidly the confidence of his patients." The goal of assuming an image of infallibility still exists with many physicians and continues to be incorporated into the training of medical students and young physicians.

In contrast, the publication of "The Care of the Patient" by Francis Weld Peabody, MD, in 1927 shortly before his death from cancer stated: "One of the essential qualities of the clinician is an interest in humanity, for the secret of the care of the patient is in caring for the patient" [2]. This quotation permeates medical literature and is an almost obligatory introductory statement in all basic textbooks. However, other than an acknowledgment of Peabody's statement, most writings fail to provide a blueprint on how to incorporate this attitude into practice. Of interest, Peabody also comments on ambulatory versus inpatient care and laments that teaching is primarily carried out on inpatient services. "Hospital practice always tends to become impersonal. The treatment of a disease may be entirely impersonal, the care of the patient must be entirely personable."

In my opinion, the most useful treatise on patient interactions and medical practice was created by Philip Tumulty, MD. In his opening lecture to third year medical students at Johns Hopkins, "What Is a Clinician and What Does He Do?" [3], the clinician is defined "as one whose prime function is to manage a sick person with the purpose of alleviating most effectively the total impact of the illness upon that person." His advice has resonated throughout the careers of many individuals: "in response to your words, you can make the sick better, and fill the dying with peace. These are great powers. Always deserve them."

Another factor that may interfere with creating and sustaining humanistic and empathetic relationships is the creation of an armor of objectivity by young physicians, a sense that "illness is for others, not for myself." This approach may become increasingly porous over time as physicians not only become increasingly aware of their own susceptibility to those conditions treated in others but also that long-term relationships with one's patients become more personal. The sense that "my patients' illnesses are starting to get to me" is a common experience in the practice of medicine that is rarely addressed and does not have easy answers [4].

Over the course of a career in the practice of medicine, one becomes aware that many of the facts learned, conditions treated, and technical skills previously acquired are no longer applicable in the current care of patients. At one time I was proficient in the use of digitalis and mercurial diuretics and the nuances of gold therapy. Fortunately, these talents are no longer needed. Technology changes and therapeutic advances occur, but patients remain the same. I am convinced that the skills and techniques used in obtaining and interpreting the patient's history, performing a physical exam and interacting effectively with patients, families, and colleagues remain unchanged and are essential to the goal of clinical excellence. They are as important now as they ever were and are almost certain to remain so.

THE INITIAL ENCOUNTER

The primary goal of the initial encounter with a patient is the creation of an atmosphere of trust and the acquisition of an understanding of the unique individual and medical characteristics of the patient. Time spent in forming this relationship is cost-effective by any criteria. It serves both parties well in dealing with the difficult times that undoubtedly will occur in the course of continuing care. The use of extraneous laboratory tests or imaging obtained solely for reassurance and needless referrals can be reduced. The patient is more likely to both comprehend and follow instructions, and less effort and time will be spent in attempting to convince patients of your competence.

A potential obstacle to the creation of trust may occur when a racial discordancy exists between you and your patient. Data based on Press Ganey surveys suggest a higher level of patient satisfaction in the encounter when racial concordance exists with the physician [5]. However, another study indicated that those patients who felt that their physician communicated shared personal beliefs and values rated these physicians higher unrelated to racial concordance [6]. I have long been aware of this issue and, in addition, suspect that a discordancy related to ethnicity, gender, or sexual orientation may also present a challenge. This demands both increased awareness and effort on the part of the physician to create trust in the relationship.

At times, unexpected challenges to the establishment of confidence occur. Several years ago, I outfitted my exam room with a fish tank assuming that it would create a warm and calming atmosphere. However, shortly thereafter, I became aware that a new patient appeared distracted while staring in the direction of the tank.

"What's up? You seem concerned."
"One of the fishes is lying on its side. Do you think it is dead?"

Assuming that a dead fish in the exam room might have a negative impact on her assessment of both my diagnostic acumen and therapeutic effectiveness, I was tempted to explain it away as a syndrome of "transient aquatic vertigo." However, honesty is essential. I confirmed her diagnosis, removed the tank shortly thereafter, and she was a loyal patient for decades.

One should obtain three pieces of data on every new patient at the time of the first encounter:

1. *What is their support system? Who are they responsible for, and who is there to support them?* This information can often best be elicited by an open-ended question such as "how do you spend your day?" as opposed to the commonly used query "tell me about yourself," a phrase that I have found to be subject to misinterpretation and uniquely unproductive. Inquiring about the typical day usually creates an entrée that can be expanded upon to obtain significant social information and provide data that are useful in quantifying function. For example, the nonspecific complaint of "fatigue" is better understood if one knows that the patient, who is employed full time, is also responsible for the care of a parent with disabilities.

2. *What is unique about individual patients? What are they famous for?* When I initially began caring for patients, I found this data helpful as a "memory trick" in that if I remembered, for example, that the patient enjoyed square dancing, it prompted me to remember other medical and social details. It also enriched the entire relationship in many ways. This information may be of great value in greeting patients on follow-up visits. Many patients have concerns as they enter a physician's office. "Do they remember me? Do they know who I am? Do they care?" The process of greeting patients with a comment about a specific unique aspect of their life tells them that you remember them, know who they are, and care about them as persons. Not only is this fun, but it takes little if any time.

3. *What are their strengths, and/or how have they dealt with adversity in the past?* Patients usually seek out medical care in difficult times. It is good to remember that illness seldom brings out the best in people. However, most

individuals have had experiences when they effectively met life's challenges. It is important to identify their strengths and use this knowledge in providing advice as they journey on the course created by their illness. This information may be uncovered whenever the patient describes an unfortunate event. Ask: "How did you deal with, or how are you dealing with this problem?" Phrasing your response in this manner also creates an empathetic atmosphere, leading to both understanding and support, in contradistinction to a somewhat hollow, more traditional "sympathetic" response such as "I am sorry to hear that." This latter reply tends to cut off the conversation and blocks the addition of much useful information.

The initial office visit should optimally begin with greeting the patient in the waiting room. Not only does it create a warm atmosphere, but it often gives insight into the patient's support system. Who, if anyone, accompanies them? How do they interact with each other at the time of introduction? Some diagnoses come to mind based on the first impression related to general appearance, mood, body signals, etc. The opportunity to observe the patient get out of the chair and walk to the exam room provides a chance to study the patient's gait and spontaneous motions. Disorders such as Parkinson's disease, myopathies, and neuropathies are often most easily detected during the walk between the waiting room and the examination area. If you defer your exam until the patient is sitting on the examination table, wearing an examination gown, many diagnoses and impressions will be missed.

Should those relatives and significant others who accompany the patient stay with them throughout the visit? Although some physicians may feel that the presence of another individual inhibits the patient's comfort and ability to relate their story and concerns, in general the presence of another set of eyes and ears is helpful both diagnostically and in the development of a management plan. They also might provide clues, particularly regarding observed changes in the patient or other subtle issues that neither the patient nor a physician seeing the individual for the first time would be aware of. The personal interactions observed may clarify the social situation and provide insight regarding why medical attention is being sought and why at this time.

Ask the individuals to define their relationship. Assume nothing, particularly based on the age and gender of the person accompanying the patient. Always ask the patient's permission to have the individual accompanying them to be present throughout the visit.

In some situations, it is wise to provide time when you are alone with the patient to allow them to express information that they might be reluctant to provide in the presence of the individual who accompanied them. One approach is to create a diversion such as asking these questions while observing the patient's gait by walking outside the exam room. Most often you will ask the companion to leave for a minute.

After the patient has sat down in the exam room, the initial focus should be on continuing to enrich the relationship. In the current era, the computer screen may be the dominant feature of the medical office. Furthermore, many physicians and virtually all physicians under age 40 have grown up with the computer and are skilled in recording their notes by typing while they talk. Many older patients, however, grew up in a different era. They often view typing and talking as rude, uncaring, and another sign that medicine has become impersonal. If you are a "typer-talker," explain at the onset that is easier and more accurate for you to type. Ask their permission to do so.

A portion of the process of taking a history may involve "thoughtless" data gathering such as listing medications, allergies, dates of surgery, etc. Physicians who are required to seek this information themselves may subconsciously change their tone of voice to a cadence that could sound harsh and rushed. Explain to the patient that you are just getting "a bit of routine information," Otherwise the patient might interpret the alteration of tone as a sign of displeasure. Always appear to have adequate time, even though you don't. Never state that you don't have time to deal with a specific matter. If you truly do not have time, develop a plan with the patient regarding the next step to deal with that issue. Do not leave a void with a statement such as "we will deal with that later." Create an atmosphere of interest and concern. Be aware of your body language, particularly in this situation.

Two studies of observed interactions between physicians and patients demonstrated that the physician interrupted the patient on an average within 11 or 12 seconds into the interview [7]. Female patients were interrupted sooner than males [8]. Other than biting your tongue, how does one avoid these interruptions, yet attempt to be more time-effective? One approach, particularly with new patients, is to start the visit by explaining your role, what information you have been able to review prior to the visit, and what you don't know and wish to learn during the visit. I believe that this avoids time wasted in the repetition by the patient of data already reviewed and allows a focus on the issues of greatest concern to the patient. An open-ended question such as "what brings you here" or an equivalent is used at the beginning. Allow patients to tell their own story. "Thinking out loud" with phrases such as "let me see if I have this correct" is often a useful technique. It describes your understanding of the problem and incorporates the patient into the process. The taking of a history should be a dialogue, not a dictation.

An additional approach that is beneficial in creating rapport is to address every concern mentioned and also develop competence regarding "little things" and interventions that are useful in the care of all patients. For example:

1. Examine every area that the patient expresses concern about.
2. As you mature, create a personal library of skills such as essentials of physical therapy, a knowledge of footwear and office orthopedics. Know the fundamentals of dermatology and the relative cost and indications for over-the-counter medications.
3. If there are no pressing concerns requiring a physical exam during a follow up-visit, examine areas that the patient cannot visualize themselves such as the feet.

Although patients seek medical care for concerns related both to pain or dysfunction, not infrequently they begin the initial visit with a complaint of pain. This may be in response to the commonly employed opening question "where do you hurt?" or even to the obligatory Pain Scale poster on the office wall. The greatest concern of many patients, particularly those with musculoskeletal issues, is the potential loss of function. They may be uncomfortable or embarrassed to reveal their fear of loss of independence. Functional concerns vary and often are not adequately defined in the patient's mind prior to the first visit. It is important at the onset of the relationship to determine the patient's unique needs and their support system. Set the expectation that the target of treatment is the preservation or restoration of function. Pain should not be ignored, but functional goals should be central to the management plan. With function as the focus, the patient is frequently a more effective partner in their treatment; the benefits of other disciplines such as surgery, orthopedics, and physical therapy are enhanced, and the tendency to employ analgesics including opiates is diminished. It has been my observation that, in the course of a long-standing chronic disease, patients whose primary objective is maintenance of function rather than relief of pain do better in every way.

Mention should be made of the approach to follow when, at the close of the examination, it seems probable that the patient's diagnosis is most compatible with a "functional disorder." This general term is used to describe syndromes without a well-defined anatomical or physiological basis that, over a prolonged period of observation, do not lead to objective changes. Patients in this category may include those with psychosomatic disorders, the "worried well" who need reassurance that they don't have a threatening condition, and individuals who seem to fit into a diagnosis of a condition such as fibromyalgia or irritable bowel syndrome.

Patients may resent the diagnosis of a functional disorder and feel that their symptoms are being passed off as "all in my mind." Although there is often a psychosomatic component to these syndromes, it is my experience that such patients seldom are malingering. They would just as soon get better. Physicians are also frequently uncomfortable and uncertain with these conditions. Office visits are characteristically lengthy events with a tendency to avoid a definitive discussion. The process may be prolonged by ordering new studies or consultations to placate the dissatisfied patient. No one is happy. Physicians' egos tend to be reinforced by observing their patient's improvement in response to an intervention. This seldom occurs early in the management of functional disorders. Avoid the tendency to allow your own frustrations and occasional associated anger to affect your care.

A reasonable approach to the care of these patients is to ask yourself the two following questions:

1. Do I have a therapeutic relationship with the patient?
2. Is the patient's view of their condition and goals for improvement in line with what I can offer as their physician?

If the answer to these questions is "yes" or "uncertain," one approach is to construct a program governed by observation over time both to confirm your initial impression and to determine the nature of the relationship. When interventions are attempted, they should be benign. Surgery, opiates, initiation of corticosteroids, and costly diagnostic imaging should be avoided. Be aware that observation is always a "harder sell" than intervention. I believe that effectiveness in the long-term management of these patients is more dependent on the creation of a supportive and cooperative relationship than on the physician's unique knowledge and technical skills in the subspecialty involved. Often a program that may be of unique value includes mind–body modalities such as yoga, exercise, and relaxation techniques. The outcome may be rewarding to both the patient and the physician. If, on the other hand, the answer to both the preceding questions is "no," it is probably wisest to seek early closure. This is never a comfortable experience for either party but is often preferable to prolonging a relationship that seems doomed to fail.

THE DISCUSSION AT THE CLOSE OF THE VISIT

This is the discussion at the end of the visit, either initial or follow-up, in which the physician advises the patient about what should be done both diagnostically and therapeutically. It can be further classified as either preliminary, in which a diagnosis has not been made, or final, in which a diagnosis has been made, and a plan of management has been developed. It is important to stress that one should never present the patient with a diagnosis or plan until the summation takes place at the end of the visit. Advice given earlier often needs to be altered based on further data obtained during the visit. If this occurs, not only does the physician have to change the advice given but also take the time to explain why. This may cause confusion for the patient.

Is it necessary to make a definite diagnosis at the end of the visit or after the initial round of tests? Many benign conditions will get better spontaneously and are diagnoses of exclusion, confirmed only by recovery of the patient. Remember that the great body of medical knowledge is based on conditions that do not get better. One sees many patients who ultimately recover for uncertain reasons. The tactic of initially considering and excluding, as best as one can, the most ominous or worst-case scenarios is a reasonable approach. The physician's mind should remain open. It is good to recall that, once you make a diagnosis, you often stop thinking. Therefore, patients tend to benefit from an uncertain, yet questioning physician.

If a program of "wait and see" is chosen, discuss the rationale with the patient, make certain that they agree, and avoid the tendency, often requested by the patient or their family, to intervene with imaging studies, further blood work, or trials of therapy. Whatever intervention you advise during the period of observation should be nontoxic, inexpensive, and readily available. Voltaire stated: "The art of medicine is to keep the patient entertained while nature effects a cure" [9].

The final summation interview takes place when a working diagnosis has been made and a management plan developed. Concerned family members and others who accompanied the patient should be invited to attend. The format that works best is when both the physician and the patient are seated. The posture of sitting implies an equal role for both the doctor and the patient and suggests that the physician is not rushed and has time to discuss the issues that arise.

It is well to stress again that people who are ill or are concerned about being ill are seldom at their best, particularly at this phase of the visit. In addition, most patients are unable to absorb more than three bits of advice at a given time. It is likely that only a fraction of what you tell the patient will be remembered, and only a fraction of your advice will be acted upon. The conversation could start off by asking the patient again what their concerns are, or "what did you hope would happen as a result of this visit," essentially a reiteration of the chief complaint. The next step is to explain how you came up with the diagnosis. On occasion it is wise to inform the patient that the working diagnosis is provisional, based on currently available information, and may be revised over time.

In presenting this information, think out loud and freely use drawings, diagrams, or any technique that clarifies your explanation. There are many reasons to consider the option of providing the patient with a copy of your note at the end of the session.

THE ROLE OF HONESTY IN THE RELATIONSHIP

Essential to establishing rapport with patients is a foundation of honesty in the relationship. What should you tell patients when there is uncertainty in either the diagnosis or management plan? This becomes increasingly more difficult when there is a possibility that a diagnosis under consideration, although unlikely, has features that are either untreatable or ominous. If the worst possible diagnosis has an available treatment, one uses clinical judgment in orchestrating the discussion and management plan. If a possible diagnosis is ominous with a prognosis that would not be altered by early diagnosis, ALS for example, the decision to inform the patient is dependent on the probability of the diagnosis and your level of comfort in being later held accountable for a "diagnosis you had missed." It is imperative to always be truthful in what you say but attempt not to needlessly worry the patient by bringing up issues that may be either improbable or untreatable. Be as positive as you can while remaining honest. "Everything said should be true, but the physician does not have to say everything" [10].

Honesty may have its challenges. Several years ago, I cared for a delightful, retired gentleman in his eighties who was doing well on a tolerable dose of prednisone for biopsy-proven giant cell arteritis. Our visits were a joy and mostly focused on the lives of his children, grandchildren, and the vagaries of our beloved Red Sox. At the close of one visit, he voiced a concern that he might not be as "sharp" mentally as he had been. His symptoms were a vague "forgetfulness" without social or functional deterioration. Due to his visual impairments, his wife did the driving. My exam was essentially negative, and his score on the Mini-Mental Status Exam was 27 out of 30. Not normal but a "passing grade." My impression was that he was not in the early stages of dementia and, given his support system and lifestyle, currently not at risk of harming himself or others.

"You did pretty well, and I don't think you have to worry about this altering your future. Continue to live the kind of life you are now enjoying."
"Thank you. This has been a tremendous worry of mine. As always, I am comforted by your words. I feel much better after each visit."
"Thank you. I also feel better myself after your visits."

At this time, we patted each other on the back, basking in the warmth of our relationship and his positive response to my advice. However, as he arose to leave, I noticed that his fly was open. What should I do? Would telling him break the spell?

I pointed it out and he thanked me. Remember, always be honest.

Giving bad news when there is certainty in the diagnosis is always a challenge. In the face of a difficult disorder with a grim prognosis, tell the patient what you know but avoid uncertain aspects of the condition such as life expectancy or anticipated mode of death. Be honest and try to focus on any positive or potentially reversible aspects of the condition. For example, patients with early dementia who are fortunate enough not to have an associated negative personality change may be comforted by being told: "You are the same person with the same wonderful human qualities that so many have grown to love over the years. You just aren't as intelligent as you were in the past. We can deal with that." It took over 30 years of medical practice before I stumbled on this approach and have found it tremendously comforting to the patient and their families. Continue to minister to the patient, be thorough, and include the care of other issues such as a rash, bowel dysfunction, etc. Remember that one of the patient's greatest fears is being abandoned. If you cease addressing these issues, the patient may sense that you have given up.

Should the physician attend the funeral, wake, or memorial services held for former patients? There is little data on this question, and the answers will vary among individual physicians and specialties [11]. Many physicians prefer to maintain a boundary between their personal and professional life and would not venture into this territory. Others feel that their presence might be a reminder of a difficult time for the family. In addition, the death of a patient may stimulate doubt about one's own competence and can be associated with guilt, albeit undeserved. On the other hand, if one has a long-term relationship with the patient and their family that spans periods of both sickness and health, attendance at the ceremony may be beneficial. When one feels that their presence would add to the "celebration of life" rather than serve as a "reminder of illness," there are reasons to attend. I have done so several times in situations in which I had a warm, long-standing relationship with the patient and their family and felt able to genuinely express sympathy, comfort the family, and relate happy stories about the deceased.

CODA

After spending many years in the practice of medicine, one should become alert to the threat of the insidious onset of complacency and a tendency to become less critical of yourself. The longer you practice, the more you tend to accumulate patients who like you, laugh at your jokes, and tolerate your inadequacies. Those that are dissatisfied with your care leave early for greener pastures. Eventually you become part of a large happy family populated by grateful patients with strains of Kumbaya playing in the background. I believe that two factors have been critical in my career to help ward off this attitude:

1. *Patients*: They are always a challenge, restorative in so many ways, and bring something new to the table with each visit. They provide perspective. When one cares for patients, you learn that you're never as bad as you fear you are when things go wrong or as great as you aspire to be when things go well. Sometimes you're the windshield and sometimes you're the bug.

2. *Involvement in the Education of Young Physicians and Relationships with Colleagues*: During my residency years, I became convinced that my goal was to become a clinician and teacher in an academic medical center. I was advised by several individuals at the time that my attraction to clinical teaching was essentially a result of my joy in the collegial relationships experienced in training. They warned me that as I became more senior and no longer shared age-specific experiences and attitudes, I would outgrow my enthusiasm for this activity. This did not happen. I believe that the fun and collegiality persist and are based on common goals, experiences, challenges, and rewards related to the care of patients.

REFERENCES

1. Osler, W. *Aequanimitas, With Other Addresses to Medical Students, Nurses and Practitioners of Medicine*. Philadelphia, PA: P. Blakiston, 1904: 3–6.
2. Peabody, FW. The care of the patient. *JAMA* 1927;88(12):877–882.
3. Tumulty PA. What is a clinician and what does he do? *N Eng J Med* 1970;283:20–24.
4. Berman N. A reason to retire? *N Eng J Med* 2023;389:1254–1255.
5. Takeshita J, Wang S, Loren AW, Mitra N, Shults J, Shin DS, Sawinski DL. Association of racial/ethnic and gender concordance between patients and physicians with patient experience ratings. *JAMA Netw Open* 2020:3(11).
6. Street RL, O'Malley KJ, Cooper LA, Haidet P. Understanding concordance in patient-physician relationships: Personal and ethnic dimensions of shared identity. *Ann Fam Med* 2008;6(3):198–205.
7. Beckman HB, Frankel RM. The effect of physician behavior on the collection of data. *Ann Intern Med* 1984;101(5):692–696.
8. Rhoades DR, McFarland KF, Finch WH, Johnson AO. Speaking and interruptions during primary care visits. *Fam Med* 2001;33(7):528–532.
9. Shaw Q. On aphorisms. *Br J Gen Pract* 2009;59(569):954–955.
10. Caplan LR, Hollander J. *The Effective Clinical Neurologist*, 3rd ed. Shelton, CT: People's Medical Publishing House-USA, 2011.
11. Zambrano SC, Chur-Hansen A, Crawford GB. Attending patient funerals: Practice and attitudes of Australian medical practitioners. *Death Stud* 2017;41:78–86.

12 Communicating a Breast Cancer Diagnosis and Treatment Plan: A Patient's Journey

Rache M. Simmons

> My name is Sallie, and I am a 53-year-old working wife and mother of two teenage children. Today was a typical day. I woke up, got the kids dressed and off to school, kissed my husband, got in the car, and drove to work. Except today, everything about my world changed. . . . My cell phone rang, and the radiologist told me, "The biopsy results came back, and you have breast cancer.
>
> I will remember that exact moment forever. . . . It was a beautiful sunny day, and I could hear my coworkers laughing in the hallway. . . . "How can the rest of the world function like everything is normal?" I stood in complete spiraling disbelief . . . this cannot be true . . . there must be a mistake. Then the fears came. Am I going to die? How am I going to tell my kids? What happens next?

"Sallie" is a fictional woman based on the conversations with thousands of my patients over decades of practice. Although the specifics of a breast cancer diagnosis individualize every patient, their stories, fears, and bravery are similar in many ways. As physicians, we are instructed over years of training in cancer treatment biology, pathology, anatomy, and biochemistry. What is not taught, however, is the method of communication with our patients during a breast cancer diagnosis and treatment journey.

In my experience, there are three vital elements in best communicating a cancer diagnosis and treatment plan to a patient:

1. Establish patient trust.
2. Have a conversation that is understandable to the patient.
3. Create a clear and definitive plan.

THE DIAGNOSIS

The initial breast cancer conversation usually begins after establishing a diagnosis with an image-directed needle biopsy. The individual who contacts the patient with this news can be the radiologist who performed the biopsy or her* primary care provider. Some primary care providers prefer to deliver this news as they have a long-standing relationship with the patient. Many radiologists, however, are quite capable of discussing a breast cancer diagnosis in an experienced way. Whoever contacts the patient should sensitively deliver the news and have the knowledge to answer general questions regarding the next steps in a referral for treatment. It is also important that this diagnosis is respectfully delivered in a fashion that allows the patient a quiet, private space. If the patient seems to be in a noisy, public environment, it is appropriate to ask them to call you back when they feel comfortable discussing their recent results. In my opinion, this communication should only be

---

*This writing refers to patients with she/her pronouns, but please know that these could also be he/him when referring to male breast cancer or gender-neutral pronouns.

DOI: 10.1201/9781003409373-12

in person or over the phone and never through electronic messaging or left on a voicemail.

TREATMENT CONSULTATION

After the patient has the breast cancer diagnosis, she is referred to a treating physician or a breast center. A referral by her primary care provider, whom she has known for many years, or by a relative or friend who has been treated by our team, immediately instills confidence.

There is often a multidisciplinary team approach with breast cancer management, which may begin with the Patient Navigator. Patient Navigators are specially trained individuals, usually nurses, who receive the initial patient call and schedule her appropriately with the team. As the first contact with the treatment team, the Patient Navigators begin by introducing themselves and their role in serving and helping the patient. They build trust and a rapport with the patient or family member by expressing empathy for the patient and acknowledging that her fears and feelings are perfectly normal. These Patient Navigators give assurance that she will be cared for by a team experienced in the treatment of her breast cancer. The Patient Navigators can answer general questions about the diagnosis and anticipated treatments, relieve many anxieties, and correct misinformation. A patient often expresses that the conversation with the Patient Navigators "makes her feel like someone has caught her in mid-air during a free fall." The Patient Navigators also ask for background information, pertinent medical history, language preferences, and any social barriers, which is essential for the consultation visit. It is crucial to promptly schedule consult appointments with treating physicians to allow the patient early access to information regarding their specific treatment plan and definitive care.

Our breast center has many online videos and media clips of our team discussing diagnosis, treatment, and new research. The Patient Navigators suggest that the patient watch these before her consultation. These videos review general treatment information, so the patient has some working knowledge of the options when she arrives for the in-person consult. It also familiarizes her with the physician she will see, building a foundation of trust. Due to this online introduction, my patients often say it feels like she already knows me when we first meet.

The in-person visit typically starts with a welcome greeting and a handshake. Then I ask to be introduced to any companions with her in the room. This action makes them feel welcome and included in the conversation. It also establishes the relationship between the patient and others, which can be necessary background for the consultation discussion.

Next, I inform the patient that I have reviewed her medical history, pathology, and breast imaging at our multidisciplinary conference that morning. This approach typically affords the patient tremendous comfort when she knows the whole team has already discussed her diagnosis at our conference. The summary might go something like this:

> Let me summarize what I know about you at this point, and you tell me if I am missing anything important. Last month, you had a routine mammogram, and they saw a spot that led to additional imaging, followed by a biopsy, which came back as breast cancer. The good news is that your cancer is tiny, and the cell type is not aggressive. So I think you have a completely treatable and curable cancer.

With this statement, the patient often takes a deep breath and relaxes. In my opinion, until the patient feels this trust, she cannot genuinely listen and effectively absorb the information and treatment recommendations of the consultation.

Unless a patient is in the medical field, I avoid medical jargon like "your Ki67 is 5%"—it is much better just to say, "Your cancer is very slow growing." My job is to explain her situation in ways she, as a layperson, and her companions can understand.

Then, if she has nothing else to add, I let her know what to expect during the consultation. I suggest performing an exam and then having a "conversation about your treatment options." The word "conversation" is preferred because it relays a two-way discussion.

Having a family member or companion as "another set of ears" during the consultation can be helpful. Patients are welcome to include a family member by phone, and I am also okay with patients recording our conversation to play back when she is home or share with others. Of course, interpreters are made available for patients if appropriate.

For the exam, providing the patient with as much privacy as she desires is crucial. I always ask if she wants me to draw a curtain or ask her companions to be seated in the waiting room during the exam. If she wishes to have them sit in the waiting room, I will then inquire whether she wishes to have them return to discuss treatment options. Occasionally, a patient does not want to have them present for the discussion, and this desire should be respected.

Typically, the conversation regarding surgery would build on the discussion of her current diagnosis and involve a review of treatment options, their benefits and risks. It is beneficial to ask the patient if she has surgical preferences or concerns *de novo*. Some patients with very small cancers desire bilateral mastectomies, and some patients with sizable cancers will do anything, regardless of the cosmetic outcome, to preserve their breasts. Occasionally, a patient has an opinion based on general misinformation or her personal, perhaps historically distant experience with a relative or friend. It is essential to politely establish the correct context regarding her specific diagnosis as well as any inaccurate reference to historical treatment options.

Surgical treatment is ultimately the patient's choice, and it is vital for the patient to feel a sense of control over her decision. My role as an oncology surgeon is to help guide her toward her optimal decision. If a patient wishes to have an inappropriate treatment, I sometimes make statements such as, "Yes, I can do that surgically, but I don't really think you want me to, and here is why . . ." In this way, my opinion and recommendation have been expressed, but it directs the decision and sense of control back to her.

Sometimes a patient selects a treatment option that conflicts with the standard of care. In that case, offering guidance based on medical knowledge and clinical trials is appropriate while also acknowledging the patient's right to autonomy. It is essential to be mindful of how cultural backgrounds and beliefs influence a patient's perspective on her cancer and treatment.

On occasion, a patient or a companion is confrontational and expresses anger toward me or my staff in this discussion. It is appropriate to recognize and acknowledge that it is normal to be upset and defensive with a new cancer diagnosis. Often this stems from feelings of fear and helplessness. Then I calmly explain that I did not cause this diagnosis and that my team and I are trying to help her proceed with treatment toward her best prognosis and to resume her normal life. Usually, this allows a rational conversation to ensue, but, if not, there are times when it is best to defer any further interaction until another day when the patient or companion are more receptive to such a discussion. If appropriate, social workers or patient care services can be included to facilitate additional supportive care.

In addition to verbal discussion of treatment options, drawing pictures to illustrate proposed surgical treatment can be very helpful in conveying a treatment plan. A blank cartoon outline of a torso with breasts is used to delineate where and how big her cancer is relative to her breast size and serves as the foundation for the discussion. Then, illustrated in this same diagram, the proposed treatment options of lumpectomy, mastectomy, sentinel lymph node biopsy, and incisions assist in clarifying her choices. Patients find this visual representation of the surgery very informative and frequently ask to keep the diagram to review at home with others. Patients often ask to speak to a patient who has undergone similar treatment. Such a patient-to-patient connection can be provided if both patients agree to contact each other. Sometimes, there are additional indicated studies such as an MRI, genetic testing, or consultations with plastic surgery or medical oncology. Another communication, either in person or over the phone, is scheduled to finalize the surgical plan once these tests or consultations are complete and make the patient feel there is continuity of the care plan.

The patient greatly appreciates an overview of what to expect in preparation for the day of surgery, the overall schedule of the surgical day, and the expected postoperative course. Our breast center has numerous handouts and online information on pre- and postoperative instructions, drain care, and additional information on the perioperative period. Giving a patient this information in writing lets her know what to anticipate and relieves anxiety. I then ask what questions I have not answered for the patient or those accompanying the patient. Giving her a name and contact method comforts the patient in the event she would like to reach out for additional questions and concerns after the visit.

AFTER THE SURGERY

The postoperative visit includes confirmation that the surgical incisions are healing well and a discussion of the pathology reports in a clear, understandable fashion. At this point, the patient is typically referred to the medical oncology and radiation oncology teams for additional adjuvant therapy. Our breast center offers information and referrals for psychological counseling, social workers, support groups, yoga and integrative care, and fertility experts as indicated.

Our Breast Cancer Survivorship Program provides long-term follow-up. This is an essential transition for a patient several years after her diagnosis and beyond active treatment. At this time a patient can feel lost or abandoned, and this type of program is very comforting. Most importantly, a patient is regularly reassured that she is not alone in her journey.

In summary, there are three vital elements in communicating a cancer diagnosis and treatment plan to a patient.

1. *Establish Patient Trust*: Personal referrals from a long-standing primary care provider or another patient can establish patient confidence. Patient Navigator communication and online videos before the first visit also encourage trust. Demonstrating knowledge of the patient's diagnosis and respectful interaction with the patient and companions during the consultation are critical.
2. *Have a Conversation That Is Understandable to the Patient*: The two-way dialogue should be in lay language and easily comprehended by the patient and companions. A drawing often assists in specific discussion of surgical options. Providing additional resources to amplify this information can be helpful.
3. *Create a Clear and Definitive Plan*: Patients find a logical and organized treatment plan extremely comforting. Explaining additional tests/consults with further finalizing discussion, outlining details of the expected perioperative period, and anticipated postoperative adjuvant therapies give the patient focus and comfort. The patient should ultimately make all treatment decisions—our job, as oncologists, is to guide her to make the best decision for her.

13 Medical Humanism

Richard M. Silver

Humanism is a core value of the medical profession and the reason most of us chose to pursue a career in medicine [1]. Humanism includes the attitudes and behaviors that demonstrate interest in and respect for patients' psychological, social, and spiritual concerns and values. Many have written about the importance of humanism in our profession. Although living and practicing in a world far different from our own, much can be learned about a humanistic approach to medicine through the life and work of Sir William Osler (1849–1919) (Figure 13.1A). Osler was a preeminent physician of the 19th and early 20th centuries, considered to be the most influential physician in the emergence of science-based medicine. Osler's influence extended far beyond the four medical schools he served (McGill, Penn, Johns Hopkins [one of its founders] and Oxford). Indeed, Osler's emphasis on clinical bedside medicine shaped the ways in which medicine has been taught ever since. Osler saw medicine in its wider scope with the right and even the duty to be concerned with the human condition as a whole. Osler's philosophy of medicine had four major components: [1] biologic reductionism about disease; [2] a scientific approach to clinical diagnosis; [3] therapeutic conservatism; and, importantly, [4] *a humanistic approach to the patient* [2].

A humanistic approach to the patient has struck some as contradictory to Osler's *"Aequanimitas"* [3], leading some to refer to Osler as "the father of cool detachment" and the originator of "Oslerian equanimity" [4]. *Aequanimitas* was the title of Osler's farewell address to the graduating medical students at the University of Pennsylvania prior to his arrival in Baltimore to open the Johns Hopkins School of Medicine. In this lecture and a subsequent essay, Osler stressed the importance of *equanimity* and *imperturbability*, imparting the following cautionary advice to the graduates [4]:

> The first essential is to have your nerves well in hand. Even under the most serious circumstances, the physician or surgeon who allows his outward action to demonstrate the native act and figure of his heart in complement extern, who shows in his face the slightest alteration, expressive of anxiety or fear, has not his medullary centres under the highest control, and is liable to disaster at any moment. I have spoken of this to you on many occasions and have urged you to educate your nerve centres so that not the slightest dilator or contractor influence shall pass to the vessels of your face under any professional trial.

Few among us have either the classical training or the gravitas to critique Sir William Osler, but one perhaps on equal footing was a rheumatologist, Dr. Gerald Weissmann (1930–2019), professor of medicine at New York University (Figure 13.1B). Weissmann made many important contributions to the field of inflammation and immunology while contributing many essays on science and society. *The Woods Hole Cantata*, a collection of Weissmann's essays, contains one of his most notable works entitled, "Against *Aequanimitas*" [5]. While referring to the

DOI: 10.1201/9781003409373-13

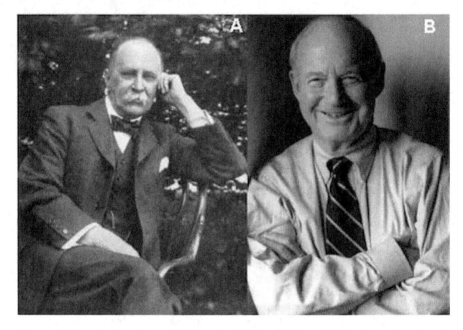

Figure 13.1 *Aequanimitas*: (A) For: Sir William Osler. (B) Against: Dr. Gerald Weissmann.

introduction of coursework in ethics, sociology, and humanism in medical school curricula, Weissmann avows:

> [I]f the goal of the new humanism is that of the old, if its aim is to lead to *aequanimitas*—to learn control over of "medullary centers"—I want no part of it.

In rebuttal to Weissmann's rejection of the "cool detachment" of Osler's *Aequanimitas*, Dr. Charles S. Bryan, a learned friend, fellow Oslerian, and perhaps the foremost authority on all things Osler [6], points to the tension between head (*detached concern*) and heart (*humanistic empathy*), placing Osler philosophically between *apatheia* and *eupatheia* [3]. Bryan goes on to provide examples of Osler's *aequanimitas* as being a philosophy not of *apatheia* nor of *eupatheia* but rather one of *metriopatheia* (emotions appropriate to the circumstance). One such example of the importance of medical humanism asserted by Osler in *Aequanimitas* reads as follows [3]:

> The physician needs a clear head and a kind heart; his work is arduous and complex, requiring the exercise of the very highest faculties of the mind, while constantly appealing to the emotions and finer feeling.

Dissimilar worldviews led Osler to profess and Weissmann to reject *aequanimitas*, yet each man held strong convictions on the imperative of medical humanism. Osler notes the importance of "constantly appealing to the emotions" [2], while Weissmann writes, "The passion of the physician may be the best part of what he has to offer his patients and his society" [5].

Sadly, the paramount position of humanism in medicine is being eroded by the "business of medicine." Osler cannily issued a warning about business and medicine [3]:

> As the practice of medicine is not a business and can never be one, the education of the heart—the moral side of man—must keep pace with the education of the head. Our fellow creatures cannot be dealt with as a man deals in corn and coal.

Osler's warning resonates even more forcefully today. Osler's entreaty that "the education of the heart—the moral side of man—" take precedence over the business of medicine is, in fact, a plea for medical humanism over and above the commercialization of our profession. In a recent commentary, Dr. Donald Berwick decries the existential threat of greed in US health care: "The grip of financial self-interest in US health care is becoming a stranglehold with dangerous and pervasive consequences" [7]. Failing to heed the words of Osler, we now find ourselves as pawns in a business model that is anything but humanistic; indeed, the present US medical paradigm is habitually *anti*humanistic. This, I believe, to be a major factor in today's crisis of professional burnout.

Our profession is devalued when technology is rewarded at the expense of time and care, favoring high-tech, low-touch encounters that rob both patient and physician of the opportunity for a meaningful relationship—a chance to recognize and celebrate psychological, social, and spiritual concerns and values. All parties lose when the essential patient interaction is reduced to a "relative value unit" (RVU). Patient and physician alike suffer at the hands of the electronic health record, efficient at capturing diagnostic codes to maximize billing but an impediment to meaningful patient–physician interaction. Patient care is now expected to be "delivered" in ever shrinking increments of time (40–60 minutes for a new patient encounter and 15–20 minutes for a follow-up patient encounter). Lines from singer-songwriter Mark Knopfler's tune memorializing Ray Kroc, the entrepreneur who made McDonald's what it is today, come to mind [8]:

> Wham bam, don't wait long
> Shake, fries, patty, you're gone.

Administrators often measure patient care in RVUs, today's coin of the realm, much as the number of burgers served or pizzas delivered are the measures of fast-food corporate success. Can anything be more *anti*humanistic? Ironically, all of this is taking place while at the same time physicians are being implored to seek understanding about and the importance of social determinants of health. The 15–20 minute patient visit leaves little room to establish a meaningful and long-lasting relationship.

I practice rheumatology in an academic setting with medical students, residents, and fellows in the clinic. One method I use to enhance the patient–physician encounter despite time constraints imposed by our system is to have all patients (except in rare situations) presented at the bedside, not outside the door or at a nearby computer terminal. I have found this approach strengthens my relationship with patient and family while at the same time affording instruction for the learners in the subtleties of medical history, physical examination, and the importance of shared decision making. Osler wrote, "The natural method of teaching the student begins with the patient, continues with the patient, and ends his studies with the patient, using books and lectures as tools, as means to an end" [9].

Manifestations of professional burnout such as mental fatigue, depersonalization, and diminished self-value are not unexpected outcomes of today's practice of medicine. Some might regard burnout as being inevitable and a preferred alternative to "fading away"—as musician Neil Young wrote in a song later infamously quoted in Kurt Cobain's suicide note [10]:

It's better to burn out than to fade away.

But is it better? I think not, nor do I plan to simply fade away. Faced with unquestionable workforce shortages, our profession cannot afford wholesale burnout. Yet data from the Centers for Disease Control and Prevention suggest that in 2022 nearly one-half of health care workers reported feelings of burnout [11]. And burnout is not limited to a particular age group or practice setting; even some first-year rheumatology fellows express symptoms of burnout [12]. One must ask the question, "Why is burnout so rampant, and why does it impact even the more junior among us?" Could it be because we have lost the humanizing aspect that first led us to our profession?

Many hospital administrators, deans, department leaders, and so-called "wellness advocates" seem to "blame the victim" rather than address what I believe to be the real issue, *i.e.*, the harmful health care environment in which we now work. In his health care blog *America's Toxic Workplace*, Dr. Nortin Hadler, one of my earliest mentors who more than anyone else steered me to a career in rheumatology, notes that "the structure we have created for practicing medicine makes taking care of patients more difficult, more stressful and, ultimately counterproductive . . . (it's) a fixing-people production line" [13] (Figure 13.2). In his book *By the Bedside*

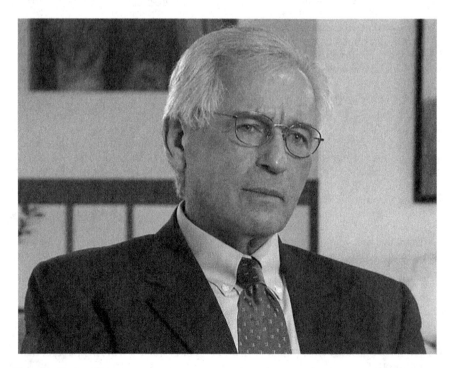

Figure 13.2   Dr. Nortin Hadler, mentor, and author of numerous books, including *By the Bedside of the Patient* [14].

of the Patient: Lessons for the Twenty-First-Century Physician, Hadler makes the truly Oslerian case for a practice of medicine that draws on the best available scientific knowledge, transmits the wisdom of experienced clinicians, and reforges an empathetic relationship between physician and patient, treating each patient as an individual [14]. For Hadler, the solution resides not in blaming the victim and instituting wellness programs but rather by recreating "a health care system that considers a rational, empathic patient–physician dialogue inviolate"—in other words, a system that truly values humanism and the doctor–patient relationship [14].

There is no simple solution to the burnout problem, or it would have been solved by now. Promoting puerile "wellness programs" like yoga and Zumba at work, dietary classes, "Mindful Mondays," team building, etc., must not be the only approach [13]. Rather, we can begin to approach the problem in a serious manner by heeding the oft-quoted advice of Dr. Frances Weld Peabody (1818–1927) [15]:

> Time, sympathy, and understanding must be lavishly dispensed, but the reward is to be found in the personal bond which forms the greatest satisfaction of the practice of medicine. One of the essential qualities of the clinician is interest in humanity, for the secret of the care of the patient is caring for the patient.

My colleague Dr. John Sergent put it more bluntly in his presidential address to the American College of Rheumatology—paraphrasing then candidate Bill Clinton's campaign slogan, "It's the economy, stupid." John declared to fellow rheumatologists, "It's the patient, stupid!" [16].

In my practice of medicine, which now extends to five decades, I have had the privilege to care for many patients suffering from serious rheumatic diseases. I have endeavored to provide *"Time, sympathy and understanding,"* as Dr. Peabody directs, and I can attest that this has been for me *"the greatest satisfaction of the practice of medicine."* I could cite many examples, but two such relationships are momentous and have provided me with utmost fulfillment. The first involves a 15-year-old daughter of a patient who suffered from and ultimately succumbed to scleroderma. Witnessing first-hand her mother's struggles and the close bond she had with me as her physician, this young lady asked to shadow me for one day on my rheumatology hospital rounds. A few years later as a college student, she asked to work in my research lab and ultimately completed medical school and then a residency and fellowship in pediatric rheumatology. I am proud to note that she now leads a vibrant pediatric rheumatology division, and I regard her as my "second daughter" (my own daughter, Kate, is a med-peds rheumatologist). The child of another severely ill patient with scleroderma led her sorority sisters to volunteer and raise awareness in a 10K walk for the Scleroderma Foundation. She (my "third daughter") is completing her medicine residency with plans to pursue fellowship training in rheumatology. Building meaningful relationships based on compassion, understanding, empathy, and trust with patients and families requires the precious gift of time and is dwarfed by the reward and fulfillment that follow.

Osler famously turned to literature, poetry, and the Bible as sources for understanding each patient as a human being. To keep myself grounded in the day-to-day world of patients and research, I developed an interest in art and literature with a particular focus on the rheumatic diseases. This provides insight into and empathy for the life experiences of my patients. It has fostered meaningful long-term relationships with my patients, one of the intrinsic motivating factors associated with physician well-being [17] and one that is threatened by "the 15-minute visit." Herein lies my joyful satisfaction in the practice of medicine, thus staving off burnout and, for the time being, averting the prospect of fading away.

A young patient whom I met during the second year of my rheumatology fellowship, Amy, suffered from lupus and its many complications including neuropsychiatric disease. At one of her clinic visits, Amy presented me with a copy of the recently published book, *The Habit of Being: Letters of Flannery O'Connor*, thus sparking my interest in the Southern Gothic author whose life was cut short tragically by systemic lupus erythematosus. O'Connor wrote, "The name of my dread disease is Lupus Erythematosus, or as we literary people prefer to call it, 'Red Wolf' " [18]. To this day, more than 40 years since I met Amy, when caring for a patient suffering from lupus and struggling with the fear and anxiety of the disease, I am reminded of O'Connor's expressive words, "The wolf, I'm afraid, is inside tearing up the place" [19].

Another literary source that shapes the way I relate to patients, in this case patients with scleroderma, comes from the Greek tragedy of Tithonus, a story that Osler alludes to in the introduction to his case series on scleroderma [20]:

> In its more aggravated form diffuse scleroderma is one of the most terrible of all human ills. Like Tithonus, to "wither slowly," and like him to be "beaten down and marred and wasted" until one is literally a mummy, encased in an ever-shrinking, slowly contracting skin of steel, is a fate not pictured in any tragedy, ancient or modern.

These words remind me that, beyond the skin score and the particular serum autoantibody, there sits before me a person whose life has been forever changed. Thankfully, outcomes for scleroderma are usually not as desperate as in Osler's time, but the myth of Tithonus recalls the toll—physical, psychological, and emotional—that a disease like scleroderma imparts on the patient and family. The story of Tithonus prompts me to address the patient's emotional suffering, not just the physical disease manifestations, and to consider the impact of the disease on the whole family.

The art world also provides insights into the rheumatic diseases and the impact disease may have on the artist as patient. This, in turn, translates to the patient I am caring for in my practice. Renoir is undoubtedly the most famous of all artists to have suffered from a rheumatic disease, i.e., rheumatoid arthritis. When the younger Matisse visited and asked why Renoir still painted when it was obvious just how much pain he suffered, Renoir replied, "*la douleur passe, la beaute reste* [pain passes, the beauty remains]." I am reminded of Susan, a dear friend and patient, who has endured arthritis for more than 50 years, yet still finds the will to paint nearly every day. A gift of one of her paintings (*Have No Fear!*) hangs on a wall outside my office where it serves as a daily reminder of the triumph of the creative will over the debilitating toll that disease can take on the human body (Figure 13.3). Many other patients have shared their art over the course of time; in each instance, the expressions contained in their art open my eyes to provide a glimpse into their world. Ansley, who was diagnosed with scleroderma when she was only ten years of age, proudly presented a drawing of a snowman notable for the blue hands that likely are a depiction of her own cold-induced Raynaud phenomenon. Now approaching graduation from college, Ansley's drawing still hangs in my office, some 12 years later. It serves as a reminder of how a serious disease is expressed in a child's innocence, while also reminding me of the beauty of a long-term doctor–patient relationship (Figure 13.4).

And then there is Paul Klee, the Swiss-German artist who suffered and died from complications of scleroderma. By delving into Klee's disease and the impact that scleroderma had on his life and art, I have gained an appreciation for the artist's suffering, as well as for the triumph of the creative will over the misfortunes of life [21]. Painted when death was inevitable, *Gefangen (Captive)* portrays a frowning face

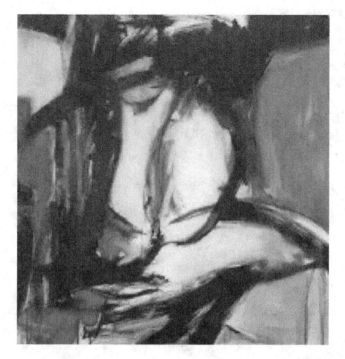

Figure 13.3 *Have No Fear!* (S. Altman, b. 1944; oil on canvas). (Reprinted with permission of the artist.)

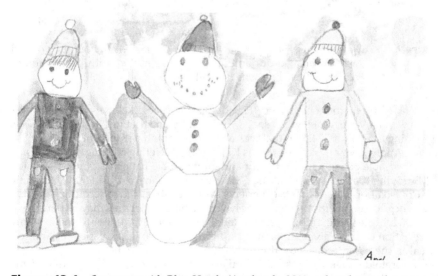

Figure 13.4 *Snowman with Blue Hands* (Ansley, b. 2011; colored pencil on paper). (Reprinted with permission of the artist.)

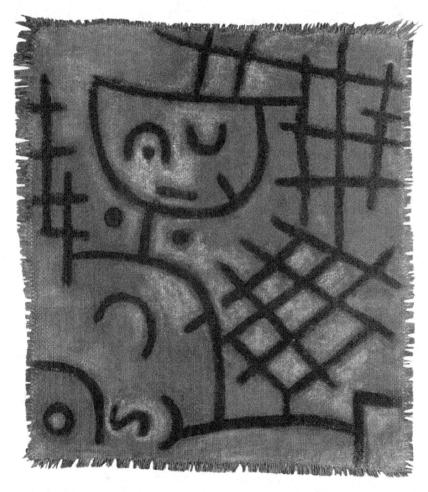

Figure 13.5 *Ohne Titel* (*Gefangen*) (c. 1940. Paul Klee [1879–1940]; oil and colored paste on primed burlap on burlap.) (Reprinted with permission of Fondation Beyeler, Riehen/Basel, Beyeler Collection.)

with a teardrop surrounded by bars (Figure 13.5). The bars likely represent the physical as well as the psychological, social, and political restrictions endured by Klee, expressing a sense of isolation that was not just geographic (Klee was forced to flee Nazi Germany), but physical as well; as Klee stated, "a feeling of being on the outside as an incurable patient; an immigrant and an incurable patient is doubly isolated" [21]. Studying Klee's art and recalling *Gefangen* prompts me to consider the lonesome sense of isolation some patients experience, as if a captive, and to recognize that my care may hopefully help the patient see beyond whatever barriers may be perceived.

Viewing literature and art from a medical perspective serves to increase my appreciation of the individual patient's suffering. Interest in the patient as an individual is the essence of medical humanity, an essential quality of the physician. Just as foretold by Dr. Peabody [12], deep and enduring relationships with patients have provided me with enormous satisfaction, serving as my touchstone and as an antidote to professional burnout. As stated by Dr. George Thibault, "Each of us has our own touchstone for humanism—an experience, a role model, an inspirational writing. It is time for each of us to draw on that touchstone and make it more real in our daily lives. Let it inform every encounter with a patient, let it inform the work within each health system to make it more humanistic" [1].

ACKNOWLEDGMENTS

The author gratefully acknowledges the insightful review and comments by Dr. Nortin Hadler, Dr. Charles Bryan, and Dr. Murray Passo—mentors, colleagues, and friends.

REFERENCES

1. Thibault GE. Humanism in medicine: What does it mean and why is it more important than ever? *Acad Med*. 2019;94(8):1074–1077.
2. Ghamei SN. In the Tradition of William Osler: A New Biohumanistic Model of Psychiatry. *Perspect Biol Med* 2023;66:520–534.
3. Osler W Sir. *Aequanimitas: With Other Addresses to Medical Students, Nurses and Practitioners of Medicine*. Philadelphia, PA: P. Blakiston, 1943.
4. Bryan CS. Aequanimitas redux. William Osler on detached concern versus humanistic empathy. *Perspect Biol Med* 2006;49:384–392.
5. Weissmann G. Against *Aequanimitas*. In *The Woods Hole Cantata. Essays on Science and Society*. New York, NY: Dodd, Mead & Company, 1985: 211–222.
6. Bryan CS, ed. *Sir William Osler: An Encyclopedia*. Novato, CA: Norman Publishing in Association with the American Osler Society, 2020.
7. Berwick DM. *Salve lucrum*: The existential threat of greed in US health care. *JAMA* 2023;329(8):629–630.
8. Knopfler M. Boom like that. Available from: https://en.wikipedia.org/wiki/Boom,_Like_That
9. Seetharam S, Gunderman R. The importance of face-to-face encounters in medical education. *Pharos* 2022:12–15.
10. Young N. My, my, hey hey (out of the blue). Available from: https://en.wikipedia.org/wiki/My_My,_Hey_Hey_(Out_of_the_Blue)
11. Available from: www.cdc.gov/vitalsigns/health-worker-mental-health/index.html
12. McGoldrick J, Molina-Ochoa D, Edwards ST, Barton JL. An evaluation of burnout among US rheumatology fellows: A national survey. *J Rheumatol* 2023;50:1185–1190.
13. Hadler N. American medicine's toxic workplace. *The Health Care Blog*. October 10, 2016.
14. Hadler NM. *By the Bedside of the Patient: Lessons for the Twenty-First-Century Physician*. Chapel Hill, NC: The University of North Carolina Press, 2016.
15. Peabody F. The care of the patient. *JAMA* 1927;88(12):877–882.
16. Sergent JS. It's the patient, stupid! *Arthritis Rheum* 1994;37(4):449–453.
17. Tak HJ, Curlin FA, Yoon JD. Association of intrinsic motivating factors and markers of physician well-being: A national physician survey. *J Gen Intern Med* 2017;32(7):739–746.
18. Silver KC and Silver RM. Peacocks and the red wolf. *Pharos* 2019:27–32.
19. Fitzgerald S, ed. *Letters of Flannery O'Connor. The Habit of Being*. New York, NY: Farrar, Strauss and Giroux, 1979.
20. Osler W. On diffuse scleroderma; with special reference to diagnosis, and to the use of the thyroid gland extract. *J Cutan Genito-Urin Dis* 1898:1–26.
21. Silver RM. Captive of art, not disease. Paul Klee and his disease, scleroderma. *Pharos* 2008:17–24.

14 Bach on the Hudson, or the Transformative Creativity of Attention

Rita Charon

> To reach an understanding in a dialogue is not merely a matter of putting oneself forward and successfully asserting one's own point of view, but being trans-formed into a communion in which we do not remain what we were.
>
> Hans-Georg Gadamer, *Truth and Method*

> there was all around not the shapes of things but oh, at last, the things themselves.
>
> Lucille Clifton, *The Death of Fred Clifton*

A MUSICAL PRELUDE

Months into my project to learn to play Bach's *Art of the Fugue*, I tackled *Contrapuntus VI*. I could not get beyond the third measure. I could read the notes. I could play the notes. I could get my left hand to play the first two measures and my right hand to play the second and third measures, but I could not put them together. Only once I took in the marks on the page as not signifying particular piano keys but as spatial and temporal patterns did I realize that the left hand takes twice as long to play the melodic theme as the right hand does. The right hand impetuously interrupts the left hand midway in the first declaration of the theme and plays it again but at double time, allowing the hands to end the third measure in unison. My piano teacher smiles as I tell him my discovery, saying softly, "This is Bach's wit."

ATTENTION IN MEDICINE AND THE ARTS

I have learned, both as a primary care internist and as a literary scholar, to pay attention. I derive pleasure in lending sharp, sustained awareness to the entity in my attention's spotlight, paying attention to landscapes, to asymmetrical pupils, to works of art, or to worlds of words. As all primary care doctors do, I allow my diagnostic mind to register a patient's shifting tone of voice, to treat incomplete sentences as subplots, and to bookmark references to things outside the health matter at hand as worthy of exploration. As a close reader, I keep track of my text's formal characteristics like metaphors and temporal shifts while not excluding from consciousness my own memories and associations activated by the reading. We all—in medicine, in the arts, and beyond—let things strike us, worry us, surprise us, and awaken us.

Scholars and investigators in fields from philosophy to the neurosciences are urgently investigating how individuals attain states of attention and why these states matter [1]. Is attention pleasure-seeking? Does it uphold cognitive or decision-making functions? Does it zero in on what needs to be done next? No consensus reigns even in foundational issues. Is consciousness necessary for attention or not? Beyond transactional or operational dimensions of attention, some scholars realize that attention illuminates ontological and phenomenological dimensions of the self, providing introspective and embodied insight as well as focusing attention on external worlds [2, 3].

                                        DOI: 10.1201/9781003409373-14

Over the years, I've realized that my doctor self and my reader self are doing the same things. The state of attention—not an ordinary, curious glance but a committed, everything-else-banished-from-mind concentration—unifies medicine and reading as countries on the same continent. Studying narrative theory and modernist fiction in graduate school triggered major changes in my clinical practice. I'd roll my chair away from the computer, stop writing, hold my hands in my lap, and invite new patients to tell me what they thought I as their new doctor should know about them. I'd listen with as wide open an ear as I could find in that cramped, Upper Manhattan clinic office, letting things register on me as the things themselves. This practice granted me surprises that would not have emerged from taking a traditional HPI and ROS. The range of subject and affect astounded me: rage at former doctors, unspent grief over decades-ago deaths, loss of a former home and language, pride at professional achievements despite failing health, exquisitely remembered dreams from childhood. Even if these details did not always inform my diagnostic or therapeutic interventions, the process itself of eliciting and paying attention to these accounts contributed to a clinical relationship that, from the start, was mutually created.

From these experiences in my practice, I started to wonder if close readers make good doctors. I wondered if teaching doctors how to read could improve their reading and their doctoring or, on the other hand, if good doctors make close readers. In medical education, we train students in how to interview patients for a medical history, how to discuss health habits with motivational interviewing techniques, and how to address patients' former life experiences in trauma-related care. Although each of these kinds of interviewing is done with specific goals in mind, the skill underlying them all is to pay attention to what their patients tell them. Clinicians can't know in the moment what will be important to the care of that patient. If they could nurture the kind of attention a close reader pays to a text, they might be able to notice and not discard things that patients say about their illnesses that might seem tangential or distracting at the moment but that turn out to be pivotal. Such skills might make the elusive "patient-centered care" more achievable in practice.

Early work in the field my colleagues and I called narrative medicine led to proposals that teaching clinical learners how to pay attention to written texts and visual images might expand their bank of attention. Whether or not the text or image deals with health or illness, the learning goals are reached through the awakening of close attention itself [4, 5]. Evidence to support these proposals accrued from studies of interprofessional teamwork in clinical settings and writing workshops for groups of patients and/or medical students [6–9]. We were learning that clinicians who are trained to pay attention to creative works grow in their capacity to pay attention to their patients' and colleagues' situations.

Attention has become a central element of our concepts of narrative medicine. The triad of Attention, Representation, and Affiliation emerged as a touchstone of our work and continues to guide new discoveries today [10]. Attention describes the donation of a listener's full concentration to a teller and their tale. Representation happens when someone pays attention to something and then captures it with words or image or movement. Affiliation connects teller and listener once attention and representation have occurred. Not static or turn-taking, the three simultaneous movements are dynamic and nonlinear, feeding one another throughout a narrative practice. These three movements intersect and expand one another and can result in what philosopher Hans-Georg Gadamer describes in the epigraph as communion—a mutual transformation of teller and listener, reader and writer, and perhaps patient and clinician.

Theorists and practitioners from both aesthetic and epistemological fields are acutely interested in the states of attention that nourish representation and that contribute to both creativity and thought [11]. Through acts of representation, the one who pays attention confers form on the phenomenon witnessed. The form could be a sonnet, a painting, a hypothesis, or an idea. It could be a note in a medical chart or a mathematical equation. Only once represented can that phenomenon be visible to the witness and shared with others. What did Van Gogh see in the night sky before creating his *Starry Night*? What did James Baldwin experience as a teenager in Greenwich Village's Calypso Café that he transformed into the final scene of his short story "Sonny's Blues"? This is, essentially, creativity's central question.

FLAWED EXPERIMENT IN ATTENTION

Around the time I was trying to play *Contrapuntus VI*, I was teaching *Let Us Now Praise Famous Men*, James Agee and Walker Evans's poetic/photographic record of Depression-era tenant farmer families in Alabama. In his previous book about the death of his father, *A Death in the Family*, Agee had displayed his heightened powers of attention to time, place, mood, and multiple conflicting points of view. He brought even more dramatic powers of attention to the study of tenant farmers. Here, he describes what happens when he is called to attention:

> This lucky situation of joy, this at least illusion of personal wholeness or integrity, can overcome one suddenly by any one of a number of unpredictable chances: the fracture of sunlight on the façade and traffic of a street; the sleaving up of chimneysmoke; the rich lifting of the voice of a train along the darkness [that stand as] strong argument[s] in favor of art which proves and asserts nothing but which exists . . . . I will be trying here to write of nothing whatever which did not in physical actuality or in the mind happen or appear; and my most serious effort will be, not to use these "materials" for art, far less for journalism, but *to give them as they were and as in my memory and regard they are* [12].

I understood Agee to be trying for that undiluted acknowledgment of a phenomenon free from preconceived meanings and independent from any interpretive formulation that later may be imposed on it. He describes his sensory experiences in seeing the sun illuminate the buildings and cars in town, noticing how smoke rises from a chimney in layers like threads of silk loosely bound, and hearing the rising Doppler pitch of an approaching train. These transient sensory experiences bring him "lucky" joy, helping me to understand one component of what I am calling attention.

I hope all of you have experienced the grace of being transfixed by an orchestral performance of a beloved composition or feeling gifted by seeing the full moon set of a dawning day. I hope you find yourselves "beside yourself" in these states where—as if by luck—you've been invited to appreciate what might be seen as mundane but is illuminated by your own capacity to behold it. I also hope that you can see that this occurs in our professional lives in medicine. Think of the sense of grandeur glimpsed in the family who brings the grandmother with dementia into their tiny Washington Heights apartment, despite the sacrifices her care will pose. Recall the sense of tragedy and heroism when a young patient diagnosed with ALS finds the means to accept and live up to such a sentence. Beyond our medical practices, the wonder can suddenly illuminate our lives as we move through our ordinary days, making transcendent a moment that could have been overlooked.

I took Agee's maxims as a challenge: what would happen if I tried to see a complex scene and represented only what occurred "in physical actuality or in the mind"? My experiment took me to lower Manhattan's Pier 46 on the banks of the Hudson River. I vowed to sit in the sun from low tide to high tide and type what I took in through my senses, doing my best to not ascribe abstract meaning to what I saw, heard, or felt. The idea was to get practice in seeing, in not letting things escape my view, in alertness, in the belief that one can find language in which to represent perceptions, and in the lifelong commitment to not let things pass me by unattended.

Here are some of the paragraphs from that morning:

The surface of the water moves in small and localized ridges that you might call ripples. It does not appear that the water moves but that its surface wrinkles as eyes squinting into the sun or a mouth smiling. Or like ocean waves where the water stands still but the impulse of the wave itself travels through the stationary water.

Stanchions sunk in the river are disappearing under the water! This one is almost submerged entirely, and I bet the others here will shorten in my view of them as the morning proceeds.

As the morning ripens, the river shows off. I see a person standing on a water board paddling with one long oar. Tall, strong-looking, oaring her way up the river, silently. Then right to the west of her comes a speedboat, spewing wake churning, but it doesn't pull her off course. They share the river, one noisy, one noiseless.

I see another group of stanchions in the process of drowning—perhaps remnants of a demolished pier which, come to think of it, must explain what my drowning stanchions are.

The New Jersey banks feature an undulating silhouette. Tall new-looking steel and glass towers of Jersey City appear to be near the Statue of Liberty and Ellis Island.

Then the skyline graph settles downward punctuated by a tall clock-and-bell tower immediately to my west. It may be connected to the startling aqueduct-like low dark-colored bridge with six bays and the word LACKAWANNA in emphatic caps. Could it be the train station? This, I think, is Hoboken.

After Hoboken, the skyline graph dips down again and the building heights shorten and the greenery announces itself to abruptly become the Palisades. It is like the eruption of the Canadian Rockies from the CP trans-continental railroad window on a small scale. As far as I can see, the banks get greener as you travel north.

Meanwhile, my stanchions are fast disappearing. At 10:00 exactly, I count only 69.

REPRESENTATION, PERCEPTION, AND INTERPRETATION

I realized only in retrospect that my experiment was poorly constructed. What my record of the morning supplied was *not* what I saw but what I represented of what I saw. It was in the representation of the scene that I *theorized* during my hours at the Hudson. Acting in turns like a scientist and a literary scholar, I was meeting unusual phenomena with either problem-solving deductive strategies or with allu-sive connections to other artworks or views. Could the aqueduct-like structure spot-ted across the river be a structural part of a railroad station, and wasn't there a Lackawanna train station in Jersey? At the same time, my literary brain was amused by the word "Lackawanna" itself—I laughed to think what Jacques Lacan would make of the funny word, a combination of *lack* and *want*, two seminal terms in Lacanian post-Freudian psychoanalysis theory.

Paying attention to my scene *and* representing what I saw and thought and felt constituted acts of interpretation. Together, my attention and my representation opened the gates of my mind's cognitive and creative wanderings. Aesthetic and cognitive theorists agree that interpretation accompanies perception: the perceiver selects, catalogues, seeks clues about the message's meanings, invents links in chains of signification, and stamps the perceived with a personal view [13]. In the same way and roughly in the same time period that attention grabbed headlines and propelled scholarly work, interpretation has become a contemporary item of heightened pur-chase. Philosopher Jean Michel's recently published encyclopedic study called *Homo Interpretans* marshals evidence and ideas from hermeneutics (philosophy's study of interpretation), anthropology, history, psychology, and neuroscience to assert that things perceived are always already shaped by their contexts and the viewer's own experience and ways of making sense of the world [14]. When automatic under-standing fails, interpretation steps in to adjudicate the trouble, calling forth prior experience and experimenting with alternative explanations to assist in decoding hard-to-understand phenomena [15]. Not only in the brain but throughout the body and into the social context do perception and interpretation occur [16].

Like narrative medicine's attention and representation, perception, and inter-pretation share a bloodstream. In the magisterial *An Introduction to the Study of Experimental Medicine*, pioneer physiologist Claude Bernard described the sequence of idea, hypothesis, and experiment: "Feelings gives rise to the experimental idea or hypothesis, *i.e.,* the previsioned interpretation of natural phenomena. The whole experimental enterprise comes from the idea, for this it is which induces experiment. Reason or reasoning serves only to deduce the consequences of this idea and to sub-mit them to experiment" [17]. Even Bernard—discoverer of the vasomotor nerves and the function of the pancreas in digestion—traced scientific breakthroughs to feelings and not findings.

Although for Bernard, interpretation may equal hypothesis, in the world beyond the laboratory, interpretation may also emerge as creative forms, metaphor, and performance. The poet exposes a perception with a haiku. The visual artist broadcasts a concept with abstract photography. The performance artist enacts a message through drama. The tectonic plates of natural creation push mountains into view. The reader, listener, or viewer approaches a creative interpretation to grasp what it might connote and to experience a personal response to the work. In a confounding and productive sense, the receiver of the creative work performs the reverse of the action it took the author or artist or natural world to create it.

AGEE IN THE CLINIC

During the weeks following my morning on the Hudson, I brought Agee's paragraph about the lucky situation of joy to two groups of clinicians—general pediatricians and clinicians on the adult palliative care service. I hold an hour-long narrative medicine teaching session on Zoom once or twice a month for these two groups. Five people attended the pediatrics class, and around 18 attended the palliative care session.

In each session, two participants in turn read Agee's paragraph aloud. We then talked about the dense text. In both cases, we understood Agee's "lucky situation of joy" as the state of being transported by viewing something that at first seems ordinary but that, with attention, becomes extraordinary. One called it a "jolt of dopamine." Others used words like transcendent, magical, focusing on beauty in chaos, and sudden awe.

After about 20 minutes of conversation about the text, I gave the groups a writing prompt, identical in both groups: "Write about a lucky situation of joy" and set my timer at 5 minutes. At the close of the writing period, I asked the groups where their writing took them. One pediatrician wrote about meeting a school classmate whom she had not seen in 40 years. His account of life in the wilderness near the Arctic Circle, worlds away from her New York wilderness, dazzled her. Another went straight to her pediatric practice, seeing a depressed patient. This physician slowed down her initially upbeat interview to meet the patient where she was, letting herself be taken into the patient's painful presence. A chaplain recognized both warmth and what he called "fraught joy" in his work with seriously ill children and with an ill member of his own family. Hearing these fragments read aloud let the rest of the participants share emotionally in the authors' own joy, however fraught, while feeling personally lucky to have heard them.

One of the palliative care doctors described a night shift in the Emergency Room where, in the midst of chaotic hyperactivity, he finds himself riveted by the view of an elderly woman on a stretcher and the tenderness of the woman's son in trying to find her some comfort. Another physician described a mountain hike in a foreboding winter storm. After the dark gray clouds parted, suddenly the blue sky appeared, and sunshine bathed the now crystalline landscape. A new member of the service wrote about a hard day caring for a very sick patient. She wrote two haikus, which she read for us. One was an interior physical description of her awareness of her body, her own breathing, and her mind. The second haiku moved from self-awareness to take in the sun hitting the trees, winter branches greeted by the light, the warmth despite the cold. The next reader read aloud a description of a scene in her apartment house's laundry room, noticing a stranger's laundry languishing in a dryer until the owner shows up to claim her clothes with a newborn baby on her shoulder. The story ends with their making a tea date and a promise of a growing friendship.

Each of these representations started with the words and concepts of Agee. This is what my participants *paid attention to*. As they each wrote in the shadow of Agee's paragraph, they found their own path toward its meaning for themselves.

They created for themselves what the paragraph of Agee described. Not expository essays, the stories and poems expressed in both form and content the authors' own connections to other persons and to the natural world. Listeners in both groups took pains to recognize what the author did with words, commenting on formal elements of the writing like temporal shifts, metaphors used, or inserted dialogue in addition to expressing gratitude to the author for having shared it.

Our hours together achieved several dividends. These stressed clinicians slowed down, paid attention to a complex description of an equally complex experience, and reflected on charged moments in their own lives. First, they sorted out together what Agee might be getting at and reached a shared awareness of the transcendence and sudden awe of these lucky moments of attention. It turned out that many present had *had* such moments but had perhaps not realized their luck in them. By capturing such personal moments in language, authors were able to fully perceive them, hail them, and acknowledge their value. The transformation for the group culminated when individuals read aloud their situations of joy, both appreciating what they themselves experienced and hearing the appreciation of their colleagues. Sharing these quickly written accounts expanded participants' views of one another's interior states. Unlike reflective writing exercises triggered by general prompts, the sequence of paying attention together to a complex work, struggling as a group to find its meaning, and then responding to colleagues' writing as creative work exceeded wellness/resilience practice to mark the session as rigorous aesthetic training, self-inquiry, team building, and collective dedication to their shared clinical task.

ATTENTION, REPRESENTATION, PERCEPTION, AND INTERPRETATION ENTWINED

I have sketched out two conceptual relationships that seem to travel in tandem: narrative medicine's relationship between attention and representation and hermeneutic theory's relationship between perception and interpretation. Although one emerged as a concept within medical practice and the other arose from philosophical analysis, they both attest to the coupling of sensing and making. They are aphorisms, if you will, about transforming what one absorbs from one's surround into a formative idea or creation.

In narrative medicine, representing one's experience for self and others *constitutes* the experience. Especially when shared with others, the words pop the experience into being. As countless writers attest, "I write to know what I think." Representation activates and manifests the ideas. Attention reaches its conclusion in representation. Without representation, attention is squandered. Without attention, there is nothing to represent. This is why clinicians write chart notes after they interact with a patient. This is why such presumed time-savers as third-party scribes and automatically transcribed voice recordings of medical encounters may seriously impair health care processes. Our writing exposes the impressions, the cautions, the ambiguities while it nails what can be said to be known about the clinical situation.

The hermeneuticists and their colleagues in psychology and neuroscience move in like manner from what is perceived to be an interpretation of that perception. They take into account the legion of influences that season what one absorbs in one's initial acts of perception, dismissing the naïve view that one can perceive anything unencumbered by opinions and experiences and biases. The medical and the hermeneutic relationships constitute parallel although distinct formulations. Not identical, the two pairs echo one another's conceptual currents. I hazard an analogy:

attention : representation :: perception : interpretation

The analogy points to structural commonalities of the pairs. Each pair aligns a sensory condition with a concept-seeking process and suggests the actions of the agent (attender, perceiver, representer, interpreter) in the scene. The first terms of the pairs, attention and perception, denote the agent's taking notice of something. The second terms, representation and interpretation, signify the creative or conceptual actions that the agent uses to incarnate impressions into words, forms, or ideas. In both cases, the process evolves from a confrontation with an unknown through a practiced method to distill the form or idea from the experience, be it with creative activity or mental activity.

The analogy clarifies what narrative medicine's attention and representation may accomplish. Perhaps this framework gives medicine tools to marshal our cognitive and affective tasks in practice. Clinicians skilled in representing both clinical data and personal introspection can harvest from the many channels of knowledge triggered during clinical experiences. Recall that the third movement of narrative medicine is "affiliation." Narrative capacities and routines equip us to fulfill our prime calling—to ally with patients in helping them to reach their goals.

CODA

Bach's *Contrapuntus VI* not only awakened me with its zany temporal joke. It also reminds me and, I hope, you of the contrapuntal nature of clinical work and aesthetic work. Multiple themes interweave, are performed in different voices, take turns, change keys, collide, and ultimately point to some layered meanings.

Clinical practice has become the locus for revolutionary experiments in bioscientific and societal exploration. Less heralded perhaps but equally foundational, clinical practice has become the crucible for creative discoveries.

I hope that this short foray into narrative medicine's principles and practices illuminates the potential for physicians' work to achieve goals beyond the diagnosis and management of patients' illnesses and collective care for the public's health. We know that the work we do in medicine comments not only on an individual patient's or community's illness but considers the human predicaments of temporariness, embodiment, and a ceaseless capacity for pleasure and suffering. We are schooled in these aspects of life through our intimate brushes with mortality, frailty, generativity, and growth. Powerful secrets are revealed to us as rewards for the hard work we do. We come to know the fraught joy of living a life.

ACKNOWLEDGMENTS

My deep gratitude to my colleagues in the Division of Narrative Medicine at Columbia who together have developed narrative medicine's principles and practices. I thank the participants of the narrative medicine teaching sessions described in this chapter. Those whose writing is reported have read my description of the teaching sessions in which they participated and have given me permission to publish this anonymized description of their work.

REFERENCES

1. Wu, Wayne. *Attention*. New York, NY: Routledge, 2014.
2. Weil, Simone. *Waiting for God*. Emma Craufurd, trans. New York, NY: Perennial Classics, 2001.
3. D'Angelo, Diego. The phenomenology of embodied attention. *Phenomenology and the Cognitive Sciences*, 2020:19:961–978. DOI: 10.1007/s11097-019-09637-2
4. Charon, Rita. Knowing, seeing, and telling in medicine. *The Lancet*, 2021:398:2068–2070.
5. Charon, Rita, Sayantani DasGupta, Nellie Hermann, Craig Irvine, Eric R. Marcus, Edgar Rivera-Colón, Danielle Spencer, and Maura Spiegel. *The Principles and Practice of Narrative Medicine*. New York, NY: Oxford University Press, 2017.

6. Sands, Stephen, Patricia Stanley, and Rita Charon. Pediatric narrative oncology: interprofessional training to promote empathy, build teams, and prevent burnout. *Journal of Supportive Oncology*, 2008:6:307–312.

7. Gowda, Deepthiman, Tayla Curran, Apurva Khedagi, Michael Mangold, Faiz Jiwani, Urmi Desai, Rita Charon, and Dorene Balmer. Implementing an interprofessional narrative medicine program in academic clinics: feasibility and program evaluation. *Perspectives in Medical Education*, 2019:8:52–59.

8. Rivlin, Katherine and Carolyn L. Westhoff. Navigating uncertainty: narrative medicine in pregnancy options counseling education. *Patient Education and Counseling*, 2019:102(3):536–541.

9. Chou, Jonathan C, Ianthe Schepel, Anne T. Vo, Suad Kapetanovic, and Pamela B. Schaff. Patient co-participation in narrative medicine curricula as a means of engaging patients as partners in healthcare: a pilot study involving medical students and patients living with HIV. *Journal of Medical Humanities*, 2021:42(4):641–657. DOI: 10.1007/s10912-019-09604-7

10. Lanphier, Elizabeth. Narrative and medicine: premises, practices, pragmatism. *Perspectives in Biology and Medicine*, 2021:64(2):211–234.

11. Otis, Laura. *Rethinking Thought: Inside the Minds of Creative Scientists and Artists*. New York, NY: Oxford, 2015.

12. Agee, James and Walker Evans. *Let Us Now Praise Famous Men*. Boston, MA: Houghton Mifflin Company, 1941/1960: 227, 231, 242.

13. Gombrich, EH. *Art and Illusion: A Study in the Psychology of Pictorial Representation, 11th Printing, with New Preface*. Princeton, NJ: Princeton University Press, 2000.

14. Michel, Johan. *Homo Interpretans*. New York, NY: Routledge, 2019.

15. Wittgenstein, Ludwig. *Philosophical Investigations*, 4th revised ed. GEM Anscombe, PMS Hacker, and J Schulte, trans. Oxford: Wiley-Blackwell, 1953/2009.

16. Johnson, Mark. The aesthetics of embodied life. In: Scarzini A, ed. *Aesthetics and the Embodied Mind*. Dordrecht: Springer-Science, 2015: 23–38.

17. Bernard, Claude. *An Introduction to the Study of Experimental Medicine*. New York, NY: Dover Publications, 1865/1957: 32.

15 Partnering with Patients

David B. Hellmann

INTRODUCTION

During my first year of medical residency training in 1977, a middle-aged man presented to our emergency department with symptoms and signs of an enigmatic, multisystem illness. All the physicians initially involved in evaluating him were completely stumped by his presentation. Then, a senior resident arrived and asked the patient one question: "What do you think you have?" Everyone nearly fell over when the patient confidently replied, "I think I have coccidiomycosis." And the evaluation proved him right! None of the residents working in my hospital located in Baltimore, Maryland, had ever seen a patient with this fungal infection, and none expected to encounter it: coccidiomycosis affects chiefly people who live in Arizona and southern California where the spore is found in the desert sand. What the initial evaluators had not appreciated is that, although the patient lived in Baltimore, he worked as an interstate truck driver and had recently driven through southern California desert soon after earthquakes had struck and had generated clouds of dust filled with fungal elements that seeded the patient's respiratory tract and ultimately caused his enigmatic (to us) systemic illness. At truck stops on the route back to Baltimore, the patient read bulletins about multiple other truckers who had developed "Valley Fever" (coccidiomycosis) after driving through California's San Joachim Valley, just as he had done.

The revelation that a doctor could team up with a patient to pull a diagnostic rabbit out of the hat immediately sold me on the value of partnering with my patients. What I only dimly perceived, 40-plus years ago, is that the rewards of partnering with patients would extend well beyond finding diagnostic gold and would influence every dimension of my relationship with patients. Aspiring to partner with my patients has helped me become a better healer and added immeasurable joy, satisfaction, meaning, and wonder to my professional life. When the truck driver said "I think I have coccidiomycosis," he not only nailed the diagnosis, but he also opened a hitherto hidden door for me and allowed me to explore what has turned out to be a magnificent medical castle of rich opportunities to develop partnerships with my patients. I will use this essay to offer a tour of the magnificent hallways and rooms in this medical castle. To illuminate the passageways, I begin by considering what a clinician does, then I will define the nature of partnering with patients. I will suggest how you can build medical castles of your own and describe some of the many benefits I have gleaned from partnering with my patients. I hope this tour will engender for you the same awe and wonder it has for me. Please come along.

WHAT DOES A PHYSICIAN DO?

When I was training in internal medicine at Johns Hopkins Hospital, the faculty member considered to be Osler incarnate was Dr. Philip Tumulty. He was renowned for his encyclopedic knowledge of medicine, charming personality, inexhaustible empathy for the suffering, and his distinguished visage adorned with thick white hair and ruddy complexion that seemed to come straight from central casting. Dr. Tumulty frequently reflected on what a clinician does, first in a classic paper, "What Is a Clinician and What Does He Do?," published in 1970 in the *New England Journal of Medicine* [1], and then in expanded fashion in a book, *The Effective Clinician* [2],

DOI: 10.1201/9781003409373-15

printed in 1977. In both publications Dr. Tumulty was quick to emphasize that the essence of being a clinician is neither diagnosis nor treatment. As Dr. Tumulty emphasized, some patients cannot be diagnosed, and some patients have an illness that has no known effective therapy. Dr. Tumulty therefore insisted that a "clinician is one whose prime function is to manage a sick person with the purpose of alleviating the total impact of his illness" [1]. The clinician, Dr. Tumulty argued, must care about the whole patient and the total impact of an illness on the patient, not just on diagnosis or treatment. Dr. Tumulty's definition of the clinician aligns well with Dr. Francis Peabody's famous observation published in *JAMA* in 1927 that "the secret of the care of the patient is in caring for the patient" [3].

PARTNERING WITH PATIENTS HAS MULTIPLE DIMENSIONS

As much as I revere the memory and teachings of Dr. Tumulty and as much as I admire his wholistic approach, I believe that the prime function of the physician is to **partner** with the patient to achieve the outcome the patient desires rather than to **manage** a sick person. I prefer the concept of "partnering" rather than "managing" for several reasons. First, "partnering" conveys that the patient is active in the process of healing and not passive. A mechanic may work on a car, a banker may manage your stock portfolio, but a physician works *with* a patient. Second, partnering also captures the mutual obligations and responsibilities of the patient and physician that managing omits. Mutual trust, respect [4], honesty, and belief in the dignity of each person, for example, are essential ingredients for success when a physician partners with a patient.

The notion of partnering is so important that it deserves further consideration. One dictionary defined "partner" as "a person who shares or is associated with another in some action or endeavor" [5]. Although partners exist in many spheres of life, including business, law, tennis, and love, the partnership between a physician and a patient requires some particular specifications. A key distinction is that doctors must always recognize that they are always the *junior* partners in this relationship with the patient. The junior status of the physician exists on two levels. First, the partnership focuses on the patient's goals, not those of the physician. Second, the physician is always the junior partner when it comes to knowing what medical care the patient wants. The doctor is not usually "junior" in terms of scientific knowledge but is always junior to the patient in terms of knowing how the patient wants to live. As much as the physician might try to understand the patient's perspective and desires, the patient is the ultimate arbiter of those decisions. Elsewhere in this book (Chapter 2), Dr. Ziegelstein writes eloquently about Personomics [6], the term he coined to describe the science of knowing the patient as a person. Great doctoring must be built on a foundation of Personomics in which the physician tries to know and understand the patient's hopes, fears, goals, barriers to care and avoids making assumptions about the patient's perspective [6, 7]. Yet, no matter how well a physician knows a patient, only the patient knows for certain what she wants; regarding choices about health care options, the patient is always the senior partner.

PARTNERING WITH PATIENTS: Checklist Not Applicable

Since each patient and physician is unique, the process of creating their partnership cannot be scripted. The physician, of course, must bring to the partnership all the virtues of the profession. While these professional qualities are essential, building the partnership with a patient resembles playing basketball or jazz in that success flows from improvisation—what should happen in one moment depends on what occurred in the previous moment. Still, my approach to partnering with patients is guided by several general guidelines.

When meeting the patient, the physician needs to be fully present. I find this both obvious and very difficult as in my typical day many things (e.g., emails, texts, phone calls, prescription refill requests, and alerts about scheduling snafus) compete for my attention. To stay focused on my patient, I have adopted the "practice of presence" advocated by Dr. Stephen McPhee, Professor of Medicine at the University of California, San Francisco, which is to use the time I spend washing my hands after entering the room to also "wash away" all other distractions. With clean hands and focused attention, I am ready to begin partnering with my patient.

When I have trainees with me, I will often ask patients to advise how best to care for them. A Wordle constructed from their responses would display "listen" in gigantic and bold font! Since studies have demonstrated that many physicians listen for less than 15 seconds before interrupting a patient, it is no wonder that patients urge doctors "to listen." After all, since the patient is not a witness on trial, the physician should not play opposing counsel demanding one-word answers! Patients plead: "let me tell my story."

In my experience, partnerships are most readily forged by a combination of listening and **caring curiosity**. I believe caring curiosity is the most effective approach to knowing the patient as a person, as detailed in the chapter on Personomics (Chapter 2).

Caring curiosity involves asking the patient open-ended questions. While the nature of the questions usually flows from the patient's medical history, some questions are so helpful that they may be routinely asked. What's most important to you? What gives you joy? How is life treating you? A pause after this question often encourages the patient to fill the silence with rich details about her true feelings. Many of my patients will initially respond "fine." But I have found that if I pause, maintain eye contact, keep my hands off my pen (or keyboard), then often the patient will expand and provide a much broader answer, one rich in the interpersonal concerns posed by her illness. The late Dr. Thomas Duffy at Yale taught me the utility of incorporating a question he found especially revealing: "Everyone is known for something in their family. Within your family, what are you known for?"

Depending on the patient's circumstances, other questions that can be prompted by caring curiosity are:

- "What most keeps you up at night?"

- "What's the biggest cause of aggravation in your life?" (This is a great question that was suggested to me by one of my patients/partners.)

- "If your spouse (partner, family member, or best friend) were here and heard our conversation, is there anything they would add about what's going on with you?" I have found this question especially helpful with patients whose stoicism or laconic style might otherwise camouflage the extent of their suffering.

- Tell me about where you grew up? (Dr. Katrina A. Armstrong, Dean of the Columbia University College of Physicians and Surgeons and a coauthor of Chapter 22 in this book, has credited one of her mentors from Johns Hopkins, Dr. Stephen Achuff, with teaching her how valuable this question is in getting to know the patient as a person.)

In pursuing caring curiosity, I often use metaphors. For example, I may explain to the patient that we have thermometers to measure temperature, and a sphygmomanometer to measure blood pressure, but we have no device to measure stress. I then hold up my pen and say, "but if this pen were a stressometer and it provided a reliable readout of stress from zero (for no stress) to 100 (the highest stress level imaginable), what level of stress would it register for you?" Their answers have often revealed important matters relating to their health that I had not detected earlier.

I almost always ask the patient what they think they have or might have and how they might have developed it. Many patients are right! Even when patients are not right, their answer can provide useful insights about their worries, which many times can be quickly dispelled—e.g., "No, your arthritis is not a sign that you have fatal ALS (amyotrophic lateral sclerosis)."

If a spouse, partner, other family member, or good friend has accompanied my patient into the exam room, I will, with the patient's permission secured first, ask that person if they have anything to add to what the patient has told me. This is an important and often overlooked step in building a partnership with the patient. Asking the opinion of a person chosen by the patient to accompany her to our appointment conveys respect for this person and acknowledges that person's importance in the life of my patient. And seeking the opinion of the friend or family member frequently adds important information about the patient's illness or adjustment to the illness.

While performing the physical examination, I will ask the patient if she has noticed any recent physical changes that were not mentioned during the history. As I examine the patient, I explain briefly what I am doing and why, e.g., "I am now looking at the back of the eye because that is the only way to see your arteritis without operating on you." An educated patient is a better partner and one who might be more likely to direct my attention to potentially important physical clues I had not noticed on my own.

When sharing my assessment and plans for additional testing or treatment, I again use simple metaphors to help explain the diagnosis and treatment—for example, "Vasculitis is like a fire in the body, and I'm trying to pick the right-sized medical fire hoses to put the fire out."

Before detailing the treatment options, I remind the patient that I work for her, that I am recommending treatments based on my knowledge of the disease and her preferences, but that I fully realize that only she knows what she wants, and, importantly, that she is the one who gets to decide. One of the most pernicious effects of illness is that it robs a person of the control she thought she had over her body. Reminding the patient that I work for her and that, ultimately, she gets to choose whether to accept my recommendations, helps restore the patient's sense of control and reminds both of us that she is the senior partner when it comes to treatment decisions. Asking if she has any questions allows me to clarify anything I have not adequately explained.

I believe an important step in strengthening our partnership is providing detailed information about how and when to contact me. I give each patient not only my office phone number and the mechanism to message me through the electronic medical record, but I also give each patient my cell phone number. I request that they call my cell phone in case of emergency, and it should not be used for routine prescriptions, appointments, or other questions. Knowing how to reach me if an emergency develops reduces her fear of the unexpected and conveys my dedication and commitment to our partnership to improve her health, as well as my commitment to journey with her through the vicissitudes of her illness and treatment.

REWARDS OF PARTNERING 1.0: Nailing Diagnoses, Improving Physical Exam

None of my patients have diagnosed coccidiomycosis, but several have partnered with me to make diagnoses I probably would not have made on my own. I offer several examples.

CPC (Not Snakes) on a Plane

About an hour into a flight from Baltimore to New Orleans, the flight attendant used the intercom to ask any physician to self-identify by pressing the call button. After doing so, I was escorted back about 20 rows where a pale, middle-aged man lay crumpled, face down in the aisle. After quickly determining he was breathing, had a pulse, and alert enough to at least mumble, and with the unforgettable experience of the truck driver just described, I asked, "What do you think is going on?" With a clear but soft voice the patient said, "I have adrenal insufficiency, and I think I have underdosed my hydrocortisone. I developed a bad cold yesterday and, in the rush to catch this flight I did not boost my morning dose of hydrocortisone as I typically would do. I also have not been drinking fluids. The combination probably explains why I just now nearly fainted." After obtaining and administering the hydrocortisone he had in his briefcase (along with several glasses of water), the patient's color, blood pressure, and seating arrangement were restored before the plane landed!

Taking the Unknown out of "Fever of Unknown Origin"

A man in his sixties was referred because he had fever of unknown origin (FUO) that had defied eight weeks of medical investigation. Appearing gaunt and tired, he was nonetheless friendly as he greeted me with the admonition that I was the 23rd physician to evaluate him. He seemed to offer this observation with a *soupçon* of hope and a larger dollop of resignation. After taking an extensive history, I started to share his resignation that I would join the long line of physicians flummoxed by his illness. As a last gasp effort, I asked him: "Is there anything you've noticed about yourself that doctors have not?" He looked at me quizzically for a moment, then pulled back the longish hair that covered his ears and said: "Yeah, why are both of my ears so red?" Reflexively, I exclaimed, "Eureka!"—the word derived from Greek meaning, "I found it." The patient had in an instant solved the mystery—he had a rare form of vasculitis known as relapsing polychondritis, about the only disease that can both cause FUO and inflame the cartilage of the ears. Inviting the patient to partner with me to solve the riddle of his disease secured for him a diagnosis (with effective treatment) and made me look better than I would have without his help.

REWARDS OF PARTNERING 2.0: The World Upside Down—Patient Teaches Doctor Physical Exam Skills

"Did you see it?" asked my patient after I had examined his nose? It was the first visit for this man who had been diagnosed previously with granulomatosis with polyangiitis (GPA), a form of vasculitis formerly known as Wegener's granulomatosis. "See what?" I asked. "The hole in my nose," he replied. Sheepishly, I admitted I had not visualized the perforation in his nasal septum, a common complication of chronic GPA. With the goodwill and confidence of a seasoned instruction, the patient explained that I was examining his nose all wrong. "Doc," he said, "you need to turn out all the lights in the room, shine the flashlight up one nostril, and then look up the other nostril to see the white light streaming across the hole." I followed his instructions and could then easily discern the white light coming through the small perforation from the pink light of the translucent septum where it was intact. Since that physical diagnosis class taught by my patient partner, I have used his technique many times to spot small and large nasal perforations and have passed on this useful maneuver to many of my trainees.

REWARDS OF PARTNERING 3.0: Patient Discovers New Marker for Monitoring Disease Activity

As a rheumatologist specializing in vasculitis, I have followed many patients with giant cell arteritis (GCA). One patient with this condition was an 80-year-old retired engineer who spent his professional career finding practical solutions to complicated mechanical problems. As he learned about the disease and my methods for monitoring his condition with, among other measures, the sedimentation rate (ESR, sed rate), he began doing what he had done all his professional life—he searched for simpler solutions for monitoring his disease. It dawned on him that his golf score might be a pretty good surrogate measure of the activity of his disease. When he had more symptoms of GCA and polymyalgia rheumatica, his golf score rose, and when he felt better, his golf score fell. He did a graphic comparison that showed that his golf score and ESR closely tracked each other! Together, the patient and I published his epiphany in a medical journal [7].

Although I usually do not coauthor papers with patients, I have learned a great deal about the impact of illness from other patient-partners. I often learn a lot when I ask patients to rate their disease activity on a scale of 0 (remission) to 10 (most active). After the patient responds, I ask them "why" or "how" they score their disease, or "what makes you rate it a 4/10?" That's when I learned that one patient assessed her disease activity by using her iPhone pedometer to measure how many steps she took when walking her dogs, and another patient judged her energy by the frequency and duration of afternoon naps. Medical training taught me how to monitor disease activity with laboratory tests; my patient-partners have taught me to identify and follow patient-discovered "sed rates" of their daily activities. Combining this information with the conventional tests has helped me better understand both the disease and the impact it has on the lives of my patients.

REWARDS OF PARTNERING 4.0: Patient Fills in Physician Knowledge Deficits

Despite all my training and my decades of medical practice, I am still regularly astounded to discover important deficits in my medical knowledge. For example, a patient I have followed for nearly 30 years for her vasculitis recently taught me how little I knew about trauma, including its frequency and how it can influence response to treatment. Although I thought I knew her well as a person, I was surprised when recently, for the first time, she revealed that her mother had disappeared for two years when the patient was four years old. The patient wanted me to know this because she had come to realize that her childhood trauma had played a large role in the difficulties she had trusting other people, including me and her other doctors. She had gained insight into all this when she recently listened to an audible version of the book, *What Happened to You?*, written and narrated by Oprah Winfrey and Bruce D. Perry, a neuroscientist at the University of Chicago, which explains how trauma can powerfully impact our response to much of life, including illness. Based on her recommendation, I too downloaded the book and found it an excellent primer on trauma. As a result, I have become more comfortable with asking other patients whether they have experienced trauma. Not surprisingly, I have been surprised at how frequently my patients have experienced trauma and how much that trauma has affected their interactions with the health care system. As a result of being able to detect and understand this side of my patients, I have become a more effective partner in promoting their whole-body health.

REWARDS OF PARTNERING 5.0: Patient Changes
Training of Medical Residents

On September 13, 2005, at 1 p.m., a patient encounter changed the way our program trains residents. At that exact time, I was conducting Chief Rounds, one of the twice-a-week sessions in which I, as Chair of the Department of Medicine, joined a handful of residents and medical students to evaluate a 70-year-old woman who had been admitted with a severe exacerbation of asthma. To my chagrin, the team did not know very much about her other than she had worked in an office. During our rounds we learned that she did not live in Baltimore (where our hospital is located) but in New York City. And to the team's great surprise, the office in which she had worked was one of the Twin Trade Towers. She was in the office on September 11, 2001, when the planes hit. What she had experienced as mild seasonal asthma prior to that date now, thanks to PTSD (posttraumatic stress disorder), worsened as each September 11 approached. In 2005, her asthma and PTSD had so worsened that she came to live with her daughter in Baltimore and was admitted to the hospital after failing outpatient therapies. In that instant on Chief Rounds, I realized that our training system had to change. The structure of our inpatient service was preventing our residents—extraordinarily talented individuals who had entered medicine to know their patients and make a difference in their lives—from knowing their patients as people and partnering with them. Thanks to the generous donations of a Greek philanthropist, Mrs. Aliki Perroti, and the creative work of multiple faculty, the Aliki Initiative redesigned our curriculum to imbue each student and resident with the importance of knowing their patients as people [8–14]. By many measures, the Aliki Initiative has been an enormous success and deeply satisfying to patients, students, residents, and faculty. One study showed that patients with heart failure admitted to the Aliki service were significantly less likely to require readmission after discharge [12]. The Aliki Initiative also received plaudits nationally for serving as an exemplary redesign of residency training that could allow residents to know their patients as people, an essential ingredient for partnering with patients [15]. The patient with asthma from New York City breathed new life into our residency training program.

REWARDS OF PARTNERING: It's about the Journey

Nearly 20 years ago, a young woman surprised me at our first meeting by saying: "I have something weird. I have gone to many different famous medical centers around the country. You are the 20th doctor I have seen. No one has figured out what I have. I don't think you will either. But I need someone to journey with me. Can you do that?" I was briefly flummoxed by her question. After thinking a few seconds more about Dr. Tumulty's teaching and reflecting on the loneliness often caused by disease, I took a deep breath, and said, "Yes. It would be my pleasure to journey with you." Lucky that I did, for journeying with this patient (and other patients) has been a great source of joy, wonder, and meaning. About seven years into the journey, thanks to other consultants, her condition was diagnosed as scleromyxedema—and responded to treatment! Along the journey I have had the great pleasure of getting to know many members of her family and friends. She partnered with me in giving Medical Grand Rounds at my hospital to educate others about her rare condition and the impact it has had on her life. My colleague at Johns Hopkins, the best-selling author, Pulitzer Prize finalist, and Professor of Psychiatry, Dr. Kay Redfield Jamison, prefers the word "accompany" rather than "journey" [16]. I'll take either. Both indicate that partnering with patients can sometimes involve being with, witnessing, encouraging, remaining curious, exploring, being available, and comforting the patient over years and decades. Doing so provides rewards that cannot be fully expressed, measured, or exceeded.

CHALLENGES OF PARTNERING

Partnering with patients enshrines the right of the patient to disagree with the treatment recommendations. While at first glance that can present challenges, I believe that on second look being explicit about the patient being the senior partner with respect to choosing treatment options makes it more likely that treatment disagreements can occur without rupturing the patient–doctor relationship. Indeed, I suspect that disagreements between patient and doctor about treatments are much more likely to induce apoptosis in the relationship if the patient does not feel free to disagree. This was brought home to me while I was caring for a patient with HIV/AIDS in 1983 when a precise diagnosis was elusive and effective treatment was nonexistent. Faced with a rapidly progressive and untreatable illness, one of my patients asked my opinion of the coffee enemas, one of the examples of quackery then being sold in a Mexican border town to young men dying rapidly from HIV/AIDS. I advised against it, but my desperate patient opted to try it. After failing to improve, the patient returned and asked me to resume caring for him until he died two months later. Recognizing his role as "senior partner" allowed me to continue the journey with him to its conclusion.

One of the additional challenges is whether partnering with patients takes more time and thus reduces the physician's ability to generate RVUs (relative value units) for billing purposes. I am sure that it takes time for medical students and residents to learn how to partner with patients just as it takes more time to play a Beethoven concerto than it does to play "Twinkle-Twinkle Little Star." Whether it takes a seasoned physician more time to develop strong partnerships with the patient is not clear to me and has never been evaluated formally. Certainly many studies demonstrate that partnering with patients leads to better outcomes in patients with heart failure, hypertension, HIV, asthma. and other conditions [12].

SUMMARY

Please don't tell the dean of my medical school that I don't work, but if you define "work"—as a teenage daughter of a good friend once did—as "what they have to pay you to do," then I don't work now and never have. I have chiefly avoided work drudgery thanks to patients who taught me early and often the joy, satisfaction, meaning, and professional growth that flows from partnering with them. I believe that partnering with patients is the soul of healing for many patients and the soul of rejuvenation for physicians and other health care providers. Partnering with patients has helped me diagnose challenging patients, taught me how to listen better, how to become more adept at physical examination, and it has added joy, wonder, and meaning to my professional life. After nearly 50 years of medical practice, I have concluded that medicine is a jewel. Partnering with patients is one of the best and most enjoyable ways to burnish the gem.

REFERENCES

1. Tumulty PA: What is a Clinician and What Does He Do? The New England Journal of Medicine 283: 20–24, 1970.
2. Tumulty PA. The Effective Clinician: His Methods and Approach to Diagnosis. WB Saunders (Philadelphia), 1973.
3. Peabody FW: The Care of the Patient. The Journal of the American Medical Association 88: 877–882, 1927.
4. Earnest M: Something for Sleep. The New England Journal of Medicine 389: 2218–2219, 2023.
5. Available from: www.dictionary.com
6. Ziegelstein RC: Personomics. Journal of the American Medical Association 175: 888–889, 2015.
7. Hellmann D and Abribat M: Golf Score as a Measure of Giant Cell Arteritis. The Journal of Rheumatology 18: 1116–1117, 1991.
8. Ratanawongsa N, Rand CS, Magill CF, Hayashi J, Brandt L, Christmas C, Record JD, Howell EE, Federowicz MA, Hellmann DB, and Ziegelstein RC: Teaching Residents to Know Their Patients as Individuals: The Aliki Initiative at Johns Hopkins Bayview Medical Center. The Pharos 72: 4–11, 2009.
9. Ziegelstein RC, Rand CS, and Hellmann DB: Redesign of Internal Medicine Teaching. The New England Journal of Medicine 363: 594, 2010.
10. Hellmann DB and Ziegelstein RC: Personomics: A Progress Report. American Journal of Medicine 136: 732–733, 2023.

11. Ratanawongsa N, Federowicz MA, Christmas C, Hanyok LA, Record JD, Hellmann DB, Ziegelstein RC, and Rand CS: Effects of a Focused Patient-Centered Care Curriculum on the Experiences of Internal Medicine Residents and Their Patients. Journal of General Internal Medicine 27(4): 473–477, 2012.

12. Record JD, Rand C, Christmas C, Hanyok L, Federowicz M, Bilderback A, Patel A, Khajuria S, Hellmann DB, and Ziegelstein RC: Reducing Heart Failure Readmissions by Teaching Patient-Centered Care to Internal Medicine Residents. Archives of Internal Medicine 171: 858–859, 2011.

13. Hanyok LA, Hellmann DB, Rand C, and Ziegelstein RC: Practicing Patient-Centered Care: The Questions Clinically Excellent Physicians Use to Get to Know Patients as Individuals. The Patient 5: 141–145, 2012.

14. Hanyok LA, Record JD, Christmas C, Hellmann DB, Rand CS, and Ziegelstein RC: The Aliki Initiative at Year 10: Changing the Culture of Medicine to Know Our Patients as Individuals. The Pharos 2018: 28–34, 2018.

15. Ludmerer KM. Let Me HEAL: The Opportunity to Preserve Excellence in American Medicine. Oxford University Press (New York), 2015.

16. Jamison KR. Fires in the Dark: Healing the Unquiet Mind. Alfred A. Knopf (New York), 2023.

16 A Medical Education

David S. Pisetsky

Like many physicians of my age (I was born in 1945), I trained in a medical education system so vastly different from that of today that any relevance to current trainees is coincidental at best. I obtained my MD and PhD degrees at the Albert Einstein College of Medicine (1967–1973) and then was an intern and resident at the Yale–New Haven Hospital (1973–1975). During that era, once classroom work was finished, medical students were thrust onto the wards to help care for the very sick. Despite decaying facilities, nasty environments, and inadequate staffing, public hospitals like Bellevue, Jacobi, and Boston City were considered prime places to train since medical students and house staff were given a lot of "autonomy."

Another way to look at autonomy is a lack of supervision, and, indeed, on many teaching services, attendings spent relatively little time overseeing the work of the ward team comprised of medical students and house staff. A common schedule for attending rounds, during my years as a trainee, was three times a week for two hours; at the end of rounds, attendings would scribble their names on notes in the chart to indicate their agreement with the plans. Cosigning sufficed for billing purposes.

One famous teaching hospital called the ward attendings "visits." I don't know the origin of this term, but it was not inaccurate. At many programs in that era, attendings would make visits, stopping by to do some teaching; involvement in the nitty-gritty of decision making, the province of the ward team, was otherwise quite limited. Rather than delving into the intricacies of patient management, attendings often quizzed trainees in a probing, even intimidating manner (e.g., "What are enzyme abnormalities associated with gout?"). Such questioning was known as "pimping," a practice that is now, thankfully, gone.

In addition to the acquisition of medical knowledge, medical education forges an attitude, mindset, and emotional frame to bolster a career for its duration. The analogy to military training is apt. The system in which I trained continuously put trainees in stressful situations to instill self-reliance and confidence often without sufficient preparation or backup. Residents taught interns, and interns taught medical students, often following the famous "See one, do one, teach one" rubric.

I know that "doing one" sometimes occurred without "seeing one," and I suspect that residents taught me procedures that they themselves had never done. Somehow, with only sparse instruction, I became adept at inserting needles, scopes, and catheters into various places in the human body. I even became skilled at intubating patients, having never practiced on a "dummy" or patient simulator. I still think back with pride (and amazement) how once, in the ER, I intubated an elderly woman struggling mightily with pulmonary edema, calmly talking her through the procedure.

As an intern, I was responsible for countless aspects of patient care. I picked up the patient in the ER, pushed the gurney to the ward (often with a stop at the X-ray department and sometimes a return trip), drew the bloods, put in an IV (as well as a Foley catheter and/or nasogastric tube as needed), did the EKG, and, depending on the circumstances, drew a blood gas and blood cultures. I had to place a PPD on every patient and perform a pelvic exam on every woman as part of routine screening. Otherwise, the chart would "bounce," which was not good; "unbouncing"

DOI: 10.1201/9781003409373-16

officially required bringing the patient back to the hospital to complete the missing tests.

In a lab on the ward (often a messy and chaotic place littered with broken and cracked glass slides), I acted as a technician. I centrifuged the urine to look for casts under the microscope. For spinal fluid, I did the cell count with my own hemocytometer that I stored in my little black bag, which had my name embossed in gold, the gift of a pharmaceutical company. For fever workups, I gram-stained the urine, sputum, or spinal fluid (sometimes all three). I also did acid fast staining, looking for the famous "red snappers" of tuberculosis. At some programs, house officers did LE cell preparations.

After preparing the labels for all of the tubes I collected, I hurried them over to the hospital laboratory for analysis, the blood gas in a plastic tray on ice. Some time thereafter, I returned to the laboratory to pick up the slips with the results, which I then wrote in the chart. Just about the only things I didn't do were making patients' beds and giving them baths, although, if asked, I probably would have complied.

As part of their clerkships in internal medicine, medical students were integral for this kind of work, which was called "scut." On my medicine rotation, as a medical student, I started each morning going around the ward drawing blood on patients, carrying with me an ensemble of tubes–blue tops, lavender tops, red tops– which I dutifully filled, often searching anxiously to find a vein; after a few weeks of this undertaking, however, I could "draw blood from a rock," as we used to say.

Another part of scut was testing the stool of patients for fecal occult blood; a small sample of stool was exposed to a dye called guaiac which turned blue if blood was present. (Such was cancer screening in the precolonoscopy era.) Suffice it to say, there was no safety equipment, and hepatitis was a genuine work hazard. Scut was so much a part of medical training that a book was written to aid students in its performance. *The Effective Scutboy* is available on Amazon for those interested in the fine points of this relic of medical education.

Given all this tiresome and time-consuming work, notes in the chart were pointed, concise, and, of course, handwritten. There was no time for anything elaborate; since word processing had not yet been invented, there was no copying and pasting to make even the most uneventful day in the hospital the subject of a three-page tome as is now common in electronic medical records.

Along with hard work came long hours. Many training programs were based on an every-other-night call schedule, although, in the program at Yale, a schedule called Black Week and White Week was used for much of the intern year; the rest was straight every third night on. There was essentially no outpatient work or weeks without hospital call. Black Week was on call on Saturday, Sunday, Tuesday, Thursday, and Friday. White Week was Monday and Wednesday. For Black Week, I calculated that the time in the hospital was 140 out of 168 hours. It was possible that an intern could go without sleep for two straight nights if by chance he had a "black cloud." On the other hand, the Black Week–White Week schedule did provide a whole weekend off.

I always remember getting ready for the long weekend on call, packing a change of clothing, a Dopp kit of toiletries (I had to shave to look neat on rounds!), and a food supply to tide me over. The stretch from midnight to the next morning is really an extra day, and calories, no matter how empty, are essential. Many interns would gain weight since they ate whatever was available at the nurses' stations, usually cookies or candy provided by families of grateful patients. In a pinch, a vending machine could supply a bag of Planters peanuts or a Mars Bar to get you through the night. Just as I learned to sleep anywhere, I learned to eat anything since the combination of hunger and sleeplessness is genuinely awful. Your stomach and brain both growl.

With an every-other-night call schedule, there was no brooding about the work–life balance since real life was not possible unless you consider that life is brushing your teeth and putting on your pajamas before going to bed. Sleep was the highest priority in a schedule ridiculously out of balance. Given the choice of a steak dinner at Delmonico's or an extra hour of sleep, I would choose the latter without hesitation. (A pizza at Sally's or Pepe's on Wooster Street in New Haven would present more of a quandary.)

One of the few efforts at improving work–life balance for house officers at Yale occurred at an event called "open library" on late Friday afternoons. Attendings and house officers would gather in the departmental library and share a highball or cocktail from the departmental liquor supply. While I appreciated the fellowship and good cheer, I usually had enough fatigue and jumbled thoughts that a glass of Chivas Regal could tip me over the edge. I also thought it was a bad idea to have liquor on your breath when interviewing a patient.

The exigencies of every-other-night on call had its share of burnouts, but, in a system geared to building toughness and stamina, there was little sympathy when a trainee found the going too hard. One of my friends at a top program tells the story of going to his department chair to explain how exhausted he had become working on the ward and was also troubled by weight loss. After hearing of my friend's travails, the chief curtly told him to get thyroid function testing and sent him on his way. Such admissions would be equivalent to an army recruit complaining to the drill sergeant that basic training is tiring.

Despite hard work and the pressure of relentless nights on call, we all got through it, and somehow had a good time and became good doctors (Whether the system then in place was necessary to produce good doctors is a discussion for another day). Some of my happiest memories of my training occurred at the nurses' stations with someone else on call, decompressing, schmoozing about people and cases, and swapping "war stories." Interns and residents have a special sensibility and sense of humor (they don't go away), and they like to reprise situations so absurd and bizarre that laughter is the only reasonable response. With embellishment, the war stories can be hilarious, and, as defenses, they are often quite effective. They distract and deflect and lighten the load that occurs when confronting the grimness that permeates every medical ward.

A few years ago, I realized that the world of my training was disappearing (intentionally so) and that I had a treasure trove of anecdotes, vignettes, and stories that I liked to share. While these stories could illuminate vital history of the medical profession, I have sensed that reminiscence about the "good old days" is discouraged at present since it could imply that the current crop has it too easy, missing some crucial learning that only happens with inexorable time spent on call.

Wanting a permanent record of a unique time in medical education as well as my own, I decided that, for posterity, I would write down stories that covered the full gamut of my experiences as a trainee; some of these writings are fragments and some are finished products. Most remain on the hard drive of my computer, although some have been published in medical journals, including fictionalized versions [1, 2]. Ensnared by the pull of memory, I visit one every so often to fiddle with the words as I seek new insights into what I learned.

My stories are in the tradition of narrative medicine, a kind of creative non-fiction growing in popularity to help explore the humanistic aspects of medicine. One definition I found online says that narrative medicine combines "narratology, phenomenology and liberatory social theory," whatever those are. But, to me, narrative medicine is good old-fashioned storytelling with language and imagery buffed and polished. At its best, narrative medicine enables the expression of the rich and varied panoply of emotions that arise in patient care. Not surprisingly, many stories in narrative medicine are serious and concern issues such as end-of-life care, giving the diagnosis of fatal illness, or making vexing patient care decisions like stopping dialysis.

My interest in writing down my stories was to explore not just the sadder and more poignant aspects of medicine but also the quirky, mundane and jolly, including my own foibles and foolish behavior. My aspiration was to someday publish a book of a collection of stories qua case histories that could be used for teaching, conversation, as well as contemplation; to the stories, I would append questions for discussion just like those found in novels popular with book groups ("Did the physician adequately respond to the patient's concerns about the treatment?"). I think that stories can add candor and honesty to understand the education of a physician, a journey with mistakes, misadventures, and mishaps, some of which are worthy of bemusement as well as reflection and regret.

So, I would like to share with you one of my favorite stories of my time as a house officer.

At Yale, like many excellent programs, a significant part of the training occurs at a hospital in the Department of Veterans Affairs system, usually known as the VA. The VA is the largest federally run health care system in the country. In addition to providing care to millions of veterans, the VA has a large footprint in medical education since a significant percentage of all physicians in the US have trained at a VA hospital at one time or another.

As a training venue, the VA is unsurpassed since it is an organized system that is mission-focused on providing care. The patient population of the VA differs from the general hospital population, however, since, until recently, it was just about only men. Furthermore, the VA patient population has a very high frequency of mental health problems and conditions like substance use disorder, post-traumatic stress disorder (PTSD), and homelessness. Trying to treat a serious medical problem in a patient with schizophrenia can frustrate and bedevil a physician at any stage of career, especially one still training.

The story I will tell is somewhat dated because of the changes in how medical students and house officers dress for work. Even though many medical schools have a white coat ceremony, today's trainees seem to prefer other garb including surgical scrubs. In my era, a dress code prevailed. Medical students wore short white coats; interns wore a short white coat and white pants; and residents wore short white coats or long white coats depending on the program. The few women who were medical students or house officers wore white skirts. (Women did not wear pants then.) Some people even wore white shoes which, while classically elegant, are perhaps too much of a good thing. Look at any house staff picture from the past and all you see is white uniforms.

Advancing the goal of "see one, do one, teach one" and the heuristic value of narrative medicine, here is a true account of an event that occurred when I was resident. I have created some details to advance, not distort the narrative. As in many other emergencies that I dealt with as a trainee, I felt on my own and had to act swiftly, propelled by instinct or intuition. Suffice it to say, there was no debriefing the next day, no sober and thoughtful discussion as would now occur with a supportive attending; any judgment about the outcome was my personal determination. Even today, as I relive this episode, I still don't know whether what I did was smart or dumb.

As you read this account, I hope that you ask yourself what you would have done in my shoes, white shoes or otherwise.

• • •

"Medic!" the man shouted, his voice shrill. "I need a medic!"

The man's eyes were fearful, his face pale and sweaty. His fist was clenched over his chest. It was a classic Levine sign except, in the man's fist, was a yellow pool ball.

The man was barricaded in a rec room at the VA. He was wearing a faded blue bathrobe, and the fingers of his left hand curled tightly around a pool stick held high over his head.

Amidst a crowd that included nurses, police officers, security guards, and an administrator in a gray polyester suit, I was the only physician. I knew I was the medic.

It was late on a Sunday night in the winter of 1975. I was the Medicine resident on call, and I did consults while supervising two admitting teams. Stressed all day, I felt my composure slipping.

Hoping to catch at least some sleep, I was miffed when, near midnight, I received a page from the psychiatry resident on call. He wanted a medical consult on a man on his service.

I took the elevator to the eighth floor of the red brick hospital that looms above the Connecticut Turnpike. I rang the bell to the locked ward and was admitted by an aide whose muscles bulged against a white T-shirt. The ward was steamy. In the corridor, an old man sat in a wheelchair, his right hand shaking rhythmically.

I went to the nurses' station and snatched a donut from a bag on the worktable. I was hungry because dinner had been take-out from McDonald's; the burger was cold, the fries were soggy, and there wasn't enough to eat.

Munching on a chocolate honey dip, I spoke to the resident about the man whose name was Tony. The resident told me that Tony had been shell shocked in the siege of Iwo Jima.

"We just discharged him two days ago," the resident said. Like mine, his face was shadowed with stubble. "He couldn't make it on the outside. He wants to stay here in his old bed, but we can't admit him again so we have to get him to leave."

"What do you need me for?" I asked, feeling uneasy.

"He had an MI last year," the resident said.

"And you want me to clear him for the eviction?"

The resident nodded with a wry smile.

I quickly reviewed the paper chart that was still on the ward.

Pushing an EKG machine that trailed a tangle of wires, I went down the floor to find Tony who was staring at the ceiling, his body tense. Tony looked about 60 years old, with gray wavy hair. His fingertips were stained yellow, and he smelled of cigarette smoke. In addition to the bed, he had commandeered a bathrobe that he wore over his street clothes.

"How are you?" I asked, trying to sound relaxed.

"OK," Tony said. He took a deep breath and exhaled loudly.

"Any chest pain?" I asked.

Tony shook his head.

"Shortness of breath? Dizziness?"

The response was again negative.

"Mind if I do an EKG?"

"Go ahead," Tony said. His mouth tightened.

I slathered some goo onto Tony's arms and his chest that were thick with dark hair. I attached the electrodes and ran the EKG. There were no acute changes, just evidence of an old infarct.

I thanked Tony for cooperating and, after detaching the machine, walked down the hall where I saw the "assault team" massing for the eviction of Tony.

"As far as I'm concerned, he's clear," I said to the psychiatry resident.

I went to the nurses' station, and, after taking off my white coat, started to write a note. As I was describing the EKG findings, I heard loud voices in the hall.

"He's gone." "Where is he?" "Look in the bathroom." "Oh, no. He's in the rec room."

I ran down the hall to the rec room, which had a thick glass window crisscrossed by silver wires. The door was closed, a chair propped under the knob. Tony was alone. His face was red, and he hissed at the crowd watching behind the glass. When one of the nurses shouted for him to come out, he heaved a pool ball in her direction. The pool ball ricocheted around the room after banging the wall.

"I'm not coming out unless you give me my bed back," Tony screamed, spit flying.

"No," the resident said, and Tony threw another ball as his face contorted in rage.

The psych resident turned to the West Haven police officer and said, "He's medically clear. You can get him out."

"This is the VA," one of the cops said, shaking his head. In this belt were a black baton and a shiny pistol. "This is federal. It's your people's responsibility."

"No, it isn't," a VA guard said angrily. He was bald and had a paunch under his blue uniform. "We never admitted him. He's yours."

Back and forth the police officer and guards went. Tony wailed. His face grew redder as he circled around the pool table, waving the pool stick in wild circles.

"Let's all go together," a nurse with a fluted white cap pleaded. "We can go behind a mattress. It's safer," she added but the lawmen continued to bicker.

Listening to the argument, I kept my eye on Tony's face. Suddenly, he winced and looked stricken. It was then he cried for the medic.

"He needs you, Doc," one of the town cops said. "You have to go in to make sure he's OK."

I looked to the VA guards and the nurses and, from their expressions, I realized I was on my own. "Will anyone help me?" I asked as they all looked away.

Behind Tony was a wall of windows that were backed with bars. Through the windows, I could see the dim lights of the city suffused by fog as water dripped down the panes.

I was the doctor on call, and, even if Tony was a maniac who might maim me with the flick of a wrist, he had chest pain, and I had to take care of him. I thought about what to do and remembered the instructions of my psychiatry attending when I was a medical student. "Violent people are often afraid. Show them you're in control, and they'll calm down."

Having no alternative, I would show Tony that I was in control. Silently, I walked back to the nurses' station to retrieve my white coat. I put it on, buttoning it completely, straightening the collar, pulling and tugging the sleeves to make sure it fit just right. On the left sleeve was a brown-red splotch, the residue from blood that had spurted from a botched IV.

I checked the pockets. I had two intracaths that I always carried, not knowing when I would need one in an emergency although I imagined that, in desperation, I could use one for self-defense. Fearing a struggle, my skin chilled, and my heart thumped.

I wiped my hand across my mouth to remove crumbs from the donut and walked to the rec room, striding as upright as I could. From the doorway to his room, a grizzled man with zombie eyes peered at me and farted.

"Star Wars" did not come out for a few years, but, in my recollection of the moment, I see a wizened old doctor floating luminously before my eyes, "Use the

Force, David. Use the Force." Suddenly, I felt sure of myself as my brain set on my mission.

Approaching the cops and guards, I felt angry because they had left me on my own and glared at them. I would show them how to handle danger even if I felt a shiver gathering in my chest.

I slowly pushed open the door to the rec room dislodging the chair as Tony's eyes widened, and he raised his arm, menacing me with the stick. I walked with measured steps. Too fast, and Tony would think I was going to rush him. Too slow, and he would know I was afraid. My pace was deliberate, and my eyes were fixed on Tony. A fluorescent light flickered, and I heard the squawk of a beeper.

I kept walking until I stopped within reach of the pool stick. I looked directly at Tony and willed my face into a visage of caring and understanding.

"Not feeling too good, are you Tony?" I asked.
Tony nodded.
"You want me to check you out?"
Tony nodded again.
"Let's go," I said.

I was in some kind of trance—maybe a delirium from lack of sleep—feeling invincible because I turned my back to Tony even though he could have split my head open with one swipe of the stick.

I heard the sound of the stick being laid on the pool table and then a pool ball being dropped and rolling on the felt. I continued walking, disdaining the police and the guards as Tony, subdued, followed me down the hall.

Tony and I went to the treatment room that had a white metal cabinet full of gauze and needles. The room had the sharp smell of antiseptic. I repeated the EKG and found what I needed. A little squiggle in AVF and some ST depression in V5—V6. It was barely perceptible but enough to call ischemia and justify an admission for unstable angina.

I then brokered a deal that satisfied everyone and admitted Tony to the CCU. The cops didn't have to arrest him. Psychiatry didn't have to admit him. And Tony could spend a few days mending whatever ailed him behind the protective walls of the VA.

After Tony was wheeled off on a gurney, I felt jazzed. I had an adrenaline rush as I realized how close to disaster I had come.

I then went back to the general medicine ward to hang out and decompress. Listening to the Supremes on the radio, I ate some Russell Stover's cherry-filled chocolates. They were a gift from a family of a man who had died of lung cancer that day. At 3 a.m., I was calm enough to go to the on-call room to sleep and, fortunately, was not awakened for the rest of the night. I don't know what happened to Tony after that. I had other patients to worry about and then rotated off the VA Medicine service.

It is over 45 years since I took care of Tony, and I still think I did good doctoring that night, whether by brilliance, luck, or folly. In remembering those events, I marvel at my composure, my resolve, and even—can I say it? —my bravery.

As a professor at a medical school, I often think about a doctor's education. The medical students and house staff are like children to me, but soon they will abound with toughness and moxie. Who knows? Maybe someday one of them will have to take care of me.

How do you teach someone to be a doctor? How do you transform people like me—otherwise ordinary except for a desire to do good and enough intelligence to pass organic chemistry—so that they can cut up patients and sew them back together, get within an eyelash of a deranged man, and tilt against mortality with faith and without despair.

The journey to being a doctor is long and arduous. It is a passage filled with ritual, myths, and mystery. The journey does not end with medical residency or fellowship. It is lifelong, continuous, and forever forges new ways of thinking, builds empathy, and, in the collaboration of patient and physician, can instill grace, equanimity, and compassion.

I am old-fashioned, and, whenever I see patients, I always put on my white coat although mine has an ink stain on one sleeve and has shrunk from too much washing. I know that a white coat is just a symbol, a garment of simple cotton, not a royal robe trimmed with ermine or a raiment of gold thread. Like all good symbols, the coat is an inspiration for the finest action, and, as I learned in taking care of Tony, it can be a vital source of strength.

REFERENCES

1. Pisetsky, D.S., The breakthrough, Ann Intern Med (1996) 124, 345–347.
2. Pisetsky, D.S., Till death do us part, J Gen Intern Med (1997) 12, 705–706.

17 At the Bedside and Beyond: Improving Health through Patient Advocacy

Michele Barry

> The idea that some lives matter less is the root of all that is wrong with the world.
>
> **—Paul Farmer**

In this profession, where physical observations can matter so greatly, something as seemingly insignificant as a patient's blanket can influence a doctor's assessment and have serious consequences for care.

In the 1980s, I saw this firsthand as a visiting professor from Yale working in Mulago Hospital in Kampala, Uganda. It was the beginning of the AIDS epidemic, and all hands were on deck. I had volunteered to assist and teach. In this resource-limited setting, where poverty and illness were deeply interconnected, we were taught to look for subtle indicators of a patient's ability to pay for medicines or tests not covered by the government. One such clue lay in the blankets patients brought with them. Those who arrived with threadbare, thin blankets were more likely to be poor—and more likely to be unable to afford medications and treatment not covered by the government. It was disheartening to witness how such indicators of poverty could signal a patient's options for care.

Years later, in 2009, I found myself in a very different setting at Stanford University, beginning a new chapter of my career as the first senior Associate Dean of Global Health. While doing rounds at Stanford Hospital, I was shocked to learn that wealthy patients and hospital donors were given special blankets. These high-quality red ones signaled not poverty but privilege. They indicated that these patients were important donors and played to a perception of perhaps better care or a different quality of care.

Both systems were unfair, each stigmatizing the patients involved but through a different mechanism. Yes, the richer patients sometimes received more attention than the typical standard of care. But it wasn't necessarily the best care, as hospital staff were often more deferential to the patient—and therefore more likely to over-test and overspend on unnecessary interventions at the patient's request. I began tearing the red blankets off beds and successfully convinced the hospital CEO to end that system.

These experiences reinforced, for me, the notion that, as physicians, we have a duty not only to diagnose and treat but also to stand up for the rights and well-being of those we serve. This is patient advocacy at its core: to ensure that each patient receives the highest quality and most appropriate care, regardless of the blanket that covers them or any other indicator of their wealth or importance.

Throughout my four decades as a tropical medicine and global health physician, I have witnessed firsthand the value of moving beyond the medical diagnosis to care for our patients holistically. As I'll discuss more later, this includes paying attention to the social—and environmental—determinants of health: listening to their stories, understanding their cultural contexts, and using that knowledge to advocate for better, more comprehensive, and compassionate care regardless of their

DOI: 10.1201/9781003409373-17

wealth or background. Recently, together with my colleague from the University of Washington, Peter Rabinowitz, I have advocated for incorporating the concept of the Social-E into a patient's record. This refers to recording not only socioeconomic determinants but also a broader suite of environmental factors that could impact health when taking a patient's social history. These factors tie into emerging global environmental challenges, such as climate change and pollution, that often disproportionately impact lower-income communities.

DEFINING PATIENT ADVOCACY

Patient advocacy has many implications, and not all of them apply to doctors. Often the term "patient advocate" describes someone working within the hospital system who serves as a liaison between patients, health care staff, and insurance companies. While this role is important, not every patient has access to such assistance, and doctors are frequently the only advocates encountered by patients. Not many of us receive formal training in patient advocacy, but there are many ways to incorporate it into our practice.

Having the mindset of a patient advocate involves bringing an open mind and a deep sense of empathy into our interactions with patients, as well as a dedication to our Hippocratic Oath—"a promise to act in the best interest of the patient and to protect patient privacy" [1]. It means taking steps to understand, and then respect, a patient's values, beliefs, and cultural background. We demonstrate our respect by providing care that aligns with patients' individual needs and preferences. One must also be able to see the larger picture beyond the symptoms a patient presents, taking steps to understand their social and environmental determinants of health.

In more concrete terms, patient advocacy may involve actions such as the following:

■ *Advocate for the best quality care, regardless of patient resources*: For example, a doctor should advocate for patients to receive the best and most appropriate testing to understand their condition, despite any financial limitations. A doctor can also go one step further to find ways to surmount those financial obstacles. For example, a Chinese visiting graduate student at Stanford, after foraging and ingesting *Amanita Phylloides* mushrooms, developed liver failure. A liver transplantation was unaffordable in the US. We convinced the hospital it was less expensive to purchase a ticket and send him back to China for liver transplantation rather than care for him until he died from liver failure.

■ *Help the patient be informed*: My first question when seeing an inpatient is, "What is your understanding of your disease, and why you're here?" In many cases, they've arrived with a frightening symptom, yet they haven't been informed of what their diagnosis might be or even what testing was ordered. Or more commonly, they have been hastily informed during the "heat" of admission but don't recall the issues the next day. Patients must be well-informed in order to be part of the decision-making process.

■ *Be aware of the power dynamic inherent in the doctor-patient relationship*: Successful patient advocacy requires trust between a physician and a patient. However, patients are often at their most vulnerable when they come into the hospital. Therefore, trust in this setting can be coercive in a nuanced manner. Patients may feel that they need to trust their doctor in order to get better. As a patient advocate, it's critical to be aware of that power dynamic and go the extra mile to engage the patient in aspects of their care. Even if they defer to your care decisions, make sure they understand the pros and cons. It's also important in such situations to be nonjudgmental of patients, especially when their background may not fit with your idea of the best way to go about pursuing a healthy life. For instance, a doctor treating a patient with IV drug use will understand the health risks of that behavior and may experience frustration when, for example, the patient comes in with their third case of endocarditis. Doctors can offer information about why the patient's choices led to the repeated life-threatening illnesses, but ultimately it's the patient's decision whether they continue using the drugs. Often, unhealthy choices may be driven by existential life threats or social determinants, which one can try to address and mitigate. Perhaps a treatable mental illness is contributing to the behavior. If a patient chooses to continue using, then a potential avenue to follow may be teaching them how to access clean needles. To some, this may sound like aiding and abetting unhealthy habits. To me, it's about respecting the patient's decision and trying to get them as healthy as possible within the parameters of their choices.

- *Advocating for changes that improve patients' determinants of health*: For instance, if a patient's health is impacted by homelessness, advocacy may be trying to get them into a shelter or helping them find employment. Rally social workers to assist you if your time is scarce or if you need additional information or resources. Advocate and promote ways to alleviate poverty.

Doctors can go one step further to promote or advocate for the social, economic, educational, and political changes that could ameliorate the suffering and threats to human health that we identify through our work. While sometimes this type of advocacy is viewed as being beyond the doctor's role, these factors closely impact the health of our patients.

These are just a few examples of the ways doctors can advocate for their patients. Beyond any specific action, however, patient advocacy is about bringing a nonjudgmental mindset and deep sense of empathy to every patient encounter.

As one modern version of the Hippocratic Oath reminds us that "there is art to medicine as well as science" [2]. We are effective patient advocates when we remember that "warmth, sympathy, and understanding may outweigh the surgeon's knife or the chemist's drug."

BEING PRESENT AT THE BEDSIDE: Listening (and Looking) for the Patient's Full Story

A core component of being a patient advocate is the willingness to be fully present at the bedside, bringing the "warmth, sympathy, and understanding" just referenced and engaging with all your senses.

I strongly believe that the vast majority of a patient's diagnosis comes from their story. Getting that complete story requires being there with the patient, talking, listening, and looking closely for clues.

Many such clues come from taking a detailed patient history. In one case, I saw a patient who came in with abnormal liver tests. The assumption was that it might be a gallstone. However, as I spoke with the patient and asked questions about their past travel, I learned that, several years ago, they had spent time in a country where the parasitic disease schistosomiasis is present in freshwater. The patient had been an avid rafter in many freshwater rivers. Based on this travel history, we obtained serology and stool for ova and parasites. We were able to diagnose and treat the parasitic infection rather than ineffectively follow a misdiagnosis.

Likewise, taking a good dietary history once helped diagnose a rare case of scurvy in patient with alcohol use disorder in Palo Alto, California, who presented with "failure-to-thrive" symptoms. I was able to make this diagnosis after noting the patient seemed malnourished and had bleeding gums. Because scurvy is so rare in the US, this diagnosis would have been difficult to make without asking detailed questions about the patient's diet, confirming that the diet had absolutely no citrus. The patient was treated with vitamin supplements and a better diet, which resolved their symptoms of fatigue and bleeding gums.

Attentive physicians can also gain a wealth of visual clues from a thorough bedside examination. While at Stanford, I treated a patient who presented with anemia, which wasn't clearly diagnosed by peripheral blood smear. We couldn't figure out the cause. When I went to the bedside and conducted a physical exam, I saw that the patient was hyperreflexic and exhibited a positive Babinski reflex, in which the big toe moves up when the sole of the foot is stroked. In adults, this physical finding can be a sign of vitamin B_{12} deficiency. When this was confirmed with a blood test, a simple B_{12} supplement cured the anemia and the hyperreflexia. Similarly, attuned doctors scouring for physical clues can identify a vitamin C deficiency as described above through abnormal corkscrewing hairs on the pretibial area of the legs, while certain facial features and eyebrow growth patterns can indicate hypothyroidism and myxedema.

A doctor's deep knowledge and experience, combined with the ability to look closely and a willingness to listen patiently, can often reveal more about a patient's condition than many diagnostic tests. One does not necessarily need CT or MRI scans. Syndromic presentations are often the first clue.

IMPORTANCE OF CULTURALLY SENSITIVE CARE

Beyond a general open mind and sense of empathy, understanding and respecting an individual's cultural background are critical to good patient advocacy. Two early experiences illuminated this point for me and shaped my career in many ways.

Understanding the Patients We Serve

I was working as a resident at Yale University School of Medicine in the late seventies when we began treating Vietnamese families escaping the war. My pediatric colleagues noticed small, round, red marks on the bodies of some young Vietnamese refugee children. Their first assumption? That the children were being abused. Some children were even turned over to child protective services.

Eventually, as I continued to care for these patients and was able to communicate with them through the help of an interpreter, I learned that this was not abuse but rather the families' attempt to provide medical care. When Vietnamese immigrant families had sick children, many would treat them with a traditional therapy called cupping, which causes marks on the child.

We then started to pay attention to the areas which had been "cupped" as clues to where the child was complaining of being ill. Cupping on the abdomen helped evince the symptom of abdominal pain. Other bodily geographic areas hinted at other symptoms.

These immigrants were forced to navigate a health system that was incomprehensible to them, while also often suffering diseases uncommon to the US. I began to see that, as physicians, we were frequently unprepared and lacked the cultural competency, knowledge of tropical diseases, and nuance to treat our refugee patients.

I realized there needed to be a specialty clinic to address the cultural problems as well as the specific diseases germane to the country of origin. I helped found the Yale New Haven Refugee Clinic to address this challenge. One of the first such clinics in the US, it allowed family members to receive care in one place at a family clinic rather than being treated separately around the hospital. At this clinic, volunteer residents, an interpreter, pediatricians, social workers, nurse practitioners, internists, and psychiatrists all worked together in an interdisciplinary fashion. Subspecialists such as dermatologists were also available.

I also saw that I needed training in the cultural nuances and diseases I was witnessing in these clinics. At the time, US medical schools were not teaching the ways in which theories of health and wellness varied by culture. For instance, the hot-cold theory of treatment of illnesses used by many traditional cultures around the world was an unknown concept to most US medical trainees. For me, overcoming these knowledge and cultural deficits meant living and working in the countries where my patients were coming from in order to better understand disease patterns and to be their best advocate. This led to my work as a tropical medical physician and subsequent efforts alongside my Yale colleague, Frank J. Bia, to provide medical students with overseas residency training. We wanted residents to see and learn from other cultures how medical care was provided, so that they could become more culturally informed as physicians. Many such residencies and similar overseas training opportunities exist today. From these overseas experiences, one often becomes acutely aware of power dynamics, as well as the legacy of colonialism. High-income countries' expertise in tropical medicine was often built as they occupied—and exploited—the countries where these diseases were common. When partnering overseas, one should strive to acknowledge this and be careful not to perpetuate historic injustices.

While not every doctor will become a global health practitioner, there is great value in seeking deeper knowledge and on-the-ground experience of the culture and background of the patients you are serving. You are likely to make many rewarding friendships in the process.

Meeting Patients Where They Are

Another early career experience underscored an important facet of culturally sensitive care: meeting patients where they are, both literally and figuratively. Many barriers prevent some of our most vulnerable patients from seeking or receiving care in traditional hospital settings. As patient advocates, we can seek to understand and eliminate those barriers.

As a young attending physician at Yale, I started speaking with colleagues working at a needle exchange program who were struggling to get their patients, often living on the streets, to come in for care.

The patients, we learned, feared receiving judgmental treatment at the hospital or clinic. This is a common obstacle to receiving hospital care for many people who use drugs [3, 4]. I thought we might have more success coming to the patients on the street—a more neutral and comfortable setting for many of them. We learned that an old mobile mammography van was going to be thrown out.

We claimed it and reequipped it to serve first unhoused people and, later, women at crisis shelters. Women in shelters were often afraid to come to the hospital for fear they'd be recognized by their abusive partner while in public. Equipped with simple tools such as blood pressure cuffs, glucometers, free samples of medications, a gynecology bed for pap smears, and testing for sexually transmitted infections, we traveled around New Haven, Connecticut, providing the best services we could. We had a set schedule, so patients knew when to show up for care. We followed the needle exchange van, offering one-stop health care. Often our patients would call us the Good Humor and Dairy Queen ice cream trucks, as we traveled side by side to soup kitchen shelters and subsidized housing neighborhoods. I once took a llama to a housing project whose residents were not seeking care. Children swarmed the van to visit the llama, and we were able to immunize these children.

I've never felt more useful than I did during these times, knowing that we were getting care to patients who needed it and may not have otherwise received it, if not for our unusual mode of outreach.

This spirit of meeting patients where they are is one all doctors can carry with them, regardless of whether they physically take their practice to the streets. Meeting each patient with an open, nonjudgmental mindset and addressing patient fears lowers barriers to accessing care, creating novel incentives to receive it. It also makes room for the trust that is the cornerstone of good medicine.

COUNTERACTING CORPORATIZATION

A modern-day barrier to patient advocacy is the limit on our time, attention, and resources that an increasingly corporate and profit-oriented health care system incurs.

The need for an electronic record is pushing against quality one-on-one patient care. We're now considerably constrained in the time we can give patients. Where, in the past, doctors easily had 45 minutes to spend with a patient, now it's closer to 15 minutes. This impacts trust: making eye contact and showing empathy with outpatients is critical, but one is really pressed to do this while meeting the requirement for exhaustive notes. It also potentially impacts the quality of patient care and the accuracy of diagnoses. Doctors can lose the opportunity to gain valuable patient information because of these constantly present time pressures. A recent study found that shorter visits are associated with potentially inappropriate prescribing of medications such as antibiotics and opioids, especially for patients of color and younger patients. Adding to the disparity, patients with Medicaid insurance coverage, dual Medicare and Medicaid coverage, or no insurance coverage received significantly shorter visits than commercially insured patients despite the latter population being healthier on average [5].

Despite these constraints, or perhaps because of them, we must remember that we are often the patient's only advocate. We can't expect the system to advocate for the patient, due to the time and financial pressures of medicine's corporatization, where the bottom line often drives health care. For instance, while there can be pressure to discharge a patient early, in order to free up a bed for another paying patient, physicians must advocate against this if they feel the patient is not ready. Or, when you see hospitals use red blankets or their equivalent to raise money from donors, shout out! Even a single voice can be effective.

PATIENT ADVOCACY ON A CHANGING PLANET

Patient advocacy is more critical now than ever in the face of climate change and environmental degradation.

We've seen myriad health impacts of extreme weather events, from massive hurricanes that destroy homes and crops while breeding disease, to scorching heat waves that threaten the young and old alike, to devastating wildfires that pollute the air with toxins. From a tropical disease perspective, climate change is shifting disease vectors, causing malaria and dengue to crop up in the US and other places unprepared to deal with them. The health care industry produces 8.5% of the carbon emissions in the US and can do better by recycling, greening, and reducing their carbon footprint with vendors [6]. The website "Health Care without Harm" offers a number of resources for achieving this [7].

Doctors can respond to this in two ways: by educating themselves and by advocating for climate mitigation and adaptations that will protect human health.

In terms of education, doctors need to understand the impact of climate and environmental changes on infectious diseases, heart and lung health, mental health, autoimmunity, and much more. They also need to understand which populations are most at risk. This has not been taught in medical schools, though we are very recently seeing medical schools begin to adopt the climate change curriculum.

To address this need, the Stanford Center for Innovation in Global Health has teamed up with the University of Washington to develop "Medicine for a Changing Planet," a series of free planetary health case studies for medical students and doctors that emphasize understanding the social, environmental, and cultural contexts for a patient's condition [8]. Often, a physician is the sentinel, or first point of notification, for an emerging disease or understanding an environmental toxin outbreak. We developed case studies, each of which includes the social and environmental aspects of a patient's health history, their exposures, their occupation, and climate factors that may be influencing their health.

Many other educational resources are available. Medical students and seasoned physicians alike should make efforts to stay informed on the research and science about the impacts of climate change on human health. The Medical Society Consortium on Climate and Health offers many educational resources [9].

In addition to educating themselves, doctors can also advocate for action and change around these environmental issues, which collectively pose the single greatest threat to human health.

They can call for adaptation and resilience measures that protect the health of the most vulnerable. This includes encouraging local cities and lawmakers to invest in resilient schools and community cooling centers, where vulnerable populations can go during extreme heat and wildfire events. Currently, I am trying to prevent the oil and fossil industry from fracking near hospitals, clinics, and schools.

At the national level, doctors can encourage their congressional representatives and senators to push for bills that protect children and vulnerable populations, along with increased funding for agencies that are responding to climate change impacting health.

Finally, doctors are still considered the most trusted profession [10]. They can leverage the trust and powerful platform granted them by the public to raise awareness of how climate change is affecting their patients.

SUMMARY

Doctors play a critical role in safeguarding patient health and dignity when they act as patient advocates. This role is needed now more than ever. I believe there is a path to patient advocacy for every physician.

Some may choose to practice patient advocacy in more intimate ways, such as taking as much time as possible at each bedside, advocating against a patient's early discharge, or helping a patient with housing insecurity access housing, food, or job resources.

Others may travel overseas or take a mobile clinic to the streets in order to build their cultural competency and overcome barriers to patients accessing care.

Yet others may leverage their platform as a trusted voice in medicine to raise awareness of social or environmental issues impacting patient health.

Each physician's journey will be unique to them, but I strongly believe we can best serve our patients with a mindset of service and advocacy. With this approach, we can do our part to ensure that every individual receives the highest quality of care and experiences the best possible health outcomes, regardless of their language, their address, or even the blanket that covers them.

REFERENCES

1. UCLA David Geffen School of Medicine. Modern Hippocratic Oath Holds the Underlying Values Of. UCLA. [Online]. Available from: https://medschool.ucla.edu/blog-post/modern-hippocratic-oath-holds-the-underlying-values-of#:~:text=Written%20in%20the%205th%20century,and%20act%20in%20patients'%20interests [Accessed: December 2023].

2. Available from: www.pbs.org/wgbh/nova/article/hippocratic-oath-today/
3. Biancarelli DL, Biello KB, Childs E, Drainoni M, Salhaney P, Edeza A, Mimiaga MJ, Saitz R, Bazzi AR. Strategies used by people who inject drugs to avoid stigma in healthcare settings. Drug Alcohol Depend. 2019;198:80–86. doi:10.1016/j.drugalcdep.2019.01.037.
4. Chan Carusone S, Guta A, Robinson S, et al. "Maybe if I stop the drugs, then maybe they'd care?"—hospital care experiences of people who use drugs. Harm Reduct J. 2019;16(1):16. doi:10.1186/s12954-019-0285-7.
5. Neprash HT, Mulcahy JF, Cross DA, Gaugler JE, Golberstein E, Ganguli I. Association of primary care visit length with potentially inappropriate prescribing. JAMA Health Forum. 2023;4(3):e230052. doi:10.1001/jamahealthforum.2023.0052.
6. Dzau VJ, Levine R, Barrett G, Witty A. Decarbonizing the U.S. health sector—a call to action. N Engl J Med. 2021;385(22):2117–2119. doi:10.1056/NEJMp2115675.
7. Available from: https://noharm.org/
8. Available from: www.medicineforachangingplanet.org/
9. Available from: https://medsocietiesforclimatehealth.org/
10. Doctors and scientists are seen as the world's most trustworthy professions. Ipsos. [Online]. Available from: www.ipsos.com/en-us/news-polls/global-trustworthiness-index-2022 [Accessed: December 11, 2023].

18 Respect

Dean L. Winslow

The *Oxford English Dictionary* has this to say about the word "respect": "a feeling of deep admiration for someone or something elicited by their abilities, qualities, or achievements." I think that is a good start, but what we need to do as doctors is much more. Sadly, in our current meritocratic society, I am concerned that many younger people inside and outside of medicine judge others (and themselves) only by what they have outwardly achieved in life. I feel that respect is, more importantly, an honest appreciation of other human beings based on their life stories and should not be focused only on "achievements" but rather on their courage, dignity, and strength as they have lived their lives.

I often think of my late maternal grandmother, Esther, who was born in rural Northern Indiana in 1893. She only had an eighth-grade education (which was common for women in those days), but she knew by heart thousands of stanzas of English and American poetry, and she rocked us to sleep in her arms when we came to visit as children. I always knew that I was deeply loved by my "Banga." I know that in God's eyes, she was just as important a human being as any billionaire or Nobel Prize winner.

I will note that medical students and residents these days are awesome. Just getting into a prestigious medical school or residency program is incredibly competitive and is much more difficult than it was when I was applying in the 1970s. Our current trainees are all excellent academically, but I am also just blown away by the many other things they have done in addition to excelling in their classes. It is not unusual to learn that many of them were also competitive athletes or volunteered for nongovernmental organizations; some even started their own similar organizations. When I pick up a new service as the attending physician, I always ask the house staff and medical students to tell me about themselves before we start rounds. Where did you grow up and go to high school? College? Med school? What are you interested in doing at this point in your career? Someone might share, "I went to Harvard for undergrad." I will then ask them what house they lived in while they were at Harvard and tell them that my wife went to Harvard, too. I will then follow up with, "What's the matter? Couldn't get into an elite school like I did at Penn State? It's good you had Harvard as your safety school!" That is guaranteed to get a laugh and put them at ease, and it lets them know that I respect and admire them.

Medicine is hard, and caring for the sickest and most complicated patients, as we do on the inpatient medicine service, is not an endeavor for the faint-hearted. Of course, it is important to teach good patient care and correct errors of knowledge and management on rounds, but I always try to do that with a smile on my face and tell stories, sometimes even about errors I made in training or as recently as the previous week. I want the trainees to know that internal medicine is, in my opinion, the toughest and most demanding specialty, and many patients will get sicker and die despite their best effort. Even the most experienced doctors don't know everything. I always remember how badly I felt at their stage in training when I made a mistake. I thus try to treat trainees as I would my own children (whom I love more than anything).

An example: just a couple years ago, our lumbar puncture kits were missing vials of lidocaine for local anesthesia (due to Covid-19 pandemic-related supply chain

DOI: 10.1201/9781003409373-18

issues), and the internal medicine trainees had to put an order into the electronic chart so that the bedside nurse could procure a vial from the pharmacy. One day, the intern (who was excellent clinically and who, before medical school, had had the unique experience of being an enlisted US Army soldier who served in Iraq, as I had done) found out that the nurse had misinterpreted the order and had injected the entire vial of lidocaine intravenously into the patient. Although the patient didn't turn a hair from this mistake, the intern felt terrible and was really beating himself up about the error. I immediately reassured him by giving him a hug and told him that this honestly wasn't his fault; this was a classic "system error," and I encouraged him to file an incident report in our quality improvement system. I also reassured him that injecting a 5 milliliter vial of 1% lidocaine intravenously would not harm the patient and that, back in the 1970s, we used much higher amounts of lidocaine to treat ventricular arrhythmias in the coronary care unit. I think that if I had been harsh in my response to this mistake, then this would have hurt the highly motivated young doctor. Treating him with kindness was exactly what he needed and showed that I respected his intellectual development, his clinical acumen, and his emotional well-being.

Over the last 30 years, I have made it a practice to introduce myself to new patients I see on the hospital wards or in clinic by smiling warmly and extending my hand. I often jokingly say something like, "Hi, Mrs. Smith, I am your attending doctor. My name is Dean L. Winslow. Dean is just my first name, not a title!" That usually gets a laugh or at least a smile. Before I ask a patient any questions about their symptoms or why they are at our hospital, I always ask them, "Where were you born and raised? Where did you go to school? What do (did) you do before you got sick?" An advantage of being older and having many life experiences is that you can honestly relate to your patients more easily. For instance, a patient may say, "I was born in New Orleans," and I will say, "Wow, I did my infectious diseases training there. What part of the city are you from? What's your favorite restaurant?" Or a patient will say, "I taught elementary school for most of my career," and I can tell them, "Cool! My mom was a public school teacher for 35 years. Since you are a teacher, we will have to give you the special VIP treatment here at Stanford!"

I also love seeing patients at our wonderful VA hospital. During World War II, more than 13 million Americans served in uniform; thus, knowledge of the military was greater among doctors of my parents' generation than it is now. With proportionally fewer people serving in the military nowadays (particularly among doctors), this has also limited knowledge of the experiences of veterans, many of whom (such as those who served in Vietnam) were never truly thanked for their service. I always ask veterans, "What was your branch of service? What years were you in? What outfit were you assigned to? What was your MOS (military operational specialty)?" Perhaps they answer, "I was a door gunner in helicopters in Vietnam assigned to the 1st CAV." I can then say, "Hey, I was a US Air Force (USAF) flight surgeon for 35 years! Did you fly Hueys (UH-1) or Chinooks (CH-47)? What part of the country were you operating in that year?"

A way to demonstrate respect for veterans and perhaps also make them laugh is to be able to tease them a bit since that is a part of military life that many of us veterans miss. One of my favorite VA patients from a few years ago was a true hero (to his primary team, he was "an 80-year-old veteran with a prosthetic joint infection due to methicillin-sensitive *Staphylococcus aureus*"). He had ejected from his burning jet fighter over the Gulf of Tonkin after being hit by enemy surface-to-air fire while returning to his aircraft carrier, the USS *Bon Homme Richard*, after flying a bombing mission in an F-8 Crusader jet over North Vietnam in 1965. After ejecting just yards offshore and coming down in his parachute through a dense cloud layer, he was captured by the crew of a North Vietnamese fishing boat. He escaped after shooting one of his captors in the face with a pistol he had concealed under his G-suit. He was eventually rescued from the water by a US Navy helicopter after two A-1E Sky Raider aircraft buzzed the vessel from just a few feet above the water. Almost 60 years after his shoot-down and escape, he still cries every time he tells someone about the guilt he feels when he remembers shooting and killing his North Vietnamese captor. When he learned that I had been a USAF flight surgeon and had flown several hundred hours in jet fighters (and had flown combat missions in C-130s and helicopters in Afghanistan and Iraq), this gave me a huge amount of credibility in his eyes. While I am careful always about appropriate physician/patient boundaries, the patient instantly knew that I was a fellow military aviator who understood in detail what his journey entailed, as nearly no one else could. After listening to his story, I gently took his arm in my hand for several minutes. After we both teared up and wiped our eyes with our sleeves, I helped break the sadness by telling him, "Willie, our team will take good care of you—even if you are a squid" (the joking term US Air Force aviators use for US Navy aviators). We both broke into laughter. We exchanged our respective fighter call signs; my call sign was Racer and his was Super Blue.

When I served as Medical Director, in the 1980s, of our HIV clinic in Delaware and several years later at our county hospital HIV Clinic in San Jose, I truly loved getting to know my patients as people and hearing about their life journeys. There was (and sadly, in many parts of our country, still is) a lot of prejudice against people based on sexual orientation and individuals with a history of substance use disorder. I truly believed that being kind and compassionate to these often marginalized people was just as important as being a skilled practitioner caring for their illnesses. In those "bad old days" before we had effective highly active antiretroviral therapy (HAART) for HIV infection, we did our best treating opportunistic infections and cancers but knew that all our patients would die (usually within two years of their AIDS diagnosis), and I, as a physician, needed to support them in the short time they had remaining in their lives. I have literally dozens of stories of these patients' bravery in the face of death; I could fill a book telling their stories. I vividly remember caring for an amazing middle-aged gay man who initially developed extensive Kaposi sarcoma, had a partial response to systemic chemotherapy, and then, unfortunately, developed a primary central nervous system lymphoma. He chose to forego aggressive treatment for his lymphoma. He had worked in a museum and had been an expert on American design. Sadly, he had been estranged from his family for many years. Friends of his offered to care for him in their home and spent hours each day listening to music with him, reading to him, and just holding his hand. On my way home from my office or the hospital, I generally made a house call to see him at least every couple of weeks. At the last house call I made on him just a few days before he died, his friend thanked me profusely for my good care and going out of my way to visit. As I broke into tears, I told them, "It's not a bother. It's an honor to come out here and make these house calls."

One of my other memorable patients with HIV in the 1980s was a lovely man in his forties who was an accomplished classical pianist. He had played as a soloist with several major symphony orchestras in the US and made several musical recordings. Sadly, he developed diffuse symmetrical polyneuropathy as a primary manifestation of HIV and lost sensation in his lower extremities. No longer having feeling in his feet meant that he could no longer use the three pedals on the piano, and his career as a musician was over. He was from a small town in Alabama, and he eventually made the decision to return to pass away at home in his mother's house. However, he did still want to have an HIV doctor in Alabama. I called Dr. William Dismukes (then the Chief of Infectious Diseases at the University of Alabama at Birmingham) to discuss his case. After hearing about him, Dr. Dismukes said in his lovely deep southern accent, "Dean, I have an outstanding young former ID fellow now running our HIV clinic in Birmingham. His name is Mike Saag. He'll take fine care of your patient."

Another part of my career illustrates how people of all walks of life, including those convicted of crimes and prisoners, are worthy of respect. Many people in prison survived sad and abusive childhoods, and being incarcerated for a crime is, in many ways, just the latest difficult episode in their lives. A great number of the prisoners for whom I have cared and have followed in clinic after their release from jail or prison often end up doing good things with their lives. Shortly after I took over as medical director of our large HIV clinic at our county hospital in San Jose in 2003, I began seeing patients with HIV at our two county jail facilities each month, so they would not have to be transported to our hospital in shackles accompanied by a dedicated Sherriff's Deputy on overtime pay (having these specialty clinics in the jail infirmary saved the county several hundreds of thousands of dollars each year). Most of the people incarcerated in county jails are there for minor, nonviolent crimes like shoplifting, forgery, minor drug possession, or parole violations. In contrast, many of the people incarcerated in state penitentiaries and prisons are there for more serious crimes.

One of my favorite friends and colleagues at our county hospital is Dr. Alex Chyorny. Alex fled the Soviet Union with his parents and came to the US when he was in high school. He later became an internist, and, in addition to attending regularly in the ICU, he also directed Santa Clara County Custody Health Program. Inmates at our county jail are cared for by our wonderful Santa Clara Valley Medical Center doctors and advanced practice providers, and they received state-of-the-art medical care just like our other patients at our county hospital. When I was working at our county hospital, Alex usually gave a didactic lecture each year to the new house staff on "Caring for Prisoners." One of the points I heard him make emphatically was, "Don't ever ask an inmate what they did to get incarcerated!" Obviously not setting a good example for my trainees, I often broke Dr. Chyorny's rule. For my incarcerated patients with HIV, knowing that someone was in for drug possession might help me get them to substance use disorder treatment. I often asked prisoners what they did to get incarcerated because I was curious, and that information frequently provided me with important insights into their lives that then informed their care.

Hopefully, without sounding like I am preaching, when on rounds, I try to teach by example a couple of important things about patients. First, don't judge a person by their appearance or life circumstances. Second, know that the core of each person is love, and try to see that in everyone you meet. For many years, my hospital gave special red blankets to wealthy donors who were hospitalized and would place these blankets on their beds to indicate that they were VIPs. This practice always bothered me as it indicated inequality, and I feel that everyone deserves the same amount of respect, kindness, and attention. One week on the wards, I had two very interesting patients at the same time: a 95-year-old retired venture capital billionaire "red blanket patient" and a 70-year-old homeless woman from East Palo Alto. I learned the 95-year-old man had flown piston-engine US Army Air Force transport aircraft during World War II on one of the most hazardous missions ever accomplished: flying "the hump" over the Himalayas in the China Burma India Theater of operations. Of course, we immediately bonded since I knew about "his war" and honored him for it (to his previous team he was "a 95-year-old man with history of hypertension, hyperlipidemia, and heart failure with preserved ejection fraction"). Despite her ragged clothes, the 70-year-old homeless woman had the loveliest sparkle in her eyes. When I met her on my first day taking over the service, I asked her where she was from, she answered, "I was born and raised in Detroit." I followed up by asking her what she did when she was younger. She replied that she was a backup singer at Motown Studios in the 1960s and early 1970s. I grew up in Dover, Delaware (south of the Mason-Dixon line), so Rhythm and Blues and especially Motown were the kinds of music we listened to and danced to at our high school gym on Friday nights. She could see my face light up with delight as I told her that she was going to get special VIP treatment from our team and that Barry Gordy (the longtime CEO of Motown Studios) would expect that of us! It was wintertime and bitter cold outside (unusual for Palo Alto), and she was to be discharged to a homeless shelter later that day. My 95-year-old venture capital billionaire and former WWII pilot buddy was in a room just down the hall from my 70-year-old ex-Motown singer. I went back to his room and asked him if I could have his red blanket to give to a sweet lady. He immediately said, "Hell yes, Doc! I must have a half dozen of these *** red blankets at home!" I walked back down the hall and placed the red blanket on the bed of my other patient, gently tucking it around her legs. My Motown singer patient took the blanket with her to the shelter when she was discharged later that afternoon.

There is a story in the Apocrypha of the New Testament that tells the story of a Roman Imperial soldier, Martin of Tours, who served as a centurion in the 4th century C.E. As he was returning to his barracks on a freezing cold night, he saw a ragged and dirty beggar shivering by the gates of the city. He initially walked by the man, but then he felt pity and turned around. He didn't have anything to give the man, so he removed his Roman Imperial military tunic and used his sword to cut the robe in half, and he gave half to the beggar and kept half to wrap himself in. The story in the Apocrypha goes on that the next night Martin had a vivid dream where he saw Jesus in Heaven wrapped in the half tunic. I haven't had any vivid dreams like that about my Motown singer patient, but I do hope to get to Heaven someday. I hope when I walk through the "pearly gates" that I see Jesus and that he has that Stanford red blanket draped over his shoulders or tied around his waist. Then he will say, "Hey Racer, welcome to Paradise! Thanks for that nifty red blanket you gave me! We always need more old football and track jocks, and Air Force guys like you up here, so glad you joined us, Racer. All your old Air Force buddies are waiting for you."

19 Communication and Collaboration

Sharon D. Solomon

INTRODUCTION

Few specialties in medicine are as sterile as ophthalmology. From measuring visual acuity "vital signs" some *distance from the patient*, to performing dilated fundoscopic examination of the retina with a 20 diopter lens delicately balanced *between the physician's hand and the patient's face*, to assessing the anterior segment of the eye with a large metal slit-lamp *separating patient skin from physician skin*, it is possible to go through the entire day in an ophthalmology clinic without physically laying hands on a single patient. Yet each day, upon entering the examination room, I am immediately aware of the fear, frustration, anxiety, or depression that may affect the patient who is suffering from loss of vision and the secondary concerns of the family members, also present, upon whom he relies for help. I touch the patient and acknowledge the presence of the family members. Despite having already been debriefed by the fellow, resident, or advanced practice provider (APP) who tries to keep one patient ahead of me in a clinic of 40–45 patients, I personally elicit the patient's reason for seeking care so that I can hear the manner with which he describes the loss of vision and the level of concern associated with the description. While washing hands and quickly pulling out lenses, I listen, looking back and forth from patient to family member to patient, again, for verification of the disease history and for subtle tensions below the surface—such as the patient's fear that he may no longer be able to support his family or the family's concern that the patient should no longer be allowed to drive.

During the examination, I make use of the patient's imaging and diagnostic tests as well as the teaching aids in the exam room to educate not only the resident or fellow but also the patient and family members. I point out normal and abnormal retinal anatomy on the color photographs, optical coherence tomography images, or fluorescein angiogram images obtained during the encounter, asking family members to look over my shoulder if I know the patient cannot see well enough to appreciate the images. In the absence of retinal imaging, I often ask the family member to look through the teaching scope attached to the slit lamp as I explain to both patient and family member what I am seeing and why I am recommending a particular therapy or, more importantly, why there is no effective therapy. I sit and provide my undivided attention as I inquire if there are more questions or concerns. I repeat the plan of management, emphasizing even in circumstances where there is no effective treatment that I am still amenable to seeing the patient in the event that treatment becomes available in the future or for the sake of monitoring the other eye that has good vision or at least to provide reassurance that disease is not progressing in the affected eye. Before completing the visit, I make sure the patient and family members know that I am accessible, often by providing my card, which has my email address, or by providing my direct office line to the patient for nonurgent issues.

To listen, to educate, to intervene with treatment when I can, and to provide reassurance and a bridge to the potential for care when nothing else can be done—this has become my mission and approach to patient care, as I *communicate and collaborate* with the patient and his family.

DOI: 10.1201/9781003409373-19

Though cliché, with each year that passes, it has become more apparent to me that the practice of medicine is an art and the ability to practice medicine a privilege. Our patients are the reason we push the frontiers of discovery through clinical trials, translational research, and basic science research. When the patient is face down with a gas bubble in his eye, confident that his retina will reattach, that his macular hole will close, and that his vision will be restored, the patient spurs the physician to work harder, to think more critically, and to think more creatively. Patients' courage and resilience in the face of disease leave an indelible mark on our hearts and souls. Our patients inspire us to go beyond what we as physicians think we can accomplish while teaching us humility and compassion.

WHO ARE YOU, AND WHAT KIND OF PHYSICIAN DO YOU WANT TO BECOME?

As a first-generation American, descended from immigrant Caribbean parents, my desire to become a physician was as much an expectation as the natural evolution and intersection of interests in science, technology, and communication. If the previous generation was able to overcome the socioeconomic inertia that had firmly rooted them in a third world country and make it to America, then the current generation should certainly aspire to greatness. The universal question asked of every first-generation child by her parents is, "What do you want to be when you grow up?" The universal answer is, "A doctor." Fortunately, if the academic stars align, then as one approaches the clinical years during medical school, that which had been a preordained professional path starts to unwind, curve, and lead toward a specialty about which you are truly passionate. This rite of passage represents the recognition and acknowledgment of what kind of person you are as well as what kind of physician you want to become.

What do I mean by what type of physician you want to become? Generally, the assumption would be that I am referencing the traditional dichotomy between choosing a medical versus a surgical career in medicine. While the decision tree of pursuing medicine or surgery is a real defining point in one's medical career, the rite of passage to which I refer is the one that unifies your values with how you will practice medicine. Equally important as the scientific and clinical body of knowledge acquired by the physician through years of training for the management of disease is the manner in which a physician communicates with her patients to develop trust and to engender a therapeutic relationship that will withstand the twists and turns of managing that disease.

> *Share who you are with your patients*: Why have I shared some of the personal details of my life journey and decision to enter medicine? Like the prologue of a book for the reader, a physician's ability to share part of her personal story with her patients provides context and background and helps to establish and solidify relationships. We all lead lives outside of medicine that influence how we practice. In much the same way that physicians are trained to elicit a good social history from the patient, patients have an innate curiosity about the social histories of their doctors. Think back to how many times patients have queried their physicians. Where did you grow up? Are you married? Do you have kids? Though more directly relevant to their care, patients rarely ask "qualifying" questions. Where did you go to medical school? How well did you do? Are you board certified? Patients desire and benefit from a human connection with the person providing their care. Recognizing the inherent inequity in the physician–patient relationship, patients unconsciously seek to find common ground and common footing during a period of relative vulnerability. They want to know that their physician is a three-dimensional human being who has interests, challenges, disappointments, and triumphs outside of practicing medicine.

As stated in the introduction, as an ophthalmologist, I typically see about 40 patients during a clinic day. The template, therefore, provides for slots that are no longer than 10 minutes, with many of those slots double-booked. So, realistically, the approach to the physician sharing her story with the patient does not take place during one intense encounter characterized by a very one-sided conversation but rather over a period of time. Identify similarities that you and the patient share, and acknowledge differences as a means to laying the foundation of a relationship. Commenting on a patient's Orioles cap and then revealing that I am a Yankees fan who at one time could recite the whole lineup in the early 1980s, far from ruffling Baltimore feathers, lets the patient know that I am an aficionado of baseball and that I see him not just his disease.

Sometimes, the physician must first overcome patients' biases in order to share her story. For example, especially as a young physician and before the prevalence of the internet, I had walked into the exam room many times and experienced frank surprise that I, a black woman, am "Dr. Solomon." Some patients boldly asked at the outset if I was Jewish or married to someone who was Jewish. Others fell silent, their discomfort palpable. Without realizing it at the time, these were opportunities to show patients who I was and what kind of physician I could be. To those patients who inquired directly, I would share the very true and very funny recollection that my sixth-grade teacher, Mr. John Wickes, was grading papers while the class was working silently. All of a sudden, he began to laugh out loud from behind his desk. When classmates asked what was so funny, Mr. Wickes stated, "When patients come to see 'Dr. Solomon,' boy are they going to be surprised!" Immediately, a connection has been formed with the patient outside of the physician–patient relationship. In relaying this very true anecdote from my childhood, I have acknowledged their curiosity without being offended and showed not only that I have a good memory but also a good sense of humor. In sharing my story with the patient, I have shown him who I am and what kind of physician I am. And what approach do I assume for patients who are uncomfortable to the point of silence? In these scenarios, I reassure them with the professionalism, patience, and willingness to educate that have become my clinical trademarks. They leave the encounter knowing they are in expert hands, and I leave the door open for a more personal exchange at a future visit.

Observe the nonclinical details and meet your patients where they are: As a physician, it is paramount to recognize the person and not just the patient that is sitting in front of you. In an academic center, a patient has typically encountered multiple health care staff during his encounter, including technicians who perform the screening and testing as well as medical students, residents, and fellows, who perform the initial clinical evaluation and report to the attending physician. I am always stunned when I finally walk into the room to find that no one has acknowledged and shared that the patient is a member of the clergy, a colleague on faculty, or someone who has chosen to prominently display some artifact that reveals his identity. A simple salutation of "sister," "father," "rabbi," "officer," or "doctor" goes a long way in meeting the patient where he is. The salutation communicates respect. There is immediate reassurance that I see you, the patient, before I focus on your diseased retina. In addition, paying attention to the nonclinical details generates conversation that can put the patient at ease, apprise the physician of the patient's values, and provide a framework for building a relationship. I have one patient who during the pandemic arrived to the clinic wearing a bright red mask marked "Trump." He was gruff with staff, and other patients in the waiting room did not want to sit near him. Upon entering the room, I immediately recognized that such a bombastic display of aggression likely suggests deep-seated insecurity. This was not someone whom I would stand over while he was seated in the examination chair. Rather, I pulled up a stool next to him so that we were face to face and on the same level. In discussing his symptoms, I repeated his words and touched his knee repeatedly to emphasize understanding. He appreciated the sense of being in control of the conversation, and I was able to provide him with appropriate care. Every now and then, there is also just a pleasant and unexpected surprise from noting the nonclinical details. Years ago, while performing indirect ophthalmoscopy on a patient, I mentioned that I had never seen a Super Bowl sweatshirt and that while I was not a football fan, my husband was. I asked the patient where he got the sweatshirt. He responded that he got the sweatshirt the same place he got the Super Bowl ring, pointing to his finger. Oh, autograph please!

Follow the patient's lead and be receptive to collaboration with friends and family: In many specialties, the patient is routinely accompanied by friends or family members to the medical encounter. This is especially true in ophthalmology where patients may have vision compromised to the point of not being able to drive. In these instances, the encounter involves not only the relationship of the physician with the patient but also of the physician with the entire support group. When walking into the examination room, greet not only the patient but also acknowledge the presence of the person the patient has identified for support. Both verbal and nonverbal cues from the patient's companion can supplement and enhance the information gathered about disease progression, response to treatment, and compliance with therapy. For example, a spouse will often candidly share safety concerns when a patient has been involved in fender benders because of difficulty seeing the road at night secondary to disease progression, while the patient may not be so forthcoming. Nonverbal responses from family and friends are also important, so pay attention to the group dynamics present in the examination room. A spouse, who has been nodding in agreement with the patient's responses, may suddenly break gaze and look away when the patient is being disingenuous about his compliance with medications.

As a retina specialist, the vast majority of the patients I encounter in clinic are being assessed for age-related macular degeneration and may receive intravitreal injections to manage their disease. The assessment involves examination as well as interpretation of diagnostic imaging of the retina. I will often use the imaging, which is projected onto a large monitor, to educate not only the patient but also the companion about the disease status. The patient benefits from visualizing either the progression or regression of his disease and better understands the adjustments in therapeutic options or therapeutic frequency. The companion, who is often younger than the patient and has taken time away from work to accompany the patient, better appreciates the severity of the disease process and is more likely to remain committed to getting the visually compromised patient to the required monthly appointments. In cases where the patient is so severely visually compromised that he cannot appreciate the retinal anatomy displayed on the projected imaging, the trusted companion acts as the surrogate who can visualize the imaging and underscore to the patient, outside of the actual encounter, the importance of adherence with the therapy and of consistent follow-up. The physician's inclusion of the trusted companion during the patient's encounter can enhance the perceived quality of care, as well as forge a collaboration that will potentially benefit patient compliance and follow-up.

Make electronic charting your ally in bolstering the doctor–patient relationship: If you are like me, the introduction of the electronic medical record (EMR) was a game changer. I went from batting a thousand in terms of maintaining eye contact with my patient and demonstrating complete engagement with my physical demeanor to striking out, with my back turned to the patient as I log into the EMR and then into the imaging. To overcome this communication barrier while still meeting the required utilization metrics for EMR, I have taken to printing a short version of the electronic note that I hold in hand while I still face the patient, jotting down pertinent history and examination findings. Of course, I have to transcribe these notes into the EMR after clinic, but face time with the patient is invaluable, especially during a 5–10 minute appointment slot, and something that I am not willing to dilute because of technology. What I find to be better with the EMR than with traditional charting is the ability to flag nonclinical information about patients that facilitates my social engagement with them. As an example, in medical school, my neurology attending insisted that the handedness of patients be included in the first sentence of the history of the present illness (HPI). Students would describe the patient as a 74-year-old right-handed man. While I did not decide to become a neurologist, a light bulb did come on, as I realized that the HPI could be utilized not only as a tool to summarize and communicate the patient's initial presentation and primary medical complaint but also to remind me at future visits of his identity. So, patient Smith is not a 67-year-old woman with macular edema secondary to central retinal vein occlusion. She is a 67-year-old school principal with macular edema secondary to central retinal vein occlusion. This small phrase in the HPI personalizes the patient in a clinic of 40 or more patients and reminds me as I enter the room that I have more than just a central retinal vein occlusion sitting in the chair who may need an intravitreal injection for her macular edema. Recalling that the patient is a school principal, a photographer, planning to hike the Appalachian trail, preparing for hip surgery, the son of an established patient, prompts me during a 10-minute encounter, and while logging into the EMR, putting the indirect on my head, and turning the lights down, to ask how the school year is progressing, to inquire about the venue of the latest photography project, whether the hike has occurred, how the postsurgical rehabilitation is coming along, and to send my regards to the family member who is also my patient. This brief but focused exchange communicates to the patient that I see and am interested in all of you and not just in your disease process. In addition, as a busy clinician, this brief but rewarding exchange with patients helps me find the joy in practicing medicine every day. I sincerely enjoy chatting with my retired geologist about how he and his colleagues utilize a network that accurately predicts where and when the next earthquake will occur—and he promises to give me a call with a heads-up! I sincerely share in the joy my barely mobile patient with diabetes feels when she recounts her days as a student in Russia and how she would ski for an hour before even starting the school day. Beyond being the physician chosen to diagnose and manage their disease, I sincerely appreciate and recognize the profound privilege of being able to participate in my patients' lives–from the excitement around the birth of their first great-grandchild to the sorrow from the loss of a spouse of 70 years.

I have even found a silver lining in the annoyance of having to enter my handwritten notes into the EMR system the next day after clinic. Running the patient roster this second time and reviewing my notes will often prompt me to make a follow-up call to a patient. Sometimes the brief call is to check in on how he is feeling after an office procedure, especially if there was a significant amount of anxiety associated with undergoing the procedure. Other times, the brief call may be to follow up on a conversation during the short clinic evaluation, especially if the patient revealed some setbacks or vulnerability. Needless to say, these small gestures are tremendously reassuring to and greatly appreciated by patients. They know that their physician cares about them on multiple levels.

Leading by example sets the tone for the entire health care team: Much in the same way that care and concern can be communicated to the patient through a combination of verbal and nonverbal cues, the physician's interaction with her patients also sets the tone for how the health care team will provide service to the patient during the encounter. For example, I wear scrubs and comfortable shoes to clinic each day not only because of the need to perform numerous procedures that involve the application of betadine but also because I choose to help patients in and out of wheelchairs and examination chairs, bending low to adjust footrests and to raise and lower adjustable steps. Given time constraints and the number of patients that need to be evaluated during a single clinic, I would be much more efficient if I passed this duty off to another member of the care team and had the patient wait for assistance after I left the room. However, in extending this basic courtesy to the patient, what I have found is that, after a few iterations, the medical student or trainee present that day in clinic begins to model my behavior. They take the patient's cane and place it against the wall for him after he transitions to the examination chair. They bring the wheelchair back into the examination room to minimize the distance the patient must walk and assist me in safeguarding the patient transfer from the examination chair. They offer to escort a patient with low vision to the lobby to facilitate scheduling an appointment and to locate transportation services that may already be waiting. Without having to verbalize expectations and preferences for how patients should be treated, staff and trainees adopt the behavior that they see me modeling.

Similarly, staff hear my conversations over multiple visits with patients and also begin to develop a rapport with the patient. During the screening process with the technician or before I enter the room for the APP who will assist me with a procedure, I will often overhear part of the conversation between the patient and staff member. Frequently, the conversation is an extension of the "social themes" they have heard me discuss with the patient in the past and as noted in the HPI. Staff may thus inquire about a patient's recent trip to attend a grandchild's graduation or extend congratulations on the milestone wedding anniversary celebrated since the last clinic visit. In addition to receiving top-notch care, patients are appreciative of the attitude and support of the entire health care team who collaborate to make the encounter an excellent experience.

Set up a path for accessibility and not a roadblock: Part of the challenge of practicing medicine is recognizing the level of care that can be provided for each patient. Of course, it is tremendously gratifying when, during the initial encounter, a definitive diagnosis can be made and a course charted to deliver immediate and efficient therapeutic intervention to stop disease progression. For example, the satisfaction in repairing a patient's macula-on retinal detachment that was picked up during clinic and fixed with surgical intervention, thereby saving his reading vision, never grows old. However, a large part of my practice also consists of patients with atrophic age-related macular degeneration, which slowly compromises reading vision and for which there is no cure. These patients are monitored for the rare instance in which neovascular leakage also occurs, at which time therapeutic intervention can be offered. Otherwise, a large part of their care is palliative and oriented toward keeping them in the health care system in the event an appropriate clinical trial becomes available that may offer some potential for therapeutic benefit. Like the patient who will clearly benefit from surgical intervention, it is just as important to be accessible and to emulate an all-in attitude with patients for whom there is currently no therapeutic intervention. The patients for whom I can offer nothing to stop their disease progression have been some of the most compliant with follow-up, often driving great distances to remain in my practice, waiting hours to be seen while I perform procedures in clinic, simply to hear me say that every-thing is stable with their examination. Over the years, I have come to under-stand that the patient, realizing that I am limited by what I can offer medically, values what I can offer—my attention, compassion, willingness to share scientific updates in the field, and promise not to dismiss or abandon them. Patients have my professional email address, which is on my business card. I respond to their queries about laymen's articles sent by relatives describing a potential new therapy for their condition and weigh in, offering an informed medical perspective. My patients know that I will intervene with treatment when possible and provide reassurance and a bridge to the potential for care when nothing else can be done.

By extension of the way I practice, my team, from front desk patient service coordinator to APP to administrative assistant, knows that I will always accept an add-on to clinic and that no patient's concern is dismissed, even if the patient has traditionally been someone for whom there is no available therapy. My adminis-trative assistant copies me in addition to sending an urgent message to the retina fellow, as she knows that I will respond to the patient if available. The retina fellow knows that if I am already on the floor seeing patients that I will want to see any emergency walk-in who is also my patient. Patients always pay compliments about how my team has followed up with them in making their next appointment, even though the front desk was closed when they left following their previous visit. They compliment us about how accommodating staff were allowing them to come earlier or later the same day for a scheduled appointment because of a conflict related to seeing another medical provider. In other words, my staff appreciate and promul-gate my preference for building a path to accessibility as opposed to presenting a roadblock when it comes to providing care to patients.

CONCLUSION

In my daily interactions with patients, I strive to be the physician from whom I would want to receive care. Beyond possessing the basic staples of superior medical fund of knowledge and currency with scientific developments in the field, that physician ought to communicate respect, compassion, consideration, flexibility, patience, and sincere humanity in an evolving relationship with her patients. She should acknowl-edge the important role that family and caretakers play in the delivery of care to her patients and value educating them, as well, about the disease process to solidify that collaboration. Finally, in addition to sharing her professional expertise with her patients, she should share part of herself. In that reciprocal exchange with her patients, she will find the joy of medicine is renewed.

20 Biosocial Medicine

Ralph I. Horwitz and Mark R. Cullen

All of medicine, its research, practice, and ethics, is directed to the care of the individual patient. The most surprising fact of that sentence is the need to write it. When a physician is engaged in diagnosis, or estimating prognosis, or selecting and monitoring treatment, her gaze is always focused on the patient at hand. Indeed, so embedded has that tradition been in medicine that we often quote medicine's most celebrated physicians for their reference to the care of the individual patient. Hippocrates, for example, wrote 2500 years ago, "It is more important to know what sort of patient has a disease than what sort of disease a patient has" [1]. Osler remarked, "To study the phenomena of disease without books is to sail an uncharted sea, while to study books without patients is not to go to sea at all" [2]. And, famously, Francis Peabody commented, "The secret to the care of the patient is caring for the patient" [3].

It is not just the humanistic features of medical practice that are focused on the individual patient. The way that physicians came to analyze the patient's clinical problem was tightly structured around the presenting complaints, physical diagnosis, and laboratory findings found uniquely in that patient. The case-based approach to clinical reasoning reinforced the patient focus. The Clinicopathologic Conference (CPC), introduced by Richard Cabot in the early 1900s, exemplified this approach [4]. In the CPC, a presenter describes a patient who is unknown to the discussant of the case. The discussant, usually a clinical expert, provides an analysis that accounts for the patient's clinical illness, physical findings, and laboratory abnormalities. Differential diagnoses are proposed by the expert discussant and narrowed with a consideration of possible diagnoses rather than a single diagnosis. At the conclusion of the discussion, the clinician typically selects from among the candidate diagnoses and proposes a final diagnosis. The pathologist then serves as the arbiter of clinical truth with an authoritative diagnosis based on examination of tissue from the patient.

Clinical research, too, has traditionally focused on the individual patient studied as an intact person. Physician scientists, like Fuller Albright, elucidated the role of the parathyroid glands and metabolic bone disease by observing patients with disorders of bone metabolism [5]; George Minot and William Murphy found that a deficiency of vitamin B_{12} was the cause of pernicious anemia and could be cured by eating abundant amounts of liver [6]; and Banting and Best isolated the hormone, insulin, that transformed the treatment of diabetes [7]. In each of these examples, and many more like them, physicians referred to "experiments of nature," where disorders of biology in an individual patient provided the opportunity for new insights into disease pathogenesis and treatment.

The modern era of therapeutics began when purified chemicals, rather than crude extracts, became the standard drugs. Morphine, the active ingredient in the plant opium, and digoxin, the chemical purified from the plant *Digitalis lanata*, were early examples. Penicillin was recognized as the active ingredient in the penicillium mold in 1928, but it took the impetus of World War II to accelerate production of the antibiotic. Soon thereafter, Gertrude Elion and George Hitchings discovered the purine drugs that act to suppress the immune system, such as azathioprine; James Black discovered beta blockers, such as propranolol; and Sir David Jack developed the first inhaled beta-2 adrenergic agonist for asthma.

DOI: 10.1201/9781003409373-20

RISE OF POPULATION SCIENCE

How would we know whether these new medicines would do more harm than good for sick patients? To answer these questions, medicine turned away from its traditional focus on the individual patient and employed approaches that estimated the benefits of treatments for *groups* of patients. The randomized controlled trial (RCT), developed in agriculture by R. A. Fisher [8], was adapted for medicine by Austin Bradford Hill to assess whether a new treatment was better *on average* than no treatment or the current standard of care [9].

The new method was used successfully in several RCTs in the late 1940s to test therapies for tuberculosis. Before long, RCTs were being readily adopted by academic investigators and especially pharmaceutical companies happy to have a method to demonstrate the safety and effectiveness of new drugs that had the endorsement of the Food and Drug Administration. The adoption of the RCT method had another notable effect: it signaled that there were significant knowledge gaps in medicine that could not be filled by the authoritative judgments of expert clinicians but rather needed the quantitative evidence that the RCT could provide.

The use of statistics to describe population level patterns of event occurrence had its antecedents hundreds of years ago, although it was not refined for clinical use until recently. John Graunt in 1661 surprised his colleagues when he made an unexpected discovery. Previous to Graunt's work, deaths in a community were understood as individual experiences, and there was no appreciation of the patterns of occurrence. In any given community of 500 persons, villagers knew that their neighbor, John, had died from fever, William from a fall, and Mary after she was kicked in the head by a mule. In his treatise, *Natural and Political Observations Made upon the Bills of Mortality,* Graunt showed he could predict the number of villagers who would die in the coming year of fever, falls, and kicks from a mule by counting how many had occurred in previous years. Graunt could not tell who would die from these conditions, but he could accurately estimate their subsequent numbers in the population [10].

Graunt's work laid the foundation for an understanding of the power of population-level data. Early probability theory and statistics soon followed and were systematized in the 19th century by social and mathematical scientists. It wasn't long before physicians were using statistics to assess the possible superiority of different therapies. Controversy over this approach reached a boiling point when a French surgeon, Jean Civiale, made claims based on statistics for the superiority of a new method to extract stones from the bladder using a crude cystoscope rather than the more widely used technique of surgically cutting to remove the stones, known as lithotomy. His numerical analysis showed that the success rate with his cystoscope was 98% compared to 78% with the open lithotomy approach. His evidence and claims attracted affluent patients and members of the aristocracy who previously would have seen surgeons who performed open operations [11].

POISSON VERSUS BERNARD

Civiale's claims were made at a time when there was growing interest in European society with the collection of numerical information about many areas of society. In Paris, the increasing focus on hospital-based methods of clinical instruction and patient care placed an emphasis on clinical observations, autopsy, and especially the analysis of statistical data, what the eminent French clinician Pierre-Charles Alexandre Louis famously referred to as the "numerical method" [12]. In response to the controversy over Civiale's claims, the French Academy of Science established a commission to assess not simply his claims but also to adjudicate the role of statistics in the research that would guide the practice of medicine. To lead the commission, the Academy called upon one of its most revered members and leading mathematicians, Simeon Poisson.

Under Poisson's leadership, the commission found numerous reasons to criticize the application of the "calculus" to medicine, but their main objection was a fundamental concern. The commission argued that the clinical practice of medicine was concerned with the diagnosis and treatment of a single individual who would present with a set of symptoms, physical signs and life circumstances that were unique to that individual. Poisson wrote that this was in direct contrast to what occurs in statistics, where "the first task is to lose sight of the individual seen in isolation, to consider him only as a fraction of the species. He must be stripped of his individuality so as to eliminate anything accidental that his individuality might introduce into the issue at hand. . . . [I]t is altogether different in the domain of medicine" [13].

Poisson's report was a clarion call in defense of the individual focus in medicine and a repudiation of the numerical method. No physician scientist of that era was more critical of the use of average results in groups of patients to support the cause or treatment of disease than Claude Bernard, the leading French physiologist. Bernard wrote [14]:

A great surgeon performs operations for stone; later he makes a statistical summary . . . and concludes from these statistics that the mortality law for this operation is two out of five. Well, I say that this ratio means literally nothing scientifically. . . . What really should be done, instead of gathering facts empirically, is to study them more accurately, each in its special determinism. We must study cases of death with great care and try to discover in them the cause of mortal accidents so as to master the cause and avoid the accidents.

Bernard ardently argued that disease was caused by a chain of events that accounted for the pathogenesis of disease and that if only we knew all the links in the chain, we could be certain both of the cause of disease and its treatment.

The view espoused by Bernard was still prevalent in the minds of many physicians when the RCT was introduced and even after it became widely accepted as the gold standard for evaluating the effectiveness of treatment. The priority given to the RCT also contributed to the rapid embrace of evidence-based medicine (EBM), an approach to evidence evaluation that placed RCTs at the top of a research hierarchy. But even as EBM was proliferating, many of the scientists who had pioneered the methods, including Austin Bradford Hill and John Tukey, were lamenting that RCTs and other group-based averages could tell you whether a treatment would work on average but not whether it would help an individual patient.

For example, in a famous paper in the journal *Science*, John Tukey wrote [15]:

It is a difficult task to drive the nearly incompatible two-horse team: On the one hand, knowledge of a most carefully evaluated kind wherever in particular questions of multiplicity are faced up to, and on the other hand, informed professional opinion, where impressions gained from statistically inadequate numbers of cases often, and so far as we can see, should control the treatment of individual patients. The same physician or surgeon must be concerned with both what is his knowledge and what is his informed professional opinion as part of treating a single patient. I wish I understood better how to help in this essentially ambivalent task.

TRANSLATIONAL SCIENCE INSPIRES BIOSOCIAL MEDICINE

The situation might have remained stuck were it not for help from an unlikely source. The emergence of "translational medicine" called for a more robust bench-to-bedside road map to bring the advances made possible by molecular and genomic medicine to clinical care. This new translational medicine approach enabled the development of targeted therapies and more accurate prediction of the patient's clinical trajectory with a disease and was ushered in with studies of diffuse large B-cell lymphoma in which gene expression profiling identified molecular subtypes of the disease with distinct prognoses [16].

The strategy was initially referred to as personalized medicine, but that term was later replaced with precision medicine. An unexpected benefit of precision medicine was to diminish the emphasis on average results in populations and instead return the focus to the patient at hand, reasoning once again about the individual patient using an individually tailored approach, albeit largely molecular and genomic.

Indeed, proponents of precision medicine heralded it as rejecting the one-size-fits-all approach of the RCT and evidence-based medicine. Precision medicine offered another underappreciated but critical innovation in knowledge generation in medicine: it sought to exploit the *variability* in medicine rather than the *average*. Rather than designing treatments based on similarities, precision medicine sought to design treatments based on differences. The focus of those differences, however, was almost exclusively the molecular and genomic differences that offered targets for drug development. Missing from the precision medicine revival were the differences in lived experience that were also fundamental contributions to our biological and biographical distinctiveness.

These conditions are part of the individual's lived experience, their biography, that emerges from the social and environmental conditions in which they live and from how they experience those conditions. *Biosocial Medicine* is focused on the lived experience of the individual and not on social categories, social ranks, or social determinants, except as they relate to the specific set of experiences in a person's life [17].

The biography of a person includes her biology in addition to her genetic predisposition to illness, any trauma occurring during development or later in life, economic circumstances, and experiences as diverse as discrimination, joy, happiness, and meaning in life. Some of these factors are in the biological body (genetic or physiological, for example), some involve the body's relationship to its physical or social context, and some relate to the affective experience of the person. The key point is that all these considerations are central to Biosocial Medicine because they are experienced by the individual and not a group or population.

We do not diminish the practice of medicine when we recognize that it is an "applied science" where the rules and principles of the science must be understood in relation to the care of one particular patient. It is true that we do not have rules or principles to guide causal inference at the level of the individual. But causal inference is less central to the approach of Biosocial Medicine than the emphasis on prediction to better anticipate the clinical trajectory of our patient. It is also true that we do not currently know the medically relevant aspects of a person's biography that are essential to an understanding of both health and disease in a particular individual.

Research over the past several decades, however, has begun to identify *Biosocial Mechanisms* that connect the patient's lived experience to her biology. Questions such as "How does social class get under the skin?" or "How does grief cause a heart attack?" begin to direct our attention to these most fundamental considerations in connecting the patient's external world, perception of experience, and internal biology. There are many biosocial mechanisms, but it is useful to consider one that has become an important focus of research to understand how a patient's biography interacts with biology to influence both the risk for disease and the response to treatment. The Biosocial Mechanism of allostasis links stress to disease in ways that explain how biology and biography are intertwined.

The understanding of the impact of individual level stress on health and disease has been enabled by a major conceptual advance in stress-related research. Allostasis, a new model of physiological regulation that complements the traditional homeostasis theory, was proposed by Sterling and Eyer in 1988 [18]. Allostasis suggests that physiological stability is achieved through variation and is marked by predictive regulation that is orchestrated by the brain. When allostasis cannot be maintained, allostatic load occurs. Allostatic load refers to the wear and tear on the body that accumulates as the individual is exposed to either repeated or chronic stress. When the individual is unable to recover to baseline from these stresses, allostatic load moves into a state of allostatic overload, a condition that often requires medical intervention to manage [19].

It is this focus on the individual's level of stress and the person's response that separates allostatic load from a population level measure of distress or disadvantage. For example, the popular Adverse Childhood Experience (ACE) scoring scale was developed using ten categories of adverse events: physical, sexual, or psychological abuse; emotional or physical neglect; divorce; mental illness; substance abuse; domestic violence; and criminality among household members. After a survey of over 17,000 subjects, the investigators determined a threshold for the sum of experiences that was associated with a high population level risk for later adverse health effects [20]. But a single event, perceived as especially traumatic, might have long-term adverse effects in one individual, even while scoring low on a population measure like ACEs. Individual experience, not population risk, is most salient for understanding the effects of these life events on our patients as the individual.

There are other important Biosocial Mechanisms. Epigenetics is emerging as a major mechanism for understanding how the external environment broadly affects the internal physiology and risk for disease of individuals. Insight into this mechanism came from the Dutch Famine study, a tragic and unplanned experiment in human health and disease. In 1944, the Nazis punished the Netherlands by imposing a total food blockade that lasted until the Dutch were liberated by the Allies in May 1945. During that time, many women carried pregnancies while experiencing severe food deprivation, and the children of these women were found to have increased rates of diabetes, obesity, and hypertension. Subsequent research explained this phenomenon by demonstrating that children who were in utero during the famine had certain genes silenced, and those genes remained silenced throughout their life [21].

Another example of the role of epigenetics comes from elegant fruit fly studies on the effects of social isolation. Employing a creative scientific approach, investigators used the fruit fly, *Drosophila melanogaster,* to explore the effects of solitude on behavior and biology. Flies were kept in groups or in isolation either for an acute interval (1–3 days) or a chronic period (5–7 days). Flies kept in groups behaved normally, but flies kept in social isolation had impaired sleep and demonstrated overeating. Remarkably, the investigators were able to identify 214 genes from these flies whose expression had changed as a result of the social isolation, and many of these genes were known to be associated with biological pathways that influence patterns of sleep. The biography of the flies had altered their biology [22].

BIOSOCIAL SCIENCE OF EVERYDAY LIFE

For all the success of precision medicine and for all the insights it provides into disease mechanisms, precision medicine's technological advances have failed to explain the cause and progression of most diseases. With the possible exception of single gene disorders, biology alone fails to account for the extraordinary interindividual variation in the risk for disease, the clinical trajectories of disease after it has developed, or the inescapable variation in response to effective treatments. The explanatory failure of biology is not limited to a single class of disease or to diseases in a certain organ system. It is a feature of the current state of medical knowledge that variation in disease risk and treatment response is beyond the capability of our current biological theories.

A possible reason for this failure may be the absence of biography—an individual's lived experience—from the scientific theory used to understand health and disease. Medicine is best practiced not solely as a biological science or as some kind of humanistic art but rather as an integration of biology and biography. In fact, this integration may better explain the many everyday life experiences that are ignored in the current conventional practice of medicine.

In the following sections, we illustrate the biology and biography of everyday life.

BIOLOGY OF FEAR

Biology of Fear: A 75-year-old woman awoke in the middle of the night after hearing a loud crash. Noticing that her husband was no longer in their bed, she got up and walked into the hallway where she found him lying on the floor unresponsive. She cried out thinking he was dead, and, when she did, she felt an overwhelming sensation of fear, followed immediately by chest pain that radiated to her back and was accompanied by shortness of breath. After arriving at the emergency department, she was given nitroglycerin with improvement in her chest pain. A cardiac catheterization showed normal coronary arteries, and a cardiac ultrasound showed multiple regional wall motion abnormalities including an akinetic apex and a newly reduced ejection fraction. The patient was diagnosed with Takotsubo cardiomyopathy [23].

The exact mechanism of this syndrome is unknown. What is known is that patients are free of the typical coronary artery obstructions associated with heart attacks. Instead, it is believed that overwhelming fear stimulates a surge of catecholamine that stuns the myocardium and leads to a drastically reduced left ventricular ejection fraction. Takotsubo is estimated to cause up to 7% of sudden cardiac admissions, and in some circumstances, it is even more frequent. For example, after a major earthquake in Japan in 2004, researchers reported a 24-fold increase in Takotsubo cases within just four weeks. A recent Ohio study reported a fourfold increase in Takotsubo during the Covid-19 pandemic.

Biology of Grief: Many of us are familiar with the following anecdote: an older couple has been together for many decades when one spouse dies; within a short time thereafter, even though the other spouse was healthy, they die as well. These stories of death occurring in persons experiencing prolonged grief are common. Parents who lose a child in war have a higher risk of death in the following year. So, too, do parents whose child is killed by gun violence or who dies from illness or accident. Why? How does grief get under the skin and lead to premature death in the grieving individual?

Recent research has shed light on the role that living with grief has on the individual's biology. Studies have shown that older mourners, compared to matched nonbereaved peers, had substantially reduced neutrophil function and elevated cortisol levels [24]. That is not the only way that grief damages the biological body. Grief is noted to aggravate physical pain [25] and increase blood pressure and clotting factors [26].

The magnitude of the experience of grief on health and well-being is remarkable. A study in 2012 [27] reported that a person's risk of a heart attack or stroke increased 21 times in the 24 hours that followed the death of a loved one and that the risk remains elevated for a prolonged period [27]. None of these results were explained by the possibly confounding effects of shared lifestyle or risk factors. The frequency of bereavement generally makes these results even more compelling. Among people at least 65 years old, 45% of women and 15% of men will become widowed with the death of their spouse. Covid-19 has, tragically, created an epidemic of grief.

We could write a book (and many have) on all the tragedies of life that create adverse effects on the body and human health. Osler said that all of life's tragedies are arterial [28]. But many of these adverse life experiences may affect other systems: endocrine, neurological, inflammatory, gastrointestinal, and so on. We haven't yet touched on job loss, divorce, pandemics, terminal illness, loneliness, and more. They too create experiences of grief and mourning, although differently than the death of a loved one. But let's turn our attention to another set of life's experiences: happy outcomes. How do they affect health?

Feeling Good versus Feeling Purpose: Feelings like gratitude, amusement, inspiration, and joy are often referred to by psychologists who study positive emotions as "hedonic" happiness. Hedonic happiness is experienced as pleasure (and pain avoidance) and exists along with another type, referred to as "eudaimonic" happiness. Many scales exist to measure hedonic happiness and include features of positive and negative affect and life satisfaction. Eudaimonic happiness is more complex. The main categories of eudaimonia are autonomy, mastery, positive relationships with others, and a sense of purpose or meaning in life.

An array of studies has suggested strong correlates between happiness and better health. But how might this occur? Investigators have sought to understand the biologic pathways that lead from happiness to health in a similar manner in which we study how stress causes disease or how persistent grief increases mortality. In one study, researchers gave questionnaires to 80 healthy volunteers and categorized their responses according to whether they reported hedonic happiness or eudaimonic purpose in life. The investigators then measured a suite of genes known as conserved transcriptional response to adversity (CTRA) that were indicators of both the degree of inflammatory and antiviral (interferon) genes that were activated. The subjects with hedonia were "happier" on the questionnaires but had worse immune profiles. A similar study was carried out on males working in a large Japanese corporation infamous for long hours and stressful work. The workers in the company who reported that they were fulfilled by their work showed a 42% better gene expression profile than workers who scored low on eudaimonia [29].

Biology and Culture: The impact on gene expression by how we live was assessed for Moroccan Amazighs, a group with distinct geographies with different cultural lifestyles such as desert nomadic, mountain agrarian, and coastal urban. Although genome-wide polymorphism analyses found evidence for limited genetic differentiation, as much as one-third of the differences in leukocyte transcriptome differentiation was attributable to differences among regions. The authors noted that there was a strong region-based variation in genome-wide expression that was associated with lifestyle issues, diet, and related features, suggesting that culture plays a prominent role (along with genetic divergence) in accounting for gene expression variation [30].

Many diseases, including asthma, obesity, and diabetes, are occurring at near epidemic rates in many countries as they transition from traditional lifestyles to more urban living lifestyles. For individuals, gene expression becomes intimately associated with how and where they live, from diet and exercise—which have been the predominant research focus—to stress, interpersonal conflict, and a loss of cultural anchors that give life purpose and ultimately are far more likely to explain the clinical observations.

PRACTICE OF BIOSOCIAL MEDICINE

Medicine is the application of biology and biography to the care of an individual patient. Scientific advances in the biology of the individual patient are enabling a form of precision, or personalized, medicine that promises to improve the care of the individual patient. But the biography of the patient can no longer be relegated to the art of medicine as understood by Osler and Peabody.

Consider what confronts the practice of medicine in the current era. The population is aging, and with that increase in elderly patients is the inevitable increase in patients with many comorbid diseases. Polypharmacy, neurodegenerative conditions like Alzheimer's dementia, and more advanced chronic disorders such as heart failure with preserved ejection fraction have increased the complexity of medical care. We need a new understanding of not just a single disease but of how diseases interact and are affected in concert with the many medicines our patients are taking.

Scientific advances in the biography of medicine are critical if precision medicine is to achieve its promise. This new focus on Biosocial Medicine is needed to discover novel explanations in the complex experiences of everyday life. Reductionist science has unraveled many disease pathways and continues to advance our understanding of human biology. But these old methods of reductionist biology alone cannot account for the new model of disease pathogenesis and Biosocial Medicine that necessarily requires a holistic integration of biology with biography.

CONCLUDING COMMENTS

Biosocial Medicine has the opportunity to transform both the science and practice of clinical medicine, while also redefining the relationship of physicians to patients. We must act now or face the possibility that medical research and care will be damaged for years to come. Large language models (LLMs) that are being developed now to guide clinical practice ignore the distinctive life experiences of patients that affect their disease risk and treatment responsiveness. Fortunately, those same LLMs can be employed to capture the patient's biography and integrate it with biology.

In the absence of Biosocial Medicine, it is likely we will cement in place an approach to the science and practice of medicine that neglects the individual patient in favor of evidence generation that is population based. It is ironic that this is happening now when genomic and molecular data enable personalized (or precision) biological signatures for each patient that guide treatment decisions. But a truly distinctive personalized patient signature requires integrating the stresses and experiences of patients that modify their disease risk and response to treatment.

The study of biosocial pathogenesis is challenging because biography remains largely undefined, in part because of the vast range, variation, and temporal complexity of individual experiences. Therefore, developing new biosocial theories is a conceptual and inferential challenge that will require a transdisciplinary approach drawing widely from biomedical, computational, and social science disciplines. Biomedicine can no longer afford to relegate nonbiological factors to mere covariates. A new integrated framework of Biosocial Medicine is the paradigm shift needed to unravel the true causes of many of the most perplexing human diseases.

How should clinicians in practice respond to this challenge of Biosocial Medicine? The good news is that high-quality medical care already includes attention to a patient's biography. Physicians typically learn about their patient's lives as a way to understand their social context and its effects on getting to the office, adhering to prescriptions, or accessing medical care. What is lacking is the scientific evidence that elucidates how biography interacts with biology in ways that are pertinent to the diagnosis, treatment selection, and management of the patient. That evidence is coming, but it is not here yet.

Three critical developments are converging to make this the right time for Biosocial Medicine. First, a trove of biographical data is now extant in the digital exhaust of our lives, including but not limited to social media. Combined with vast data stores of clinical, genomic, imaging, sensor, microbiome, proteomic, epigenomic, environmental, and other data available at the granularity of the individual, we are poised to be able to cross-reference biology and biography as never before.

Second, advances in machine learning and causal reasoning are providing increasingly powerful tools for making sense of the complex, multidimensional, time-varying, qualitative, and quantitative data that is biography. Biosocial pathogenesis will leverage ongoing public investment in artificial intelligence and computation in areas such as natural language processing, multimodal in silico modeling, uncertainty reasoning, and temporal reasoning. LLMs fueled by advances in artificial intelligence are beginning to alter our understanding of what may be possible with these new tools. Finally, important advances have occurred in conceptualizing and understanding the role of social determinants of health. For example, the National Academy of Medicine proposed 12 social and behavioral measures (e.g., education, social isolation, financial strain) that should be routinely included in electronic health records. In the field of geography, scholars have recently proposed a framework for investigating the relationship between the body and its environment that emphasizes how affective, hard-to-capture features of lived experience may explain different health outcomes [31].

Now is the time to leverage the large-scale availability of biography in computable form, advances in machine learning and causal inference, and the deepening appreciation of and commitment to incorporating social determinants into precision medicine to braid together a new medical science that centers our humanity with our bodies to understand health and disease more deeply.

REFERENCES

1. John M. HSR Proceedings in Intensive Care and Cardiovascular Anesthesia. 2013;5(1):52–58.
2. Osler W Sir. Books and men. Boston Med Surg J. 1901;144:60–61.
3. Peabody FW. JAMA. 1927;88(12):877–882. doi:10.1001/jama.1927.02680380001001.
4. Horwitz RI, Lobitz G, Mawn M, Conroy AH, Cullen MR, Sim I, Singer BH. Biosocial medicine: Biology, biography, and the tailored care of the patient. SSM Popul Health. 2021;15:100863. doi: 10.1016/j.ssmph.2021.
5. Albright F, Smith PH, Richardson AM. Postmenopausal osteoporosis: Its clinical features. JAMA. 1941;116(22):2465–2474. doi:10.1001/jama.1941.02820220007002
6. Scott JM, Molloy AM. The discovery of vitamin B(12). Ann Nutr Metab. 2012;61(3):239–245. doi: 10.1159/000343114.
7. Banting FG. An address on diabetes and insulin: Being the Nobel lecture delivered at Stockholm September 15th 1925. Can Med Association J. 1926;16(3):221–232.
8. Armitage P. Fisher, Bradford Hill, and randomization. Int J Epidemiol. 2003;32(6):925–928.
9. Marshall G, Blacklock JS, Cameron C, Capon NB, Cruickshank R, Gaddis JH, Heaf F, Hill AB, Houghton L, Hoyle J, Raistrick H. Streptomycin treatment of tuberculous meningitis. Lancet. 1948;254:582–596.
10. Boyce N. Bills of Mortality: Tracking disease in early modern London. Lancet. 2020;395(10231):1186–1187.
11. Herr HW. Civiale, stones and statistics: The dawn of evidence-based medicine. BJU Int. 2009;104(3):300–302. doi: 10.1111/j.1464-410X.2009.08529.x.
12. Shimkin MS. The numerical method in therapeutic medicine: 43d James M. Anders Lecture. Public Health Rep (1896–1970). 1964;79(1):1–12. doi:10.2307/4592038.
13. Matthews JR. Commentary: The Paris Academy of Science report on Jean Civiale's statistical research and the 19th century background to evidence-based medicine. Int J Epidemiol 2001;30(6):1249–1250. doi: 10.1093/ije/30.6.1249.

14. Bernard C. An Introduction to the Study of Experimental Medicine (Dover ed. 1957; originally published in 1865; first English translation by Henry Copley Greene, published by New York, NY: Macmillan and Company, 1927).
15. Tukey JW. Some thoughts on clinical trials, especially problems of multiplicity. Science. 1977;198:679–684.
16. Alizadeh AA, Eisen MB, Davis RE, Ma C, Lossos IS, Rosenwald A, Boldrick JC, Sabet H, Tran T, Yu X, Powell JI, Yang L, Marti GE, Moore T, Hudson J Jr, Lu L, Lewis DB, Tibshirani R, Sherlock G, Chan WC, Greiner TC, Weisenburger DD, Armitage JO, Warnke R, Levy R, Wilson W, Grever MR, Byrd JC, Botstein D, Brown PO, Staudt LM. Distinct types of diffuse large B-cell lymphoma identified by gene expression profiling. Nature. 2000;403(6769):503–511. doi: 10.1038/35000501.
17. Lobitz G, Armstrong K, Concato J, Singer BH, Horwitz RI. The biological and biographical basis of precision medicine. Psychother Psychosom. 2019;88(6):333–340. doi: 10.1159/000502486.
18. Sterling P, Eyer J. Allostasis: A new paradigm to explain arousal pathology. In Fisher S, Reason J (Eds.), Handbook of Life Stress, Cognition and Health. Hoboken, NJ: John Wiley & Sons; 1988:629–649.
19. Horwitz RI, Singer BH. Clinimetrics and allostatic load. Psychother Psychosom. 2023;92(5):283–286. doi: 10.1159/000534257.
20. Felitti VJ, Anda RF, Nordenberg D, Williamson DF, Spitz AM, Edwards V, Koss MP, Marks JS. Relationship of childhood abuse and household dysfunction to many of the leading causes of death in adults. The Adverse Childhood Experiences (ACE) study. Am J Prev Med. 1998;14(4):245–258. doi: 10.1016/s0749-3797(98)00017-8.
21. Horwitz RI, Singer BH, Hayes-Conroy A, Cullen MR, Mawn M, Colella K, Sim I. Biosocial pathogenesis. Psychother Psychosom. 2022;91(2):73–77. doi: 10.1159/000521567.
22. Kerrigan D, Dwyer K. Brown Sound: (Almost) Scared to Death by Takotsubo Cardiomyopathy. Brown Emergency Medicine Blog, 2021.
23. Vitlic A, Khanfer R, Lord JM, Carroll D, Phillips AC. Bereavement reduces neutrophil oxidative burst only in older adults: Role of the HPA axis and immune senescence. Immun Ageing. 2014;11:13. doi: 10.1186/1742-4933-11-13.
24. Bradbeer M, Helme RD, Yong H-H, Kendig HL, Gibson SJ. Widowhood and other demographic associations of pain in independent older people. Clin J Pain. 2003;19:247–254.
25. Buckley T, Sunari D, Marshall A, Bartrop R, McKinley S, Tofler G. Physiological correlates of bereavement and the impact of bereavement interventions. Dialog Clin Neurosci. 2012;14(2):129–139. doi: 10.31887/DCNS.2012.14.2/tbuckley
26. Mostofsky E, Maclure M, Sherwood JB, Tofler GH, Muller JE, Mittleman MA. Risk of acute myocardial infarction after the death of a significant person in one's life: The Determinants of Myocardial Infarction Onset Study. Circulation. 2012;125(3):491–496. doi: 10.1161/CIRCULATIONAHA.111.061770.
27. Carey IM, Shah SM, DeWilde S, Harris T, Victor CR, Cook DG. Increased risk of acute cardiovascular events after partner bereavement: A matched cohort study. JAMA Intern Med. 2014;174(4):598–605. doi:10.1001/jamainternmed.2013.14558.
28. Silverman ME, Murray TJ, Bryan CS, eds. The Quotable Osler. Philadelphia, PA: American College of Physicians; 2003:114.
29. Cole SW, Levine ME, Arevalo JM, Ma J, Weir DR, Crimmins EM. Loneliness, eudaimonia, and the human conserved transcriptional response to adversity. Psychoneuroendocrinology. 2015;62:11–17. doi: 10.1016/j.psyneuen.2015.07.001.
30. Idaghdour Y, Storey JD, Jadallah SJ, Gibson G. A genome-wide gene expression signature of environmental geography in leukocytes of Moroccan Amazighs. PLoS Genet. 2008;4(4):e1000052. doi: 10.1371/journal.pgen.10000529
31. Shantz, E., & Elliott, S. J. (2021). From social determinants to social epigenetics: Health geographies of chronic disease. *Health & Place*, 69, 102561.

21 Professionalism and Ethics in Medicine

Robert G. Lahita

PROFESSIONALISM

It is frequently said that medicine is a "noble" profession, even a calling beyond just a job. The reason for this righteous label is the fact that the cornerstones of the medical profession are professionalism and ethical behavior. People tell their doctors things they would never tell their lawyers, investment advisors, or even religious leaders in their communities. As physicians, we care for people at some of the worst times in their lives, and we may often be responsible for delivering bad news. Patients rely on our professional knowledge and expertise, and we seek to maintain each patient's well-being and trust. We do this for our fellow human beings regardless of political views, socioeconomic background, or any other individual characteristics of each patient. Our job is to keep the patient alive and well and, if possible, free of pain and discomfort [1, 2]. Medicine should, at all times, be dedicated to the concept of *"pro bono humani generis"* (for the good of the human race), the motto that, many years ago, was on my Rockefeller lab coat throughout my fellowship training.

Health care providers must be well trained and have the necessary knowledge, skills, and abilities to provide high-quality care, regardless of external conditions. Emergency department physicians in large urban hospitals or physicians on the front lines of battle in field hospitals learn to make good with limited resources, all the while keeping up-to-date with the latest medical advances and using that knowledge with confidence.

Professionalism may be difficult for some physicians. Monitoring integrity may be challenging, especially when politics or financial status influence medical care. We must hold honesty, transparency, and ethical conduct as crucial for medical practice, and we must, at all times, prioritize the patient's interests, maintain confidentiality, and avoid conflicts of interest. This is not always possible, and physicians face challenges when a practice has financial interests or a bottom line to maintain. Moral principles should be established and enhanced by medical schools prior to a student's graduation and further reinforced during residency training.

Many medical schools have students recite the Hippocratic Oath at graduation, an explicit expression of the ethical duties carried by physicians. Students are also meant to learn ethical and professional behavior while observing the work of residents, fellows, and more senior clinicians in the hospital and in the clinic. One hopes that examples of integrity, protection of patient privacy, and an overall respect for a patient's time are organically plentiful, though this is not always a guarantee. I would argue strongly that professional codes of conduct should be taught early in the young doctor's education; just as we expect medical students to learn the fundamentals of basic science and clinical medicine, so too the topics of ethics and professionalism must be taught and studied. Throughout this chapter, I will return many times to the concept of trust between health care providers and their patients. One has to be honest, transparent, and ethical with all clinical decisions and make sure that the patient is kept at the heart of any and all decisions. Doing so will best ensure a strong, therapeutic relationship between the patient and doctor, one that is built on integrity, understanding, and trust.

DOI: 10.1201/9781003409373-21

ETHICS

Ethical behavior is intimately tied to professionalism. It means that decisions and actions of doctors must prioritize the well-being of patients. My hospital has an ad hoc ethics committee that meets once per month and responds to acute ethical issues. This committee is an essential part of the hospital's day-to-day operations. Ethics deals with "rubber meets the road" issues like informed consent, confidentiality, beneficence and nonmaleficence, and justice. Many physicians who educate residents and medical students feel strongly that ethical practice should be included in the medical school curriculum. I, for one, strongly agree with this sentiment [3, 4].

Informed consent is probably one of the most important issues that physicians deal with in caring for patients. We must communicate with patients about their conditions, treatment options, and the risks and benefits of certain procedures or therapies, and throughout this we ought always to retain respect for patient autonomy. Many patients tell me that their doctor fails to listen to them, that they were given medicines without an explanation of side effects, and, in some cases, they were never told of the prognosis of their condition. In other words, patients may feel that they do not have the information they need to make informed decisions about their care. Patient adherence depends on informed consent. It is obvious to most doctors that social media may explain the patient's diagnosis and prognosis to them erroneously or cause much anxiety when the physician fails to be clear about a patient's state of health. Having a patient absorb inaccurate information through Googling is worse than telling the patient the truth about their condition, even when that truth may be hard to hear. Family members must never hide the prognosis or diagnosis from a patient unless the patient explicitly identifies reasons for such a decision.

Confidentiality is stressed in the relationship between doctor and patient. It must never be compromised. Patients confide in us, knowing that a breach of confidence is not only unethical but also unprofessional. Sensitive information that patients regard as highly personal is held in strict confidence. Disregard of patient confidentiality in many hospitals is a reason for employee job termination. The HIPAA (Health Insurance Portability and Accountability Act) underscores the fact that the patient–doctor relationship is sacred. Confidentiality is also enforced by the law [5].

Beneficence and nonmaleficence refer to acting with the patient's best interests in mind. Prescribing a drug that helps the patient and does no harm is central to this ethical premise, though in practice the ability to estimate risk versus benefit may be quite challenging. Perhaps less frequently but often over the course of a career, a physician may be responsible for counseling a patient and the family on when palliative care should be incorporated into their treatment. The physician should use their knowledge to explain the many facets of end-of-life issues for both patient and family and recommend hospice care when needed. These ethical actions, while not easy, require the judgment and knowledge that comes with appropriate training and experience. It is also a major aspect of professionalism.

Given that the writing of this chapter comes not long after the US Supreme Court decision in *Dobbs v. Jackson Women's Health Organization*, in which the court ruled that the Constitution does not confer a right to abortion, it is important to touch on this sensitive subject. Medical ethics places a strong emphasis on respecting patient autonomy, confidentiality, and the provision of nonjudgmental care. At the same time, individual physicians may feel that the act of performing an abortion is unethical based on their personal beliefs, cultural, religious, or professional values. It goes without saying that there is a wide range of opinions on this matter; some physicians believe that women should have the right to choose abortion as a valid medical procedure, others do not. After the *Dobbs* decision, the legality of abortion now differs widely from state to state. It is my personal opinion that, in those states that permit abortion, physicians have the ethical duty to refer patients to other health care providers if they do not feel that they themselves can perform the procedure in good conscience. My own views and the context in which I practice demonstrate the complexities of this ethical topic (the hospital in which I work is Catholic and such procedures are prohibited).

TEACHING ETHICS IN MEDICAL TRAINING

Ethics can profoundly affect the professional and personal development of medical students and residents in training. In 2015, The Romanell Report was published in the journal *Academic Medicine* and sought to explore the essential role that medical ethics plays in cultivating professionalism among medical learners. The authors noted that medical schools seek to recruit and select students with the "right" character and attitudes, but such selection is exceedingly difficult; it some cases, you may "know it when you see it," but this is not always the case. Since changing the essence of a student's character is at best very difficult and at worst not entirely possible, the authors suggest that medical schools seek to cultivate behaviors that embody ethical and professional virtues [6]. I agree with this approach, and my hope is that doing so will help medical graduates make ethical decisions when they are faced with moral quandaries in their careers. Let me reflect on a few specific topics in this regard:

- *Personal Health and Wellness*: Physicians have an ethical obligation to maintain their own health and wellness. This includes preventing or treating acute or chronic diseases including mental illness, occupational stress, illicit drug use, or alcohol use disorder. This was paramount during the Covid-19 pandemic when many physicians were challenged with their own infections and had to make the hard choice of becoming well themselves prior to rendering care to others.

- *Social Media*: The use of social media can support a doctor's personal interests, allow the physician to advertise online, and communicate with colleagues within the profession. However, these interactions create potential new challenges to the physician–patient relationship. Patients find it convenient to express their concerns after contact by email even though this mode of communication does not afford maximum security for patient confidentiality. Moreover, interactions between patients and physicians through social media can create tricky situations with regard to professional boundaries.

- *Physician Self-Regulation*: The concept of self-regulation for physicians is, according to the American Medical Association (AMA), "based on physicians' enduring commitment to safeguard the welfare of patients and the trust of the public" [7]. The AMA code requires that physicians report incompetent or unethical conduct of other professionals that may put patients at risk of harm. It is part of our ethical standards and also of the law. Physicians who do not meet competency expectations must be reported without fear of loss of favor by colleagues or institutions.

- *Health Disparities*: All physicians should be aware of and reject inequities in health care. There should be no prejudice or bias based on gender or other arbitrary evaluations of any individual. Bias regarding race, ethnicity, or gender are not appropriate when rendering care. In today's culture where gender selection is an issue, physicians must not base their care on preordained opinion. Physicians who believe that they are unable to care for such patients should voluntarily withdraw from providing care to that patient and refer the patient to a provider who can be of help in this regard.

- *Handling of Gifts*: Accepting gifts from patients is a challenging subject. Holiday gifts from patients should never influence the quality of care provided. Modest gifts from grateful patients are common around the holidays and, in my view, are acceptable, whereas cash gifts from patients are not appropriate and should not be accepted. Instead, donations to an institution on behalf of a grateful patient may be both an ethical and reasonable alternative, one that provides benefits in advancing research and care for many patients.

As someone who has long been active in medical education, I will note that involving medical students and residents in the care of patients is important yet sometimes complicated. Patients have the right to know whether their caregiver is a resident or medical student. When a patient receives care from a medical student or resident, the patient should be informed by the attending of record that the student or resident is under their supervision. Residents have a great amount of autonomy, whereas students must be directly supervised or observed in everything they do. A teaching hospital affiliated with a university has a hierarchy of instruction and responsibility. Fellows are physicians in advanced specialty training and will generally have greater independence but still practice under the supervision of a certified specialist. When a resident or fellow is to be involved in performing surgery and other procedures, the patient must have knowledge of their participation. My take-home message: transparency is key when learners are involved in direct clinical care.

IMPACT ON PATIENT CARE

Professionalism and ethical behavior are fundamental to the delivery of excellent patient care. Trust and confidence are the bulwarks of care provided by physicians and other health care providers. Such care should be taught in medical schools and be a central area of focus of residency training. People trust physicians who are professional and ethical. From basic conduct, like spending time with patients, listening to their concerns, and dressing and conducting oneself appropriately, physicians can imbue their relationships with patients with ample trust. In turn, trust allows open communication, encourages patient engagement, and has a positive effect on the outcomes of treatments. Professionalism ensures that patients' needs and preferences are at the front of one's medical practice. Ethical behavior promotes shared decision-making, a respect for the patient's autonomy, and the delivery of personalized care.

Professionalism and ethical conduct are intertwined with quality of care and patient safety. If we adhere to professional standards and ethical guidelines, we will improve patient safety and enhance the quality of care. Medical errors can be prevented when evidence-based medicine and a culture of continuous improvement is the way we practice medicine. Patients quickly become aware of a physician's talents when the patient and doctor establish a firm relationship based on trust and the patient believes that their doctor is choosing the correct treatment for them or selecting the best consulting specialist to best treat their disease.

Finally, let me summarize by saying that embracing professionalism and ethical conduct reminds us that we are in a most noble profession. It is noble because of our cherished values and principles, which we seek at all costs to uphold in order to improve and save lives. If we hold these values dear, we will ensure the provision of high-quality care and maintain the public trust in health care delivery. Our ultimate tasks are to alleviate suffering, preserve dignity, and promote the well-being of those entrusted to our care. In doing so, we honor the sanctity of our professional calling and ensure that we do right by our patients.

REFERENCES

1. Abbasi K: Health, wellbeing, and equity: the tenets of health professionalism. *J R Soc Med* 2023, 116(8):259.
2. Loxterkamp DA: An exploration of professionalism in everyday practice. *J Am Board Fam Med* 2023, 36(3):515–519.

3. AMA code of medical ethics opinion on resident physician training. *Virtual Mentor* 2009, 11(11):874–875. doi: 10.1001/virtualmentor.2009.11.11.code1-0911
4. The AMA's code of medical ethics serves as "gold standard." *Virtual Mentor* 2002, 4(11):329–330. doi: 10.1001/virtualmentor.2002.4.11.code1-0211
5. Walters RJ: What's a nurse to do? How the Health Insurance Portability and Accountability Act of 1996 impacts a nurse's (or any other healthcare provider's) ex parte discussion of protected health information in medical malpractice cases. *JONAS Healthc Law Ethics Regul* 2005, 7(1):21–32; quiz 33–24.
6. Carrese JA, Malek J, Watson K, Lehmann LS, Green MJ, McCullough LB, Geller G, Braddock CH, 3rd, Doukas DJ: The essential role of medical ethics education in achieving professionalism: the Romanell Report. *Acad Med* 2015, 90(6):744–752.
7. American Medical Association. "Professional Self-Regulation: AMA-Code." *Code-Medical-Ethics.ama-Assn.org*. Accessed 16 Feb. 2024.

22 Dealing with Uncertainty

Arabella S. Begin and Katrina A. Armstrong

> Doubt is not a pleasant condition, but certainty is an absurd one.
>
> —Voltaire

As we continue to emerge from the global Covid-19 pandemic, the impact of uncertainty in medicine has been brought into sharp focus across all domains and from multiple sources: professional and personal, emotional and financial. Covid-19's trajectory was defined by uncertainty: estimates of disease severity suffered from an uncertain denominator, making true mortality figures hard to quantify; individual reactions were highly variable and largely unpredictable; estimates of health system capacity and sustainability of preventive strategies fluctuated daily; and there was little sense of control over what was going to happen to loved ones and our nation. While the importance of managing uncertainty has been understood for generations, the Covid-19 pandemic catalyzed an urgent need for modern medical systems and practitioners to develop ways to better understand and embrace uncertainty. In this chapter, we review the presence of uncertainty in the health care environment, the consequences of reactions to uncertainty for both physicians and patients, and strategies to help physicians manage uncertainty in medicine.

UNCERTAINTY IN MEDICINE

Understanding the impact and management of uncertainty in medical practice includes recognizing, and paying attention to, the different dimensions of uncertainty that exist in health care—for both patient and provider. The reality is that doctors continually have to make decisions on the basis of imperfect data and limited knowledge, which leads to diagnostic uncertainty, coupled with the uncertainty that arises from unpredictable patient responses to treatment and from health care outcomes that are far from binary [1].

Dimensions of Uncertainty

Despite decades of research into uncertainty in a multitude of disciplines, it has proven challenging to develop a unified definition of uncertainty that encompasses the numerous types, sources, and manifestations of uncertainty. Broadly, uncertainty can be thought of as "the conscious awareness of being unsure, of having doubt, of not fully knowing" [2]. It is not simply the absence of knowledge as it often can include the company of an abundance of information. All medical decision-making occurs under conditions of varying levels of uncertainty about diagnoses, optimal treatments, and prognoses—it is ubiquitous in health care.

Uncertainty has been recognized to have two major dimensions:

1. *Aleatoric Uncertainty* (from the Latin root *alea* for "dice and gaming"), relating to chance uncertainty, i.e., the inherent uncertainty due to random variability
2. *Epistemic Uncertainty* (from the Greek root *episteme*, meaning "knowledge"), relating to our incomplete knowledge that arises both from limitations in existing scientific knowledge about a medical question and from limitations in the decision maker's ability to access and effectively process existing scientific knowledge

DOI: 10.1201/9781003409373-22

Any scenario has a combination of these two dimensions. As an example, there is inherent variability in whether a patient develops a certain disease (aleatoric uncertainty) and inherent limitations in the provider's ability to diagnose the disease—in part because scientific knowledge about the disease is imperfect and in part because of imperfections in the provider's access to and use of the existing knowledge (epistemic uncertainty). Understanding these dimensions can be helpful for both physicians and patients as they seek to manage the impact of uncertainty on their experience in the health care environment.

Sources of Uncertainty in Medical Practice

Uncertainty exists with essentially every question that arises in the care of a patient: whether a patient has or will develop a particular condition, how a condition will evolve, to what extent a particular treatment is beneficial, what complications might occur from a given treatment, and whether a patient is receiving the right care, in the right place, at the right time, from the right people [2]. Paradoxically, the complexity of preventive, diagnostic, and treatment options over the last century has dramatically increased, not lessened, the degree of uncertainty involved in any given clinical scenario. A hundred years ago, a physician caring for a patient with a set of symptoms would face substantial uncertainty about the patient's course, perhaps about whether there was anything to offer that could improve that course. Today, that same scenario also includes uncertainty about which tests to order, how to interpret the results of the test, whether to consult other physicians, what treatments to order, what can be done to minimize treatment interactions or complications, what frequency of follow-up testing should be done, and when treatment should be stopped or changed. The list of decisions that a modern physician faces, each with its inherent uncertainty, can be never-ending.

In addition to the explosion in the number of decisions involved in the care of patients, changes in several other aspects of medical practice have further exacerbated the level of uncertainty experienced by many providers. The increasingly rapid emergence of new medical technologies has outpaced the development of evidence regarding benefits, harms, and implications, often resulting in physicians being asked to make recommendations about treatments in the absence of evidence to guide those recommendations [2]. At the same time, the exponential increase of knowledge in health sciences about the widening array of therapies and diagnostics makes it harder and harder for providers to stay up-to-date and more and more likely for a provider not to have access to the needed information, even when it does exist, to guide a recommendation. On top of the dramatic increase in available tests and treatments for all patients, the average patient now has more coexisting illnesses, takes more medications, sees more specialists, and undergoes more diagnostic testing. As a patient's complexity of care increases, electronic medical record data accumulates exponentially, making it harder and harder to find the information needed for any given decision. As many patients become a big data challenge, with vast amounts of information on past trajectories and current states, uncertainty about what is "signal" and what is "noise" increases.

The advent of personalized or precision medicine has also increased the uncertainty a provider faces in medical practice. With major advances in immunology, genetics, and systems biology, we now recognize the complexity of biological pathways that underlie any given clinical presentation and the level of individual variation that can be hidden by phenotypic similarity. This recognition adds a level of uncertainty about our ability to predict an individual's course or response to treatment, given that the results of population-based studies like randomized clinical trials provide only average effects that mask substantial variation across patients.

Reaction to—or Tolerance of—Uncertainty by the Health Care System

Although few doctors would argue against the intrinsic uncertainty in medical care, the modern health care environment largely positions uncertainty as an enemy that must be overcome, striving to minimize and even eliminate its existence [1]. This quest is evident in the major areas of biomedical research over the past 50 years, including evidence-based medicine, precision medicine, and, most recently, artificial intelligence. Each of these areas explicitly seeks to reduce one aspect of epistemic uncertainty by increasing knowledge about average effects across groups (evidence-based medicine), individual variation in effects (precision medicine), and future probabilities (artificial intelligence). New knowledge is translated into guidelines that can be applied uniformly to patients to minimize variation in practice if not in outcome. At the same time, the implementation of electronic medical records and decision support in clinical practices seeks to reduce the other aspect of epistemic uncertainty by increasing the ability to access knowledge once it is created. Altogether, the modern health care system emphasizes a paradigm where uncertainty means failure, and a physician is at the front lines in the fight against that failure.

Reaction to—or Tolerance of—Uncertainty by Individuals

While there are limited data on the reaction of physicians to uncertainty, it is widely accepted that human reactions to uncertainty are generally uncomfortable and unpleasant. The human brain is hardwired to perceive reward from certainty and discomfort from increasing levels of uncertainty [3]. Large bodies of research have demonstrated that uncertainty provokes fear, worry and anxiety, perceptions of vulnerability, and avoidance of decision making. The drive for certainty makes sense from an evolutionary standpoint. Natural discomfort with uncertainty is a legacy of survival instincts: we are more comfortable with what is familiar and certain (it hasn't killed us yet) than the unknown, which could be dangerous. Certainty is rewarding, and so we have evolved to steer toward it. Though we are now far from life-threatening situations in most of the spaces when we face uncertainty, our response is the same as that which our ancestors evolved to avoid long ago. Embracing uncertainty is counter to our evolutionary instincts.

In addition to the biological drive to avoid uncertainty, most modern societies are still strongly influenced by a rationalist tradition that seeks to provide a world of apparent security where both aleatoric and epistemic uncertainty are controlled by rational thought and behavior. This world view has created an educational system and societal norms that reward the appearance of certainty, whether in answering questions in school, providing financial advice, or holding political positions. Tolerance of uncertainty is devalued, and natural tendencies to avoid uncertainty are reinforced.

Although biological and societal pressures lead to general discomfort with uncertainty, tolerance of it also varies across individuals, and the factors driving that variation are just beginning to be understood. As with many states, heritable personality traits and environmental exposures may predispose individuals to specific psychological responses, including the reaction to uncertainty. However, tolerance of uncertainty can also be influenced by situational or contextual factors [4], suggesting that it may be amenable to change through an educational and/or experiential process.

Reaction to—or Tolerance of—Uncertainty by Physicians

Physicians may be particularly intolerant of uncertainty, both because the profession selects individuals who gravitate toward the concept of scientific truth and because medical education and training have traditionally prioritized the ability to acquire and replay "facts" over critical thinking or managing uncertainty. Of course, an individual physician's response to uncertainty may depend on the specifics of the clinical situation, previous experiences, support from peers and other colleagues, and norms of the local organization or practice. Tolerance of uncertainty may be lowest when there is no need for urgent decision making, perceived adverse consequences from not adequately reducing uncertainty in the past, and little support from the environment for acknowledging limited knowledge. Too often, doctors in unsupportive environments fear that, by expressing uncertainty, they will project ignorance to patients and colleagues. Thus, they internalize and mask it.

Consequences of Reactions to Uncertainty
Burnout

Given that humans are programmed to want to reduce uncertainty in a world full of irreducible uncertainty, it is not surprising that the failure to effectively manage that conflict can have a negative impact on well-being and contribute to burnout and depression [5]. An intolerance of uncertainty has been shown to be a characteristic involved in excessive worry, to be strongly associated with generalized anxiety disorder, as well as depression and obsessive compulsive disorder [6]. Burnout has been described as "the index of the dislocation between what people are and what they have to do" [7]. It makes intuitive sense that burnout could follow from the "dislocation" caused by consistently facing substantial uncertainty in medical decision making without the ability or tools to manage or even recognize that uncertainty [1, 5]. This situation is likely exacerbated by traditional approaches to medical education and training and the "anti-uncertainty" stance of the health care environment. High levels of burnout seen among health care providers coming out of the Covid-19 pandemic may, in part, reflect the extraordinary levels of uncertainty they faced during the pandemic. At a time when concern about physician well-being is high, with much speculation about the causes of burnout, we have found a strong relationship between tolerance of uncertainty and physician well-being across specialties [8]. The psychological distress associated with an intolerance of uncertainty not only has consequences for the physical and mental well-being of physicians but also has a detrimental impact on their ability to perform well academically. Particular attention likely needs to be paid to those with less experience, those in specialties with high rates of undifferentiated illness and uncertainty, such as primary care, and ensuring all physicians have access to a trusted advisor [8]. As we think about the urgent call to alleviate burnout, efforts focused on understanding and embracing uncertainty seem vital.

Team Functioning

Confidently exposing uncertainties without fear of judgment or perceived incompetence is at the core of successful team functioning. It has been described as psychological safety, defined as "being able to show and employ one's self without fear of negative consequences of self-image, status or career" [9]. Too often, however, it is missing from the health care environment, where a salient hierarchical structure and powerful professional norms may threaten an ability to speak up or openly voice uncertainty. An inability to tolerate uncertainty means that clinical practitioners boldly wear a mask of self-assurance and control, hiding their internal sea of uncertainty. Aside from improving physicians' sense of comraderie and community, which is likely to positively impact well-being, psychological safety has been shown to be a crucial element in organizational efforts to detect and prevent patient harm by errors and process failures [10]. Inculcating a culture of psychological safety that embraces the discussion of uncertainty, thereby ensuring community members feel respected and included while striving for high performance, is essential for high-quality health care.

Physician–Patient Relationship

Open, honest, and respectful communication with patients is impeded when physicians who are intolerant to uncertainty are unable to disclose uncertainties to their patients [11]. The inability to communicate uncertainty creates a false sense of certainty among patients, which can lead to substantial distrust when that certainty proves to be overstated. An increasing emphasis on precision medicine and artificial intelligence—terms that undoubtedly connote certainty—risks widening this gap between expectation and reality for patients and physicians. In the long run, inadequate discussion and management of uncertainty may cause unnecessary concern and distress to patients, undercut the patient–provider relationship, and decrease trust.

In addition, a focus on reducing uncertainty can lead physicians to spend less and less time at the bedside and more and more time in front of a screen trying to retrieve and process data. The human connection central to the physician–patient relationship frays as computers replace conversation. Furthermore, computers may reinforce a sense of a black-and-white world where certainty is readily achievable— the antithesis of the grayscale perspective that physicians need in order to tolerate the uncertainty inherent to 21st-century medicine [1]. As technology increasingly performs many routine tasks of medicine, it will become evermore essential that physicians learn to embrace and communicate uncertainty to their patients—human connection will always be central to the physician-patient relationship.

MANAGING UNCERTAINTY IN MEDICINE

Recently the medical profession has begun to recognize the need to identify and address clinical uncertainty, acknowledging its impact on patient safety as well as wellness among working physicians and trainees. Understanding and acknowledging uncertainty and acquiring proper coping strategies is now regarded as one of the core clinical competencies for medical graduates and trainees in the UK, US, Australia, and much of Europe.

Strategies to Enable Physicians to Help Themselves

Recognizing that uncertainty is rife in the health care environment, there is much that the individual physician can do on a day-to-day basis to help embrace uncertainty in their clinical practice. Acknowledgment and acceptance of uncertainty is an essential shift in the revolution to embrace uncertainty in clinical practice. Empowering individual physicians to help themselves sit comfortably with uncertainty begins the process of reframing uncertainty as a surmountable challenge rather than as a threat. By reflecting on the emotions and thoughts that uncertainty triggers within us, we can begin to gain more control over our automatic behaviors and actions. This allows us to respond mindfully and choose more functional rather than dysfunctional ways to deal with uncertainty. By identifying areas where physicians can anticipate feeling uncertain, individuals can prepare themselves to face these situations rather than being blindsided by them [12].

What may be most relevant and practical for the everyday practitioner is making the distinction between "knowable" and "unknowable" forms of knowledge underlying uncertainty. Identifying, articulating, and prioritizing the minimization of "unnecessary uncertainties" (that is, the knowable forms of knowledge) can enable a constructive approach to assessing and managing the multiple sources of uncertainty in any given decision. By deconstructing the sources of uncertainty, the physician can take specific actions to address each source, recognizing that acceptance can be a beneficial and important strategy. For instance, a knowledge gap can be addressed by seeking consultation with a more knowledgeable colleague, while the aleatory uncertainty of random variation may require a more humanistic or spiritual approach.

Recognizing uncertainty can also improve decision processes as our desire for certainty leaves us open to the influence of cognitive biases. To prosper in the face of increasing knowledge and a busy workplace, well-versed experts learn to recognize patterns that allow them to think and act quickly. Such quick-thinking heuristics, first identified by Tversky and Kahneman [13], serve a useful purpose—recognizing the cardinal signs of an acute stroke or myocardial infarction and initiating appropriate therapy and organizing the appropriate personnel—yet they leave clinicians vulnerable to cognitive bias and, in turn, false assumptions, misdiagnosis, and errors. Physicians would do well to pause when making medical decisions and ask themselves if there is any uncertainty that they are avoiding: Do they feel confident in their reasoning? What else have they left out? "Holding uncertainty" can allow more possibilities to remain "in play." It is wise to proactively include a role for uncertainty in management plans. By creating safety nets and following up, physicians can reduce the potential harms of uncertainty and more quickly catch outcomes that run the risk of veering off course. Physicians can specifically ask themselves: "If I'm right, what do I expect to happen? How will I know if I'm wrong? What would I do then?" Particularly important is for senior and experienced physicians to explicitly reassure junior colleagues that uncertainty is not only appropriate but also an expected component of medical practice. With clinical experience and over time, physicians evolve to recognize that clinical problems most often have poorly defined borders, evolving characteristics, and multiple legitimate treatment approaches rather than a single correct one [14]. Early stages of medical training—with a predominance of multiple-choice questions with "right" answers—inculcate a notion that there is one absolute truth or single best answer in medicine, suggesting an element of certainty that does not translate from the textbook and classroom to the real world at the bedside. Students and trainees need to be supported and encouraged to express and embrace the uncertainty inherent to medicine.

Strategies to Help Physicians Work with Patients

Authentic disclosures and communication of uncertainty in meaningful ways has been shown to enhance trust in the patient–provider relationship and to improve decision making and health care outcomes [15]. This is often challenging for physicians, trained in a culture that prioritizes certainty and views it as a form of ignorance or failure. Normalizing uncertainty is important as it seeks to reset expectations. Patients are bombarded in the lay media with the notion that high-tech advances in imaging and genomics have resulted in definitive answers to clinical questions, such as prognosis. Clinicians should be honest with patients about the boundaries of knowledge, saying, for example: "I understand that you want more accurate information about the future. The reality is that it's like predicting the weather—we can never be absolutely certain about the future. I wish I could be more certain" [16]. Saying "I don't know exactly what is going on, but I will be with you and will support you" goes a long way in reassuring the patient even if the clinical "answer" is unclear. Open discussion, including admitting vulnerability and acknowledging our limitations, builds trust and shared responsibility when it is grounded in the mutual recognition of the inevitable uncertainty of clinical medicine. To help a patient refocus on the here and now, clinicians might ask, "What can we do to help you now, given that we are unsure of exactly what the future will bring?" This can help ground both doctor and patient in the present and prevent rumination about a future that cannot be predicted with complete accuracy or control.

Strategies to Help Physicians Guide Students, Trainees, and Less Experienced Colleagues

Talking openly about uncertainty in the clinical environment helps normalize the experience of uncertainty not only for colleagues but also for learners, modeling that it is "safe" and necessary to express uncertainty and setting a new culture that embraces uncertainty. One way to prioritize learners' open-ended thinking is by asking questions that begin with "how" or "why" rather than "what" or "when" [1]. Questions that start with "what" or "when" suggest a specific answer is expected that is either known or not—further inculcating the notion that there is a right answer and thus rewarding certainty. Questions that start with "how" or "why" promote higher-order skills, such as synthesis and evaluation, and allow for answers that can more easily acknowledge and embrace uncertainty. Role modeling that embraces the inherent uncertainty of clinical medicine helps set a new culture that normalizes the experience of admitting "I don't know" [17]. These simple words welcome input and curiosity, a fundamental motivator for learning that are pivotal to the development of sound clinical reasoning.

Physicians can increase a trainee's mastery of probability-based logic by explicitly discussing thresholds to test and treat as well as how such thresholds may change from patient to patient (i.e., Bayesian reasoning). This strategy brings discussion of the individualized nature of uncertainty to the clinical learning environment. To help shift the culture, physicians should consider adding an explicit discussion about the level of uncertainty during clinical handover and transitions in care. By embedding these discussions into clinical practice and the health care environment, physicians help reinforce that what matters is not the absence of uncertainty but rather the processes and thinking patterns one uses to manage it.

Strategies for the Health Care System

In striving for certainty, the health care field widens a gap between expectation and reality. Unfortunately, the health care system's infrastructure is not currently set up to easily embrace uncertainty. In particular, few incentives encourage embracing clinical uncertainty. Certainty is valued implicitly and explicitly in health care institutions, policies, and the learning environment. In many hospitals, admission from the emergency department to the inpatient ward requires a formal diagnosis to be entered in the patient's chart; electronic health record systems require laboratory testing, imaging, and prescriptions to be associated with specific diagnoses in the record; and billing for an encounter is often stratified according to the final diagnosis or the treatments offered without crediting, recognizing, or valuing the work and time required for clinical reasoning, patient education, shared decision-making, and the consideration and communication of uncertainty. Amid the 87,000 ICD codes, there is none for "I don't know." Many physicians eschew tasks they feel are time-consuming, including discussions of goals of care, patient education, evaluating health literacy, or uncertainty. Yet these are the components of a clinical encounter that patients and providers both find valuable, and such conversations may serve to reduce readmissions, improve adherence, and improve the quality of a patient's health and wellness over time [18].

Changes to support uncertainty could include more flexible diagnostic codes and treatment algorithms that build in uncertainty and room for modification over time, as well as clinical decision support tools and electronic medical record systems that offer provisional diagnoses or, better and more flexibly, capture how diagnostic knowledge and certainty evolve over time, enabling tolerance of uncertainty rather than undermining it. We do not reimburse physicians for their "thinking time" or for the important but nuanced work of carefully and compassionately communicating uncertainty. But perhaps we should. We must advocate for better ways to measure, assess, and train the management of uncertainty.

A final means to thrive in the face of uncertainty is to see it as a natural starting point for system quality improvement in health care. Clinical uncertainty may unveil unnecessary variation, inconsistent practices, safety errors or near misses, or areas in which new knowledge or new processes are necessary. This is a natural precursor for improvement—health systems would do well to draw on the observations, questions, and ideas of trainees and physicians in practice to identify areas for future research, clinical practice or guideline development, or organizational process improvement [19].

The Future

Health care is a breeding ground for uncertainty. Although advances in biomedical research will continue to improve the accuracy of information available for clinical decision making, uncertainty in medicine will always be present. Responding to the plethora of uncertainties that arise in the health care environment in an adaptive way is one of the most important challenges facing clinicians and patients. We know how prevalent uncertainty is in health care and the negative impact that it can have on a provider's cognitive, emotional, and behavioral outcomes, with consequences for the delivery of high-quality patient care. William Osler famously and aptly recognized medicine to be "a science of uncertainty and an art of probability." For too long, uncertainty has been an unwelcome guest. Perhaps this next era will see us eliminate the fear and anxiety that has been fueled by our unhealthy reaction to uncertainty. Uncertainty is, after all, a certainty in medicine [1]. We must ensure we are resting, not wrestling, with it.

REFERENCES

1. Simpkin AL, Schwartzstein RM. Tolerating Uncertainty—The Next Medical Revolution? N Engl J Med 2016;375(18):1713–1715. DOI: 10.1056/NEJMp1606402.
2. Hillen MA, Gutheil CM, Strout TD, Smets EMA, Han PKJ. Tolerance of Uncertainty: Conceptual Analysis, Integrative Model, and Implications for Healthcare. Soc Sci Med 2017;180:62–75. DOI: 10.1016/j.socscimed.2017.03.024.
3. Hsu M, Bhatt M, Adolphs R, Tranel D, Camerer CF. Neural Systems Responding to Degrees of Uncertainty in Human Decision-Making. Science 2005;310(5754): 1680–1683. DOI: 10.1126/science.1115327.
4. Durrheim K, Foster D. Tolerance of Ambiguity as a Content Specific Construct. Perso Individ Diff 1997;22:741–750.
5. Simpkin AL, Khan A, West DC, et al. Stress From Uncertainty and Resilience among Depressed and Burned Out Residents: A Cross-Sectional Study. Acad Pediatr 2018;18(6):698–704. DOI: 10.1016/j.acap.2018.03.002.
6. Gentes EL, Ruscio AM. A Meta-Analysis of the Relation of Intolerance of Uncertainty to Symptoms of Generalized Anxiety Disorder, Major Depressive Disorder, and Obsessive-Compulsive Disorder. Clin Psychol Rev 2011;31(6): 923–933. DOI: 10.1016/j.cpr.2011.05.001.
7. Maslach C, Jackson SE, Leiter MP. Maslach Burnout Inventory Manual. 3rd ed. Menlo Park, CA: Mind Garden Inc, 1996.
8. Begin AS, Hidrue M, Lehrhoff S, Del Carmen MG, Armstrong K, Wasfy JH. Factors Associated with Physician Tolerance of Uncertainty: An Observational Study. J Gen Intern Med 2022;37(6):1415–1421. DOI: 10.1007/s11606-021-06776-8.
9. Kahn WA. Psychological Conditions of Personal Engagement and Disengagement at Work. Academy of Management Journal 1990;33(4):692–724.
10. Edmondson AC. The Kinds of Teams Health Care Needs. Harvard Bus Rev 2015:2–5.
11. Katz J. Why Doctors Don't Disclose Uncertainty. Hastings Cent Rep 1984;14(1): 35–44. Available from: www.ncbi.nlm.nih.gov/pubmed/6715153.
12. John CC. The Art of Constructive Worrying. JAMA 2018;319(22):2273–2274. DOI: 10.1001/jama.2018.6670.
13. Tversky A, Kahneman D. Judgment under Uncertainty: Heuristics and Biases. Science 1974;185(4157):1124–1131. DOI: 10.1126/science.185.4157.1124.

14. Benbassat J. Role Modeling in Medical Education: The Importance of a Reflective Imitation. Acad Med 2014;89(4):550–554. DOI: 10.1097/ACM.0000000000000189.

15. Simpkin AL, Armstrong KA. Communicating Uncertainty: A Narrative Review and Framework for Future Research. J Gen Intern Med 2019;34(11):2586–2591. DOI: 10.1007/s11606-019-04860-8.

16. Smith AK, White DB, Arnold RM. Uncertainty—The Other Side of Prognosis. N Engl J Med 2013;368(26):2448–2450. DOI: 10.1056/NEJMp1303295.

17. Gheihman G, Johnson M, Simpkin AL. Twelve Tips for Thriving in the Face of Clinical Uncertainty. Med Teach 2019:1–7. DOI: 10.1080/0142159X.2019.1579308.

18. Arora NK. Interacting with Cancer Patients: The Significance of Physicians' Communication Behavior. Soc Sci Med 2003;57(5):791–806. DOI: 10.1016/s0277-9536(02)00449-5.

19. Blumenthal D. Performance Improvement in Health Care—Seizing the Moment. N Engl J Med 2012;366(21):1953–1955. DOI: 10.1056/NEJMp1203427.

23 Falling Short

Daniel Shalev and Vicki A. Jackson

Our profession, like many others, is filled with those with incredibly high standards and little tolerance for mistakes, missteps, or falling short. Yet none of us was born a surgeon, pediatrician, or palliative care doctor. We gain knowledge and skills, allowing us to carry out our professional roles. This skill acquisition took years and countless hours of painstaking work. Becoming a competent clinician, researcher, or educator takes practice and *always* involves mistakes. These experiences run the gamut: giving a patient the wrong medication, failing to secure an important research grant, acting unsupportively toward a trainee, and so forth. But regardless of the context, falling short—whether through mistakes, failing to bring our best selves to an endeavor, or simply not getting the outcome we had hoped for—is a universal experience. Falling short can be profoundly painful. And yet, by approaching the times we fall short with self-compassion, curiosity, and a growth mindset [1], these can be among the most powerful moments of learning and connection in our lives.

In this chapter, Vicki and Dan will offer their approach to managing times when we fall short. Dan is earlier in his career, and Vicki is at a later stage in her career, which we hope will help a variety of readers in relating to this content. In this chapter, we offer some of our learning from mistakes we have made throughout our careers. It is also the result of learning from various important scholars in psychology, education, leadership, management, and mindfulness. We are indebted to the work of Amy Edmonson, Adam Grant, Carol Dweck, Angela Duckworth, and Pema Chodron. We will pepper important concepts from their work throughout this chapter but encourage you to read their work for deeper learning.

Though this chapter is nominally about *mistakes*, we use the term "falling short" to encapsulate a broader experience. Falling short of what we had hoped is where the learning is. We selected this term because we believe mistakes are only one part of falling short. The term "mistake" implies that the agency lies entirely with the mistaken person. Rather, when we fall short, there are often multiple loci of control. Engaging with and growing from such experiences entails cultivating a nuanced perspective that allows us to cope with disappointment, vulnerability, and sometimes shame. Only when we can cultivate a generosity toward ourselves can we recognize and differentiate the factors over which we may have had control while also understanding those over which we may not have had control. Learning can only happen when we reframe our falling short as a humble path toward growth. We'll come back to this idea later.

FALLING SHORT IN MEDICINE: From Shame to Growth

Our goal for this chapter is to help reframe the experience of falling short as an opportunity for learning. We would be remiss to begin the discussion without acknowledging that the perfectionism we are conditioned to manifest as clinicians often precludes us from learning when we fall short. This conditioning process starts early in our medical training. Clinical clerkship students are meant to be learning, yet they are also under evaluation from their first day on the wards. Students experience immense pressure to answer each question on rounds correctly, to achieve clinical competence immediately, and to succeed at each academic endeavor. The

 DOI: 10.1201/9781003409373-23

clinical language we use around poor outcomes reinforces this: *preventable* errors, *never* events.

The *never event* attitude in medicine stems from our shared mission as clinicians to provide the best possible care. But when we approach our lives as though poor patient outcomes, grant or manuscript rejections, romantic breakups, and other challenges are *never events*, we stymy our capacity to learn, take risks, and grow. When we believe something should never happen, we experience shame when it does. Shame is a powerful emotional response in which, rather than feeling bad about a decision or outcome, individuals internalize a negative sense of themselves; if we fall short, we are bad doctors, parents, partners, and people. Shame is a particularly powerful inhibitor to learning and growth. When we conceptualize our falling short as a reflection of immutable characteristics about ourselves, we close the door on a lifelong process of transformative growth. However, our ability to persevere despite our negative feelings about ourselves when we fall short, sometimes called grit or tenacity, ties more into success than our inherent abilities [2]. To that end, we advocate for approaching experiences of falling short as part of a continuous improvement process fueled by the growth opportunities that come with falling short.

By not only accepting but expecting that sometimes we will fall short, we can devote the energy to considering how to learn from such experiences. Medical students who show up every morning on rounds, read when they miss a question, try again when they cannot complete a procedure, and resubmit when their paper is rejected are better prepared to be excellent clinicians and lead meaningful lives than those who answer 99 consecutive questions correctly but find it so intolerable to get the 100th question wrong that they cannot learn from the experience. This is all to say that, even if we do not invite failure into the space of our lives, we must prepare for the certainty that it will sometimes be a guest—and a teacher—there.

LEARNING FROM FALLING SHORT: Reframing, Containing, Examining, and Growing

To learn from falling short, we need to be able to reframe the experience as a pathway to growth, not a window into our inadequacy. But that is certainly easier said than done. Committing to reframing painful experiences of falling short as opportunities for growth is a lifelong process. Work by psychologist Carol Dweck [1] has identified the importance of a *growth mindset*—the belief that our abilities and intelligence can be developed through effort rather than their being static and unchangeable. The growth mindset allows us to embrace challenges, persist in the face of setbacks, recognize the link between effort and success, and learn from our mistakes and those of others. A growing body of evidence from various disciplines shows that a growth mindset is closely linked to success and well-being. This doesn't mean that falling short feels good or that we are glad about the outcome. But the act of sitting with the experience of falling short, of not looking away, and of refusing to accept that the outcome is a reflection of our flawed personhood is a radical first step that we have to take to ensure that our pain serves our growth.

We're going to first share Dan's experience of falling short during his residency training and then use this as a window to talk about a process for turning falling short into an opportunity for growth.

When Dan was a second-year resident on the psychiatric consult service, he was assigned to conduct a psychiatric consult for depression and suicidality for a woman admitted to the neurology service with a progressive neurological disorder that had rendered her legs paralyzed and left her with only limited strength in her arms. At the time, Dan was a confident psychiatry resident who had done well on his consult rotation and prided himself on working collaboratively with multiple disciplines in

175

the hospital, including nursing, physical therapy, and other specialties. Dan completed the consult and agreed that the woman was indeed very depressed. During the consultation, the woman explained to Dan that when she was able to leave the hospital, she was going to procure a firearm and end her life. However, the woman also reassured Dan that she would never "disrespect" her clinicians by trying to harm herself in the hospital itself. Dan was worried by the conviction and specificity of the woman's plan to kill herself but was reassured that the woman was not mobile enough to be able to leave the hospital of her own volition. Dan considered instituting a sitter to observe the patient, but, because he wanted to support the nurses who were worried about staffing a constant sitter, he decided it would be okay to leave the patient unattended.

The following morning, when Dan was reviewing his patients' charts, he noted with alarm that the woman was no longer listed as admitted. Dan felt pangs of dread as he opened the chart and read multiple event notes stating that the patient had eloped overnight, apparently crawling to a wheelchair and using that to leave. Dan was so overcome with shame and fear that he had a difficult time even looking at the chart, at one point putting his fingers over his eyes and reading only a few words at a time. His feelings were overlaid with thoughts that he was a terrible physician who would be fired.

In complete shock, Dan walked into the office of his mentor—the chief of the psychiatric consultation service. Dan's mentor saw immediately that Dan was extremely upset and sat him down, gently encouraging him to share what had happened. Dan explained the situation as well as he could, and his mentor listened thoughtfully. After hearing what had happened, Dan's mentor told Dan to take a few deep breaths and reminded him that many, perhaps most psychiatrists lose patients to suicide at some point in their careers. He reassured Dan that they would do everything they could to find the patient safely, that Dan would not be fired for making a mistake, and that this incident would make him a better physician for countless future patients in his career.

Once Dan had calmed down sufficiently, his mentor suggested they think through the case together and asked Dan to reflect on how this outcome may have happened. Dan immediately began to rattle off things he had done wrong—not being careful enough, not being thoughtful enough. But his mentor stopped him and pulled a worn copy of The Myth of Sisyphus by Albert Camus [3], reading the introductory sentences: "There is but one truly serious philosophical problem and that is suicide. Judging whether life is or is not worth living amounts to answering the fundamental question of philosophy." Dan's mentor reminded him that he was not omnipotent or omniscient. With his mentor's guidance, Dan realized that to understand what had happened, he had to recognize the factors over which he had control and those over which he didn't. With that in mind, Dan and his mentor considered the internal factors that had led to this event, such as Dan's acquiescence on a sitter because of his desire to support staff and Dan's incorrect assumption that the patient's weakness made her immobile. But they also considered the external factors that may have shaped the outcome: the woman's agency over her own life and the burdened staffing system that made obtaining sitters difficult.

Finally, once Dan and his mentor had alerted the police, debriefed with the teams, and explored the factors that led to this outcome, Dan's mentor asked Dan to consolidate the experience and think about how it would shape his practice. Though still very painful, Dan could recognize what he had learned: the importance of following his clinical intuition, the risk of allowing colleagues' approval to trump patient care, and the need to be careful about his perceptions regarding patients' functional status. These insights comforted Dan, who knew that he would be a more capable clinician the next time he evaluated psychiatric risks in a hospitalized patient.

Committing to a growth mindset allows us to ask how to turn the pain of falling short into growth. We approach experiences of falling short through a three-step process—one that you might recognize in the preceding narrative.

ACKNOWLEDGING AND MANAGING OUR EMOTIONS

We need to manage our emotions before we can learn, grow, or even fix. An experience of falling short—particularly when the stakes are high, as in clinical care—can be crushing. Without giving ourselves a chance to experience the intense emotions that often accompany the experience of falling short, we cannot be psychologically prepared to learn from the experience. These emotions are not merely by products of an experience; they are profound indicators of the depth of our engagement and investment in our work.

In Dan's situation, he would not have been able to learn from his experience when he first walked into his mentor's office in a panic, assuming he would be fired on the spot. Learning requires us to attend to the emotions first, so we can then do the important cognitive work of reflecting on the experience.

Leadership expert, Leonard Marcus, and his colleagues note that, when we are dealing with the emotional surge of a crisis, we are in our "mental basement," a place of shelter and survival amid the storm of emotions [4]. In this mental basement, our primary focus is weathering the emotional surge, akin to how one might hunker down in a physical basement during a tumultuous storm. In this state, our responses are geared toward immediate survival and shielding ourselves from further humiliation rather than reflective thinking or creative problem solving.

To ascend from this "basement," it is crucial first to acknowledge and understand these intense emotions. This process requires not just self-awareness but also self-compassion. It involves recognizing the normalcy of these emotional responses and allowing oneself the space and time to experience and process them. This step is not about suppressing emotions but understanding them as natural responses to challenging situations.

Over the years, Vicki has found that a sense of humor can also be very helpful in this process. Anyone who has worked with her knows that she has a saying she uses for the work of managing the emotions associated with falling short. She calls it an AFGO—"another flipping growth opportunity." She has no idea where she heard this but finds that the concept of an AFGO can be a shorthand that eases the tendency to catastrophize and adds a welcomed lightheartedness. An AFGO signals that the experience is important enough to do the work of reframing and acknowledges that the experience doesn't feel great in the moment.

Managing our emotions with humor and self-compassion calms the physiological and psychological activation that accompanies these emotions. It is foundational for doing the higher-order cognitive work of reflecting and learning from the times we fall short. The more strategies we have in our toolbox to climb out of the emotional basement, the better. These strategies increase the likelihood of showing up for ourselves in difficult moments. Experiment with what works for you. Some effective strategies we use include:

- Sharing and discharging the experience—and our feelings—with a supportive mentor, colleague, friend, or family member where you can let it all out. For Vicki, this often involves swearing.

- Engaging in physical activities such as running, walking, or stretching.

- Getting out in nature.

- Partaking in something that provides physical comfort, like a nourishing meal or a warm drink. Vicki and Dan both love dogs and find great physical comfort in a snuggle with a pooch.

- Deep breathing, meditation, mindfulness, or prayer activities. Even a few deep breaths can help soothe the fight-or-flight response that may accompany the experience of falling short.

- Reading a positive or comforting passage or poem.

While the feasibility of each of these strategies depends on the context, one or more are almost always accessible to us. These techniques are powerful not because they make us numb or neutral but because they allow us to reach a state in which we can think clearly, reflect deeply, and learn effectively.

When the Emotions Persist

Often, as we begin to process a difficult situation and figure out how to move forward, the intensity of our emotions gradually calms. These techniques are helpful ways of caring for ourselves amid emotional intensity and preparing to move forward. But for various reasons, sometimes the negative feelings we experience when we fall short persist and make it difficult to grow.

Being trapped in an activated and negative emotional state prevents us from learning from our mistakes and harms our overall well-being. When the intense pain, shame, self-doubt, and fear that can accompany falling short persists over days or weeks, that's a sign that we may need more support. When this happens, we think about several potential causes and paths forward.

First, working in a professional setting in which falling short is met with humiliation or punishment rather than with a growth mindset can make it difficult to emerge from the emotional activation associated with these experiences. While it may not be possible to change environments in the short term, falling short in a harsh or unsupportive environment makes it even more important to obtain external support from peers, mentors, family, and friends who are unequivocally "on your side" with a commitment to your personal growth rather than amplifying or delighting in your misstep.

Second, sometimes difficult experiences can precipitate or worsen underlying challenges with mood, anxiety, and sense of self that extend beyond just the isolated pain of a poor outcome. In situations when we or our colleagues have fallen short and have struggled to recover emotionally or have experienced persistent feelings that impair our quality of life, we identify the value in seeking the support of a mental health professional who can help address underlying issues that can impair our capacity to manage difficult emotions successfully.

When we can reframe and manage our emotions with generosity and self-compassion, we can then begin to learn from the experience through our own reflection and asking others for feedback. With practice, these skills can become second nature, and the time spent in intense negative emotion often lessens.

WORKING TO UNDERSTAND HOW AND WHY WE FELL SHORT

Once we have managed the emotional response to falling short, we can take the second step of thoughtfully examining the intrinsic and extrinsic factors that may have contributed to the outcome. In the basement, we focus on survival at the expense of self-reflection and observation. In contrast, Vicki uses the image of "going to the balcony" to achieve a state of mind where one can replay the experience as a compassionate, keen observer. Often with this new vantage point, objectivity is easier to harness.

Getting to the balcony is a key step in achieving personal growth from the complex experiences of falling short. Most of the time, when we fall short, there is not a single factor but rather an interplay of intrinsic and extrinsic factors. The term "intrinsic factors" refers to personal attributes or factors such as our decision-making processes, skill levels, emotional responses, personal experiences, and behavioral patterns. Vicki remembers a time when her children were quite small and sleep felt like a luxury. It was also a time when her mother had just died and another close family member was diagnosed with advanced pancreatic cancer. She found herself struggling to manage her typical clinical panel, often completing her charts late. She also noted that she didn't have the emotional reserve to cope with the complicated patients for whom she was caring. She felt as though she was falling short. As Vicki reflected on the experience, she was able to identify her sleep deficit and personal losses as intrinsic factors contributing to her experience. Identifying the intrinsic factors was the first step in developing creative solutions.

Conversely, extrinsic factors encompass environmental conditions, systemic issues, team dynamics, and other factors often beyond our control. Recognizing these external elements helps us understand the broader context of our actions and decisions, providing a more comprehensive view of the situation. In Dan's preceding experience, the hospital being short-staffed was an extrinsic factor that contributed to his falling short.

Understanding intrinsic and extrinsic factors requires examining ourselves and our situation honestly and holding on to both the ways in which we shoulder responsibility for an outcome and those factors out of our control. It is a challenging task, even for the wisest. Fortunately, a support system of friends, coworkers, mentors, spouses, and/or family members that you can trust with your worries and "warts" can help you. Just as we all make mistakes, it is not possible for any one of us to "know" ourselves completely.

The work of psychologists Joseph Luft and Harry Ingham can help us understand why a challenge network (more on this shortly) is so critical to continued growth. Luft and Ingham conceptualized the dynamics of self-awareness as a four-quadrant framework called the *Johari Window* [5] (Table 23.1). The model supposes that if we were to have a clear view through the four quadrants, we would achieve full self-awareness. In the first quadrant are the parts of ourselves known to us and to others. In the second quadrant are the hidden parts of ourselves of which we are aware but may keep from others. In the third quadrant—also known as the blind area—are the parts of ourselves that others may see but that we may not see about ourselves. And finally, in the fourth quadrant are those parts of ourselves that are not perceivable to us or to others around us. Without accessing the parts of ourselves that are perceived by others but not by us, we may become stalled and repeat the behaviors that led to falling short. Conversely, by tapping into the help of others, we can make an entire additional quadrant available to us for leveraging toward learning and growth.

So, who are the right people to help us explore those blind areas? We want people who care about us and can simultaneously support us while challenging our thinking and providing genuine feedback with transparency. We want people who can help us do the work of learning from situations where we've fallen short. While

Table 23.1 Johari's Window

Open Area: Known to self and others, representing shared knowledge.	*Blind Area*: Unknown to self but known to others. Our support network can recognize and help us explore these parts of ourselves, but we may not be able to access ourselves.
Hidden Area: Known to self but hidden from others, encompassing aspects we choose not to reveal.	*Unknown Area*: Unknown to self and others, representing undiscovered potential and behaviors.

these individuals may overlap with those in our lives who support us through step one—managing our emotions—they may not all overlap in such a way. For example, a doting parent may offer calm and comfort when upset but may not be the right person to obtain feedback about areas for professional improvement. We respect these people for their skill and expertise and know that they have our best interests at heart. They want us to grow and get better. They are not reveling in our mistakes.

In Dan's experience, his mentor was pivotal in exploring the negative outcome. This is a key component of learning from falling short: without a network to help us, we may miss the more valuable lessons in the experience.

The individuals we call upon to help us with this process are called a *Challenge Network* by organizational psychologist, Adam Grant [6]. Grant identifies that these networks have two key characteristics: they are radically transparent and process focused. Radical transparency refers to the capacity of our network to express their belief in us by pushing us, providing honest feedback, and empowering us to be our best. Process focused refers to the precedence of improvement and growth over any specific outcome. Having a challenge network is critical at all career stages. But as we work with our challenge networks and learn to see ourselves through the eyes of our colleagues, peers, mentors, and mentees, our capacity for self-exploration and assessment is also enhanced, and how we relate to our challenge network may deepen and evolve. Vicki notes that it is often quite difficult to get true feedback as one advances in a career. Hierarchy can make many wary to give feedback to senior faculty. If true excellence is the goal, a growth mindset coupled with the cultivation of a trusted challenge network is necessary at every stage in one's career.

Learning from falling short involves a dual process of self-exploration and external feedback. In this way, the process helps us understand the current situation and equips us with a deeper understanding of ourselves and our professional context. In a way, the duality of the exploration process parallels what we often find about falling short: that it is an interplay between intrinsic factors (internal to ourselves) and extrinsic ones (aspects of the outcome over which we do not have control). Part of the challenge of effectively learning from times when we fall short is the need to recognize our role's impact and limitations simultaneously. Though the balance may differ across situations, it is uncommon that the experience of falling short can be fully assigned to intrinsic or extrinsic factors. When we approach these experiences from the perspective that we are not responsible (hubris) or bear the entire burden (shame), we significantly hinder our ability to learn.

The Risk of Hubris

Hubris—excessive and reckless self-confidence—can lead to dismissive attitudes toward falling short. Most concretely, it can lead us to neglect our role when we have fallen short in favor of externalizing blame. With overconfidence, there can be an exclusive focus on extrinsic factors rather than an ability to see how any intrinsic factors might have contributed. Many years ago, Vicki was supervising a trainee who made an opioid prescribing error. These kinds of errors are something clinicians must guard against as they can pose a great risk to the patient. When discussing the medical error with the trainee, he stated that he was excellent in math. He did acknowledge that he may have used the wrong medication dose conversion but that it wasn't his fault. He noted that the print was very small in the handbook he was using, making it difficult to clearly distinguish the different medication doses. He also stated that it was ultimately the pharmacist's and nurse's fault for not catching his error in prescribing the medication. He struggled to see that his inattention to detail might have been a contributing intrinsic factor. Such an attitude inherently creates a barrier to self-reflection of growth; there is no sense in looking inward if nothing is our fault. Inpatient care and hubris are particularly dangerous. If we cannot recognize gaps in our knowledge and skills, we are unlikely to seek help and thus may put patients at risk.

Some degree of externalization is a common response to falling short. When we identify this thought process in ourselves or others, strategies that we use to make self-reflection safer and more accessible include:

- Opening a dialogue with others that normalizes falling short and reinforces using such experiences for learning and growth.

- Having senior team members or mentors share their experiences of falling short.

- Reframing self-reflection as an opportunity for improvement and action.

The Risk of Catastrophizing

Paradoxically, overly negative self-evaluations and self-blaming can be as dangerous as hubris. Once, Vicki was supervising an intern who incorrectly assessed a patient's fluid status by evaluating his neck veins as indicating he was volume depleted. The trainee gave the patient fluid instead of a diuretic. The patient quickly became short of breath. The trainee reassessed the patient, this time noting fluid overload and prescribing a diuretic, which quickly treated the issue. This trainee experienced falling short as a complete catastrophe, something from which she would not be able to recover. She was unable to manage her emotions and could only identify intrinsic factors that contributed to this error. She could not see that her entire team also contributed to the error and that there may have been other approaches to assess the patient's fluid status other than a physical exam, which can be unreliable.

When we reframe a complex situation with many contributing factors entirely driven by our behavior, it becomes impossible to identify the more limited and actionable ways we have contributed to the situation (and through which we can learn and grow). When we feel that things are "all our fault," we are driven toward an avoidance mentality that makes it impossible to safely self-reflect, hinders using our Challenge Network, and ultimately prevents us from learning both from intrinsic and extrinsic factors involved in the experience of falling short.

Overcoming shame involves cultivating a culture of compassion and support. Strategies include:

- Creating an environment in which mistakes are viewed as learning opportunities (AFGO).

- Encouraging open discussions about failures.

- Self-compassion and mindfulness exercises.

When we build up a practice of self-reflection and feedback around falling short, we can honor the pain of these experiences by translating them into learning and growth. Creating professional environments and mentorship relationships in which mistakes are identified as learning opportunities can help foster such a practice—and allow us to mentor others toward these approaches.

INTEGRATION OF LEARNING ON THE PATH TO FUTURE GROWTH

In her work on failing well, organizational leadership expert Amy Edmonson writes about *intelligent failure* [7]. She argues that when we fall short, we are often able to learn more about ourselves and our goal than we could have possibly known without having experienced the outcome that we did. The journey of learning from falling short in the medical profession is not just about introspection and understanding; it culminates in the crucial phase of consolidation and moving forward. Consolidation is an active process of synthesizing the insights from introspection and feedback. It involves distilling the complex interplay of factors that led to a shortfall into actionable knowledge. This process transforms setbacks into valuable lessons, fundamentally shaping our approach to patient care, decision making, and professional interactions.

Going back to Dan's experience, after Dan and his mentor had managed Dan's emotions and explored the extrinsic and intrinsic contributors to his falling short, Dan's mentor helped Dan distill actionable points from experience: the importance of following clinical intuition, recognizing the risks of prioritizing colleague approval over patient care, and being cautious about assumptions regarding a patient's functional status. These insights were not just theoretical; they became integral to how Dan approached his future patients, shaping him into a more capable and empathetic clinician.

Practically, consolidation entails making a conscious step to take what we learn and to identify actionable points. We have found several helpful tools to facilitate this process:

- *Reflective Practice*: Reflective practice is a vital tool in the consolidation process. We encourage journaling or reflective writing, focusing on the lessons learned and the next steps. This practice isn't just a record of events; it's a deliberate process of distilling experiences into wisdom and future action plans. After falling short, Vicki often asks herself, "What is there for me to learn here? How can that inform my work in the future?"

- *Traditional and Peer Mentoring Relationships*: Engaging in scheduled mentorship sessions or peer group discussions with a specific focus on integrating learnings from our experiences of falling short is invaluable for sustained learning and growth.

- *SMART (Specific, Measurable, Achievable, Relevant, and Time-Bound) Goal Setting*: SMART is a powerful way to consolidate the learning from an experience of falling short. Goal setting is particularly useful when an action item that emerges from falling short involves increasing, decreasing, or altering a given behavior. This method ensures that the changes we aim to make are well-defined and realistically attainable within a set time frame.

Integrating learning from falling short has a ripple effect beyond individual growth. As medical professionals, when we apply these learnings, we contribute to a culture of continuous improvement where we strive for and can achieve true excellence in our professional work.

WHEN WE LEARN TO FALL SHORT, WE BECOME MORE CAPABLE MENTORS, TEACHERS, AND LEADERS

Sharing these experiences of falling short and the lessons learned with colleagues and mentees not only reinforces our own learning but also fosters a more open, learning-focused environment in medical practice. When starting a new project with a team, Vicki often reminds the team that this is a "learning lab." She encourages them to remember that we won't get it all right. Despite our hard work to develop a thoughtful approach to a new clinical program or teaching session, we won't know how this will go until we test it out and see where we fall short. Paying attention to those bumps in the road will be key to growth and learning.

When doing this work in teams, we can learn a great deal from Amy Edmonson's writings about how to develop psychological safety in teams. She writes about how high-functioning medical teams make more errors than worse-performing teams [7]. High-performing teams have a culture of psychological safety that normalizes mistakes and promotes discussion of those mistakes. When a culture is created where fear and shame are lessened, teams can learn from places where they fall short, allowing for creative problem solving and improved performance. This requires generosity with others when things don't go as planned.

Adam Grant writes about how high-performing teams have high task-related conflict but low interpersonal conflict [8]. If team members feel safe to challenge ways of doing the work, they examine mistakes. The conflict is about the task and not about the person's attributes. Sometimes in the moment, it can be easier to "blame the person" rather than do the hard work that is required to unpack what is complicated about the task or the system that might be contributing to challenge.

CONCLUSION

What's the take-home message? First, the bad news: you will fall short. It will happen at every stage of your career. It will happen in big and small ways. Sometimes, it will be because of a choice you made. Sometimes, you will have no control over the outcome. Often, it will be a combination.

The good news is that the skills needed to navigate the times we fall short can be learned. Healthy, high-functioning professional environments are comprised of individuals who have learned these skills. They know that falling short is part of being human, that life is one big learning lab. They show up with generosity for themselves and others when an AFGO presents itself. They take the time to identify the intrinsic and extrinsic factors that contributed to the problem and integrate them into their approach moving forward. When we gain skill in being able to manage our own experiences of falling short, we are in a position to help others in our work environment thrive.

REFERENCES

1. Dweck CS. *Mindset: The New Psychology of Success.* Random House Publishing Group; 2006.
2. Duckworth A. *Grit: The Power of Passion and Perseverance.* Scribner; 2016.
3. Camus A. *The Myth of Sisyphus.* Knopf Doubleday Publishing Group; 2018.
4. Marcus LJ, McNulty EJ, Henderson JM, Dorn BC. *You're It: Crisis, Change, and How to Lead When It Matters Most.* Public Affairs; 2019.
5. Luft J, Ingham H. The Johari window, a graphic model of interpersonal awareness. In *Proceedings of the Western Training Laboratory in Group Development.* University of California; 1955.
6. Grant A. *Think Again: The Power of Knowing What You Don't Know.* Ebury Publishing; 2021.
7. Edmondson AC. *Right Kind of Wrong: The Science of Failing Well.* Atria Books; 2023.
8. Grant A. *Originals: How Non-Conformists Move the World.* Penguin; 2016.

24 Physician Burnout

Marcela G. del Carmen

Physician burnout has been described extensively in the peer-reviewed literature and is increasingly becoming a larger challenge to the practice of medicine globally [1, 2]. Freudenberger first described the concept of staff burnout in terms of physical signs and behavioral indicators [1]. Maslach defined burnout as a syndrome characterized by depersonalization, emotional exhaustion, and sense of low personal accomplishment [2]. Three separate degrees of burnout have been described: first degree: failure to keep up and gradual loss of reality; second degree: accelerated physical and emotional deterioration; and third degree: major physical and psychological breakdown [1, 2].

Burnout rates among physicians vary between countries, across time, by specialty, age, and gender [3]. It is estimated that at least 35% of physicians in the developing world and 50% in the US suffer from burnout, now considered by many experts to be an epidemic and exacerbated by Covid-19 [4]. In the US, an estimated 63% of physicians reported at least one manifestation of burnout in 2021 compared to 38% in 2020 [4]. Burnout is also more prevalent among physicians than other US workers. According to the 2021 Medscape National Physician Burnout and Suicide Report, almost two-thirds (64%) of US physicians surveyed, reported that Covid intensified their feelings of burnout [5]. Burnout rates are higher for physicians engaged in the front lines of care, including primary care, family medicine, emergency medicine, and general neurology [6, 7].

Burnout carries significant professional and personal consequences [6–9]. Physician burnout negatively impacts altruism, professionalism, and quality and safety of care [9–11]. At the personal level, physician burnout has been associated with cardiovascular disease, alcohol use, depression, suicide, broken relationships, and shorter life expectancy [12–19]. Burnout is also associated with an increase in medical errors, physician turnover, decreased patient satisfaction, and decreased productivity [12–19]. Higher burnout rates also correlate with an increased number of absences, greater intention to leave a practice or medicine, and decreased workability—ability to handle the demands of the job [17]. Burnout has also been implicated as having an adverse financial impact on practices and organizations [17]. The estimated cost to replace one physician due to turnover is USD$500,000–1,000,000 [6]. For each 1-point increase in burnout, the correlating reduction in professional work effort by physicians decreases 30–50% for the subsequent 24 months [6]. Medical errors are three times more likely to occur in medical units with high levels of physician burnout, even those ranked as "extremely safe" [6]. The increased error rates may also result in increased litigation and payout activities.

I was born and raised in Nicaragua and fled the country in 1979, at the age of ten, during the revolution. I learned resilience from my parents, who immigrated to the US, leaving behind a comfortable and familiar life, with three young children, and having to build and imagine a completely new life from the one they had planned. To consider resilience as the remedy or counterforce to manage burnout risks misinterpreting the fundamental challenge facing physicians and the practice of medicine today. Burnout is not alleviated or remedied by higher levels of resilience. Burnout needs to be addressed by increasing support for clinicians, assuring that everyone is practicing "at the top of their license, "restoring the joy back into the practice

DOI: 10.1201/9781003409373-24

of medicine, and not by expecting higher levels of resilience in a profession where resilience lies at its very core.

Personally, for me, resilience has allowed me to get through 17 years of medical education and training to become a gynecologic oncologist and has given me the discipline to appropriately meet the demands of caring surgically and medically for women with cancer. But the day-to-day, minute-to-minute demands of the job, which can lead to burnout, are not eased by higher levels of resilience.

I was first educated in burnout among gynecologist oncologists in 2014, at our professional society annual meeting. Data from a survey conducted among gynecologic oncologists were presented. I was shocked to learn about the experience of colleagues practicing in my specialty. The survey showed that 32% of respondents scored above clinical cutoffs indicating burnout. A reported 33% of gynecologic oncologists screened positive for depression, 13% endorsed a history of suicidal ideation, 15% screened positive for alcohol abuse, and 34% reported impaired quality of life [20]. Physicians with high burnout scores were less likely to choose a career in medicine now, become a physician again ($p = 0.002$), or encourage a child to enter medicine ($p < 0.001$) and were more likely to screen positive for depression ($p < 0.001$), alcohol abuse ($p = 0.006$), history of suicidal ideation ($p < 0.001$), and impaired quality of life ($p < 0.001$) [20].

As I sat in the audience listening to the alarming facts reported by colleagues who had similarly elected to dedicate their professional lives to caring for women with gynecologic malignancies and had competed for coveted training positions to learn the required competencies, I could not really connect. The consequent discomfort in the realization that my own experience was foreign to the one on the screen made me realize that having found meaning in the practice of medicine had protected me from the perversity of the burdensome parts of my work, which erodes into the profound sense of purpose that brings such joy and fuels my desire to continue to serve as a physician. Although I have found strategies to mitigate these burdensome tasks; a continued renewal of the meaning of the practice of medicine and remembering the privilege we have to serve others in this dimension continue to be my most effective strategy not only to keep me from feeling burned out but also to allow me to experience the joy of being a physician.

My mother recalls that I first expressed an interest in medicine at age five or six. Her father was a urologist, trained at Johns Hopkins University, and I vividly remember how my grandfather was transformed every time he ran into a patient or family member while running errands with my older brother and me. He went from what I perceived to be a serious and contemplative man to an engaged, kind, and, most of all, joyful being. I wanted to do what he did! Mark Twain said, "The two most important days in your life are the day you are born and the day you find out why." Witnessing my grandfather's joy for the practice of medicine facilitated for me the discovery of my life's purpose. I cannot imagine a different calling, and so much of what defines me is tied to my identity as a physician.

I have always understood the charge to practice medicine as a sacrosanct calling, a life of service and responsibility. This sense of purpose that I experience multiple times a day—in that first encounter in the office with a patient just diagnosed with cancer, in the terrified look of her husband clenching her purse as he listens intently to every word I say, holding on to phrases like "this cancer is curable," "we will go over your treatment plan and what you can expect and how you will soon start to feel better." This is truly a renewal of the Hippocratic Oath and the compass that never fails to center me on what matters, what is important and the privilege of being in the office, the operating room, on the telephone, or even in answering a patient message sent via the electronic medical record. I find renewed energy in those parts of my calling that are directly centered in the care of the patient, and in the activities that are further removed, I understand my responsibility in participating in them because they are all part of someone's care. I have experienced burnout like others in medicine, but, for me, the most effective management tool remains the meaning in all of it, the joy I find in being someone's physician, and the deep gratitude for the privilege of being allowed to care for a patient, to remain committed to relieving human suffering through the practice of medicine. There is joy in sitting with patients and listening to their ailments, as we try to identify ways to alleviate their suffering, in holding a patient's hand before she goes under anesthesia prior to an operation, in the sharing of a family picture with loved ones, or in receiving a holiday card expressing gratitude for the surgery done years ago that has allowed those memories to continue to accumulate over the years. In those exchanges, I have found the realization of the most perfect form of love and trust I know. It is that experience that drives me and energizes me to continue to serve as a physician and to do so with all the compassion, empathy, dignity, expertise, and respect I can bring to the relationship. I have a personal commitment, irrespective of the daily pressures and demands of the job, never to miss the opportunity to connect with patients, to learn from them, and to be humbled by the privilege they invest in me in allowing me to be part of the care at a time of their vulnerability, such as when someone faces a cancer diagnosis.

All relationships define us, bring us meaning, purpose, and joy, but they can also be challenging and demanding. The ones that endure are the ones that remain aspirational in the search for that perfect realization of love; medicine has been such a relationship for me. Like all relationships, renewing commitment vows can be helpful. It is inspiring to consider the enthusiasm in the faces of medical students and trainees, eager to engage in the full practice of medicine and in remembering excerpts from the Hippocratic Oath: "May I always act so as to preserve the finest traditions of my calling and may I long experience the joy of healing those who seek my help."

Over the years, and after becoming educated on the incidence and risk of burnout, as an academic physician, I have studied the literature, have evaluated my own risk factors, and have sought remedies to protect myself against losing meaning in my professional life. It is estimated that physicians spending less than 20% of their time engaged in activities that they find most meaningful are three times more likely to experience burnout when compared to colleagues spending at least 20% of their time engaged in meaningful work [8]. Over the course of my 24 years in academic practice, I have focused most of my time on clinical care but have also engaged in research and remained committed to the education of students, residents, and subspecialty fellows. Over the last six years, I have also assumed institutional leadership roles, including service first as chief medical officer and most recently as president of our academic practice, overseeing over 3,300 academic physicians and 250 ambulatory practices. Most recently, I have also assumed the presidency of the hospital. This diverse portfolio of responsibilities has facilitated different experiences, allowing me to continue to learn and educate myself in domains where I had little to no previous expertise and to apply myself in very distinct areas and spaces. It has allowed me to meet colleagues outside my specialty of gynecologic oncology, and, in all those experiences, I have often reinvented myself and, in turn, renewed my indefatigable commitment to clinical medicine.

One of the most significant transitions I have experienced in my professional career has been the conversion from paper medical records to the electronic platform. I am the first to admit the benefits of the latter, not the least of which are ready access to records, ease of communication with colleagues and patients, reduced duplication of tests, reduced incidence of medical errors, and reduced delays in treatment. However, this significant improvement in how we care for patients comes at the cost of a different way to document the clinical encounter, a different way to order studies, to review results, and to submit billing. In order to manage what may not be more but certainly different responsibilities in maintaining the health records, I have found several management tools helpful. I have built into my day at least three time slots to review results, call patients, and manage the electronic health record workflow. I also inform patients from the time of our first visit that the patient portal should be used to communicate issues that truly cannot wait until the next time we meet or connect. I spend time in the office trying to anticipate and manage questions that would otherwise be asked through the portal at a later time.

I have also changed the way I document. I still take a full history and do an examination on every new patient and a directed one in all follow-up care visits. As an oncologist, I think it is important to fully engage with the patient, and I personally find it distracting to carry out the clinical encounter with the computer system open. I still take notes but have found significant efficiencies in dictating my notes and tailoring the encounter to the events and plan of care most relevant to the oncologic care of the patient. I also have become more efficient during the time that I am in the office so that I can get most if not all my clinical work completed during scheduled sessions. I huddle with the nurse and medical assistant who support my practice before and after each session so that we have a team approach to the care of each patient, and follow-up care is discussed before the end of each clinic session.

Continuing to connect with trainees and colleagues remains another source of support and engagement for me. I try to find time each day to teach and learn from our trainees, to review a case with a colleague, and to attend as many social gatherings organized by our faculty practice as my schedule permits. I find joy in my relationship with family and friends and try to spend time on weekends connecting with loved ones and truly being present in those events and conversations. I am committed to not bring home too much work and have found it helpful as a strategy in self-care to sign out my practice when I am not on call and to have some dedicated time off every week, even if only during part of the weekend. I exert the same discipline that has characterized my clinical and academic career to self-care and engaging in lifetime hobbies such as literature, travel, and music.

Over the course of my administrative career, I have had the privilege of building programs to support physicians and mitigate the impact of burnout in their lives. Institutional support focused on establishing programs to manage administrative burdensome tasks can improve the experience of physicians and reduce burnout.

The Massachusetts General Physicians Organization (MGPO) conducts a biennial survey of active members of this multispecialty academic faculty practice. The biannual survey was started in 2004, and since 2014, it includes the Maslach Burnout Inventory and the Utrecht Workplace Engagement Scale (UWES). The survey data are used to inform initiatives to address and mitigate physician burnout. In 2021, the time of the last assessment, the survey was informed, with a 92% response rate, by the experience of 2,079 physician respondents. When compared to 2019, fewer physicians reported being either satisfied or very satisfied with their careers (83% versus 88% in 2019, $p < 0.0001$). Burnout rates were higher (43% in 2019 versus 50% in 2021, $p < 0.001$). Physicians' report of engagement declined (56% in 2019 and 49% in 2021; $p < 0.001$).

Physicians identified clinical note documentation, patient-related messaging, and fewer opportunities to connect with colleagues as the primary drivers of burnout and loss of engagement.

Under my leadership, first as MGPO Chief Medical Officer, then as president, data from the survey have been used to design and implement programs to support physicians and have shown promising results in decreasing burnout. In order to address the reported administrative burden of clinical documentation and patient messaging, we created a 24-hour, 7-days per week support "hotline" that can, in real time, address any challenges physicians may have with the electronic health record platform. We have also facilitated in-person and virtual scribes to assist with clinical documentation. We are piloting deployment of additional clinical staff to primary care practices to assist with the management of patient messaging. This effort has already resulted in higher clinician and patient satisfaction.

In order to engage physicians themselves in solutions to the burnout challenge, we have conducted a series of rapid-session engagements that bring together clinicians from across our institution to identify and solve an issue identified as impacting burnout. One of these sessions focused on facilitating prior authorization approvals for medications. We have also instituted a process through which any staff member can submit a request for problems or barriers they encounter in their clinical domain of work. These submissions are reviewed and managed in real time via a working group composed of both physician and nonphysician stakeholders and experts from across the institution.

Engagement and participation in generating solutions to burnout were also encouraged through a grant program aimed at supporting local solutions for local problems, with the potential opportunity to scale successful and impactful initiatives across the organization. One of these grants resulted in the successful implementation of a peer coaching program that has now been made available to interested faculty. Another such grant led to the implementation of an organization-wide parental wellness program. The program aims to improve wellness and productivity and to reduce burnout of expectant and new parents. The program includes feeding and lactation stipends, parental wellness advocate pairings, access to lactation resources, and the opportunity to join virtual new parent affinity groups. The parental wellness advocate allows participants to connect with a more experienced parent who provides guidance and practical strategies on issues such as navigating parental leave as well as the transition back to work.

In order to address the need for increased connectivity among physicians, we have launched several programs. One of these initiatives focuses on career planning and developing leadership skills. Physicians meet quarterly over dinner and review a curriculum designed to address competencies in these domains. Another collaborative was designed with a physician coach who advises on skills and strategies to improve work–life balance and group-generated discussions, facilitating sharing experiences and best practices. Connectivity is also the focus of bimonthly lunches for all faculty, and we also offer monthly breakfast and lunch events, with administrative leadership, for groups of 10–12 faculty members.

In summary, the association of physician burnout with detrimental personal and professional outcomes, patient experience, quality of care, and decreased health care system productivity underscores the importance of continuing to explore solutions and mitigating strategies to restore joy and meaning to the practice of medicine. Solutions to address physician burnout will entail shared commitment from physicians and organizations, as well as clinician-, practice-, and institutional-level initiatives. For me, when all these tools and strategies threaten to fail, I remind myself of the fact that I volunteer to take these responsibilities on, that it is indeed a sacrosanct charge that each of us choosing to be physicians has assumed, and that in this privilege I have found a lifetime of meaning and have experienced joy. I remind myself of David Brooks's reflections of the difference between happiness and joy: "Happiness involves a victory for self. Joy involves the transcendence of self" [21].

REFERENCES

1. Freudenberger HJ. Staff burn-out. *J Social Issues*. 1974;30(2):159–165.
2. Maslach C, Jackson SE, Leiter MP. *Maslach burnout inventory manual*, 3rd ed. Palo Alto, CA: Consulting Psychologists Press, 1996.

3. West CP, Dyrbye LN, Erwin, PJ, Shanafelt TD. Interventions to prevent and reduce physician burnout: a systematic review and meta-analysis. *Lancet*. 2016;388(10057):2272–2281.

4. Shanefelt TD, West CP, Lotte N, Dyrbye LN, Wang H, Carlasare LE, Sinsky C. Changes in burnout and satisfaction with work-life integration in physicians during the first 2 years of the COVID-19 pandemic. *Mayo Clin Proc*. 2022;97:2248–2258.

5. Available from: www.medscape.com/slideshow/2021-lifestyle-burnout-6013456#1 (accessed December 14, 2023).

6. Shanafelt T, Goh J, Sinski C. The business case for investing in physician wellbeing. *JAMA Intern Med*. 2017;177(12):1826–1832.

7. Shanafelt TD, Boone S, Tan L, Dyrbye LN, Sotile W, Satele D, West CP, Sloan J, Oreskovich MR. Burnout and satisfaction with work-life balance among US physicians relative to the general US population. *Arch Intern Med*. 2012;172(18):1377–1385.

8. Shanafelt T, West CP, Sinsky C, Trockel M, Tutty M, Satele DV, Carlasare LE, Dyrbye LN. Changes in burnout and satisfaction with work–life integration in physicians and the general U.S. working population between 2011 and 2017. *Mayo Clin Proc*. 2019;94(9):1681–1694.

9. Dyrbye LN, Massie FS Jr, Eacker A, Harper W, Power D, Durning SJ, Thomas MR, Moutier C, Satele D, Sloan J, Shanafelt TD. Harper W, Power D, Durning SJ, Thomas MR, Moutier C, Satele D, Sloan J, Shanafelt TD. Relationship between burnout and professional conduct and attitudes among US medical students. *JAMA*. 2010;304(11):1173–1180.

10. Jager AJ, Tutty MA, Kao AC. Association between physician burnout and identification with medicine as a calling. *Mayo Clin Proc*. 2017;92(3):415–422.

11. Shanafelt TD, Balch, Bechamps B, Russell T, Dyrbye L, Satele D, Collicott P, Novotny PJ, Sloan J, Freischlag J. Burnout and medical errors among American surgeons. *Ann Surg*. 2010;251(6):995–1000.

12. Ahola K, Väänänen A, Koskinen A, Kouvonen A, Shirom A. Burnout as a predictor of all-cause mortality among industrial employees: a 10-year prospective register-linkage study. *J Psychosom Res*. 2010;69(1):51–57.

13. Oreskovich MR, Kaups KL, Balch CM, Hanks JB, Satele D, Sloan J, Meredith C, Buhl A, Dyrbye LN, Shanafelt TD. Prevalence of alcohol use disorders among American surgeons. *Arch Surg*. 2012;147(2):168–174.

14. Oreskovich MR, Shanafelt T, Dyrbye LN, Tan L, Sotile W, Satele D, West CP, Sloan J, Boone S. The prevalence of substance use disorders in American physicians. *Am J Addict*. 2015;24(1):30–38.

15. Pompili M, Innamorati M, Narciso V, Kotzalidis GD, Dominici G, Talamo A, Girardi P, Lester D, Tatarelli R. Burnout, hopelessness and suicide risk in medical doctors. *Clin Ter*. 2010;161(6):511–514.

16. Shanafelt TD, Balch CM, Dyrbye L, Bechamps G, Russell T, Satele D, Rummans T, Swartz K, Novotny PJ, Sloan J, Oreskovich MR. Special report: suicidal ideation among American surgeons. *Arch Surg*. 2011;146(1):54–62.

17. Shanafelt TD, Dyrbye LN, Sinsky C, Hasan O, Satele D, Sloan J, West CP. Relationship between clerical burden and characteristics of the electronic environment with physician burnout and professional satisfaction. *Mayo Clin Proc*. 2016;91(7):836–348.

18. Aiken LH, Sermeus W, Van Den Heede K, Sloane DM, Busse, R, Mckee M, Bruyneel L, Rafferty AM, Griffiths P, Moreno-Casbas MT, Tishelman C, Scott A, Brzostek T, Kinnunen J, Schwendimann R, Heinen M, Zikos D, Sjetne IS, Smith HL, Kutney-Lee A. Patient safety, satisfaction, and quality of hospital care: cross sectional surveys of nurses and patients in 12 countries in Europe and the United States. *BMJ*. 2012;344(1):1717–1721.

19. Salyers MP, Bonfils KA, Luther L, Firmin RL, White DA, Adams EL, Rollins AL. The relationship between professional burnout and quality and safety in healthcare: a meta-analysis. *J Gen Intern Med.* 2017;32(4):475–482.

20. Rath KS, Huffman LB, Phillips GS, Carpenter KM, Fowler JM. Burnout and associated factors among members of the Society of Gynecologic Oncology. *Am J Obstet Gynecol.* 2015;213(6):824.e1–824.e9.

21. Brooks D. The difference between happiness and joy. 2019. Available from: www.bibme.org/citation-guide/apa/newspaper (accessed December 26, 2023).

25 Saying Goodbye

Nancy B. Allen

> Goodbye: taking a leave; originally used in 1565–1575 AD as a contraction of "God be with ye"
>
> **—www.Dictionary.com**

In our lives, we all say "goodbye" many thousands of times—to our family and friends, to our teachers, students and colleagues, to our pets. Presumably, we learned how to do this as young children, just as we learned to say "hello" or "please" and "thank you," all part of our early socialization. Our parents, grandparents, and teachers reminded us to use these phrases when we forgot to say them. We practiced often, and, by the time we finished kindergarten, most of us were pretty good at it. We said goodbye to our parents with a smile, hug, and/or kiss when we boarded the bus to school or walked down the block to play with friends, knowing we would return in a few hours. Sometimes, however, goodbyes were more permanent when a relative, friend, or pet died.

Early memories of my goodbyes include a young friend, whom I met 56 years later at a Duke Parents' Weekend when our sons were fraternity brothers. At age four, I said goodbye to my maternal grandmother Clara who passed away on Christmas Day; her memory has remained a strong influence and guiding light in my life. When I was six years old, I said goodbye to my older sister's hamster as I buried it in the backyard, wrapped in aluminum foil and placed inside a glass jar, a method I made up since I had no prior experience; my sister was too distraught to handle this herself.

In 1960, I accompanied my father to visit my paternal grandfather, who was in an oxygen tent after a heart attack. Papa was short of breath, so talking was difficult. I recall holding his hand, telling him I loved him and then waiting outside his hospital room while Dad and Papa shared quiet moments. At home, Gran joined us for Sunday midday dinner. Thirty minutes later, the phone rang, and even though I couldn't hear the conversation, I knew that my grandfather had just died. Gran tearfully told us, "Papa loved you." I had said my last goodbye to him that morning, grateful that I had that opportunity, a foreshadowing of doing this innumerable times as a physician, daughter, sister, and friend.

As teens, we said goodbye to classmates who moved away, to new acquaintances at the conclusion of camp, to teachers each day and at the end of the school year, to friends as we scattered after high school graduation. Sometimes we accompanied these goodbyes with parties, gifts, and/or cards. During the pandemic, frequent Zoom sessions with eight of my high school girlfriends brought us back together until we could meet in person.

As college and professional students, we had countless opportunities to say goodbye to new friends and to our professors, administrative and staff members who supported our learning and social environments. We said goodbye at the end of the academic year or after summer work experiences. In 1972, I spent ten weeks working in a Karolinska Institute laboratory in Stockholm and was welcomed warmly by the Swedish people with whom I worked. Saying goodbye, not knowing if I would ever see them again, was particularly poignant.

DOI: 10.1201/9781003409373-25

191

As physicians and providers of care to others, we say goodbye to our patients in many settings—in the clinic or at the conclusion of a telehealth visit, in the hospital when we discharge patients or hold their hand when they die. We also say goodbye to patients' relatives after discussions of treatment plans or end-of-life concerns. Handling these interactions with listening, patience, and gratitude makes a difference in our relationship with patients and their families.

In academic settings, we face many goodbyes to colleagues, students, trainees, and staff during our careers. For me, saying goodbye, often at the end of June, was always bittersweet. I took time to get to know each trainee, and, by the end of a rotation, I considered them a friend and colleague. When I joined the Duke faculty in 1982, I wanted to develop my own style of teaching based on mutual trust, respect, and partnership, just as I partnered with patients in their medical care. A few years later, one of the editors of this book, Dr. Marcy B. Bolster, rounded with me on the Rheumatology Consult service when she was a medical student. Dr. Bolster vigorously pursued her interest in rheumatology, and I am so proud that she has become a distinguished teacher, clinician, and leader in our field.

In the remainder of this chapter, I expand on the topics of saying goodbye to *patients*; to *students, trainees, colleagues, and staff*; to *family members* while continuing professional obligations; to *patients, colleagues, and career at retirement*. For each topic, I conclude with *Lessons Learned*.

SAYING GOODBYE TO PATIENTS

There are many opportunities for clinicians to say goodbye to patients. We introduce ourselves at the beginning of a visit with new patients in the clinic or hospital and then spend time getting to know them. We listen, acquire pertinent history, perform a physical exam, consider differential diagnoses for their health issues, discuss diagnostic studies and treatment options, and come to a shared agreement about the path forward. At the end of the visit, we ask whether they have questions or additional concerns and express gratitude for their coming to our clinic. We shake hands or bump elbows (a pandemic behavior), give a smile, wave or make some other kind gesture. We ask patients to contact us if additional questions or concerns arise. Then we say goodbye.

I practiced medicine at Duke University for 42 years, starting with Internal Medicine residency and followed by a rheumatology fellowship. I joined the faculty in 1982 with a pretenure track title in a "temporary position," as "I was not the kind of faculty member they needed long-term at Duke," according to the Department Chair at the time. I interpreted the reasons as [1] I am a woman, among only four other female faculty out of 125 in Internal Medicine at the time, and [2] my primary goals were clinical care and education, not bench research, the prime rewarded professional activity. Although I felt devastated by the comment, I believe I worked even harder in the ensuing decades to do the best I could in all areas of my career: clinical, education, clinical research, administration, and advocacy.

I was fortunate to have my own private practice within Duke University Medical Center, along with teaching fellows, residents, and students in the hospital and clinics. I spent two to five days per month at outreach clinics in smaller cities or rural communities throughout my career. That meant that I said goodbye at the end of thousands of patient visits, with the knowledge that we would see each other again in three, six, or twelve months.

I developed strong relationships with my patients. I was drawn to the field of rheumatology for several reasons, including influential mentors, chronic care of patients with multisystem disease, fascinating diagnostic puzzles, evolving science and treatments, and the desire to care for the whole patient, not just one organ system. My younger sister developed rheumatoid arthritis at age 13, and her rheumatologist's care for her and my family impressed me. These human relationships are powerful.

In the early years of my career, I shared my home phone number (long before cell phones and electronic medical records) so that patients could contact me outside office hours. Sometimes the comfort of having a number to call was all they needed to reduce anxiety and to know that I cared and would help at any time. Patients called me from the emergency room, from their room in another hospital, or with a medical concern while traveling. I answered their questions and helped create a plan of action. Then we said goodbye until our next encounter.

Not all goodbyes were happy. When patients were not satisfied with the diagnoses or treatments I suggested, I tried to understand their concerns and find constructive resolutions, eventually accepting that they did not wish to continue in my care. I was grateful that only a few patients "fired" me during my 42 years of practice. Only a handful of times did I initiate a severance of care with a nonrespectful patient. Both types of goodbyes were painful.

Sometimes goodbyes were sad, even tearful, when a patient relocated due to family or work obligations. I provided appropriate referrals and told them I had enjoyed our professional relationship, would miss them, and wished them well as we said goodbye. Rarely, a former patient moved back to NC and returned to my care, and those were happy reunions indeed.

By the mid-1990s, Duke jumped on the managed care bandwagon, hoping to curb rapidly rising medical costs by reducing referrals and expensive diagnostic studies through primary care "gatekeepers." Other upheavals in the insurance business related to "in-network" coverage so that many patients were forced to change providers, clinics, and hospitals to those approved by their insurer. Even more frustrating, the patient's insurance provider or network often changed again a year or two later. Establishing strong working relationships with patients takes time. To break those bonds is anxiety-producing for patients and disruptive to their care. These situations also profoundly affected and concerned me, as losing those relationships took a toll. So those goodbyes were especially difficult for the patients and for me.

In 2013, I reluctantly said goodbye to one of my outreach clinics when management announced closure of all Duke specialty clinics at that hospital for purported economic reasons. For 26 years, my fellows and I had provided continuity of care to hundreds of patients at that location. The clinic ran efficiently, had an infusion clinic for infliximab and cyclophosphamide, and free parking was literally steps away from the front door. Fellows enjoyed this valuable educational experience, contrasting the rural, small hospital setting to the tertiary care referral center. We saw many undiagnosed patients with early rheumatic disease and some whose diseases had progressed severely over many years with a lack of prior adequate therapy.

When I learned of the planned clinic closure, I met with the CEO to no avail other than persuading him to keep our clinic open for an additional three months to assure appropriate transitions of care and proper goodbyes. I wrote a passionate Letter to the Editor of the local newspaper to point out the benefits of our clinics to the patients and community and the anticipated harms to those patients if the clinics closed. Unfortunately, that didn't convince the business leadership. Some patients did transfer their care to Duke Clinics, though it was a hardship in terms of travel, time, cost, and anxiety; others established themselves with a private practice or, I'm afraid, got lost in the shuffle. That was difficult—for them and for me. The goodbyes were heartfelt on the part of the patients, our fellows, and me. Not to mention saying goodbye to the dedicated clinic staff; one of the nurses had been with me for the entire 26 years and had taught me everything I needed to know about the

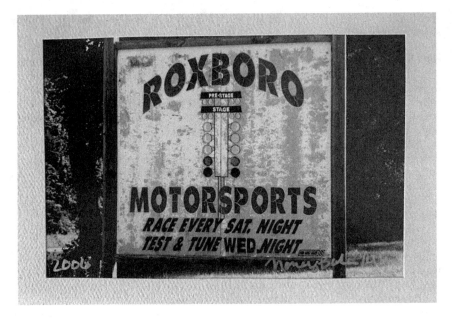

Figure 25.1 "Speedway Sign."

(Source: Photo by Nancy Bates Allen [2006].)

operations of that clinic within the hospital. I attended her retirement party a few years later and her memorial service in 2023.

At the same time, I bid goodbye to my series of large framed black-and-white photographs hanging on the walls of the clinic waiting room. Six years before the clinic closed, I drove 120 miles in the rural county, stopping to photograph barns, schools, churches, rural roads, fields, even the local Speedway. The images inspired my patients to share memories. One gentleman with rheumatoid arthritis met his future wife at the Speedway; he was watching while she drove a race car! (Figure 25.1). Many years later, upon seeing her husband's obituary, I sent his wife a condolence card; she responded with a kind note of appreciation. That is another powerful way of sharing goodbyes.

Saying goodbye to hospitalized patients evolved over time. Prior to the early 1990s, our division had an inpatient Rheumatology unit along with the hospital ward, our clinics, and offices all in the same building. Then our inpatient service moved to the new Duke North Hospital, a 5–10 minute walk away from our clinics, making rounding more complicated. Sometimes, I found that my patients were off the floor for radiology studies or specialty procedures, so I needed to go back later in the day to see them. I occasionally had to say goodbye to patients over the phone before they were discharged.

Eventually, due to increased clinic volumes and outpatient time commitments, we reluctantly turned over care for our own inpatients to General Medicine. Our Rheumatology consult service, staffed by one attending and a fellow, would follow the patients. I missed the continuity of care from clinic to hospital, so, whenever possible, I visited my own patients even when I wasn't the consult attending. I wanted to say goodbye to my patients, especially when they were seriously ill or dying.

By choice, I cared for hundreds of patients with complex multisystem diseases such as lupus, antiphospholipid syndrome, scleroderma, and vasculitis. Sometimes I first met them when they arrived via Duke's Life Flight helicopter service: a patient with scleroderma renal crisis during Hurricane Hugo 1989; a woman with acute renal failure and breast and lung masses due to granulomatosis with polyangiitis; a young woman with pulmonary hemorrhage due to severe lupus. I cited their and other cases in a Medicine Grand Rounds titled "Life-Flight Rheumatology." Since these patients lived beyond their hospitalizations, I had opportunities to say goodbye many times at later clinic visits.

My patients aged with me. My definition of "old" changed as I aged, as yours undoubtedly will or has over time. Earlier in my career, "elderly-onset lupus" was defined as onset after age 50, which is now two decades in my own rearview mirror! Because of the length of my career, I followed many people from their forties or fifties into their eighties. When one of my patients entered the hospital or hospice with a terminal illness, I wanted to be with them and their family through that journey. I want to say goodbye in a meaningful way.

As rheumatologists, we have fewer opportunities to say goodbye to our patients at end-of-life than our colleagues in oncology, pulmonary/critical care, cardiology, nephrology, and palliative care. Because of time spent as an Internal Medicine resident, as an attending on General Medicine and on the inpatient Rheumatology consult service, I cared for many seriously or critically ill patients in the hospital and intensive care units. I led or participated in numerous multidisciplinary conversations with family members and patients about their wishes, provided support and a realistic assessment of what our care was able to accomplish. Palliative Care and Hospice services have taught us a lot about how best to say goodbye at end of life.

One lesson I shared with trainees is the importance of extending condolences to the family of a patient after their death in a phone call or a card. Because of my interest in photography (inherited from my Dad), I made condolence photo cards for the family or for my patients when one of their close relatives passed away (Figure 25.2). They were grateful for those gestures. When possible, I also attended visitations, funerals, or memorial services. As examples, I cared for a husband and wife for several decades. When he passed away of heart disease, I sent her a condolence card and attended his visitation. Several years later, I visited her while she was receiving hospice care at home for Stage IV breast cancer. We shared good conversation, expressed our gratitude to each other, and said our goodbyes. After her death, I sent a personal, handmade photo card with my condolences to her family and attended her memorial service. A decade later, their daughter still sends me an annual holiday card.

LESSONS LEARNED

- Pair your goodbyes at the end of a clinic visit with gratitude for the patient coming to see you.

- When visiting a dying patient, be present, kind, and gentle; listen, answer the patient's questions and those of their family members; reflect on the life of the patient and your relationship.

- Appreciate end-of-life care support (Palliative Care, Hospice).

- Send personal condolences after your patient dies, and/or attend services if possible.

- Learn from each experience; teach, model, and reinforce your behavior.

- Take time to process the experience and your care of the patient.

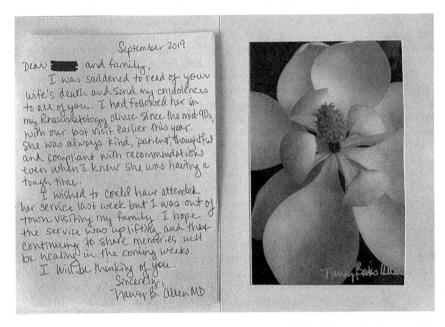

September 2019

Dear ▮▮▮ and family,

I was saddened to read of your wife's death and send my condolences to all of you. I had followed her in my Rheumatology clinic since the mid-90s, with our last visit earlier this year. She was always kind, patient, thoughtful and compliant with recommendations even when I knew she was having a tough time.

I wished to could have attended her service last week but I was out of town visiting my family. I hope the service was uplifting and that continuing to share memories will be healing in the coming weeks.

I will be thinking of you.

Sincerely,
Nancy B. Allen MD

Figure 25.2 Example of condolence card message (2019); "Magnolia Blossom." (Source: Photo by Nancy Bates Allen [2023].)

SAYING GOODBYE TO STUDENTS, TRAINEES, COLLEAGUES, AND STAFF

Academic life is rich and varied—and full of rituals and timetables. In medicine, the academic year runs from July 1 to June 30, which means that the end of June is full of goodbyes. Knowing that our trainees are heading to a new adventure can be rewarding to us as scholars and teachers, especially when we learn later that they are pleased with their decisions. Sometimes, when things didn't work out, former fellows called, emailed, or texted me for advice. Some eventually returned to Duke to further their career goals. When connections with colleagues continue throughout our careers, through any communication means or personal visits, we all benefit.

Before the pandemic (and my retirement), seeing former fellows and colleagues at national meetings was always a joy. Continuing the mentoring relationships and friendships was important to all of us. During the pandemic, Zoom meetings, emails, and text messages had to substitute for in-person communications. Over the years, many former rheumatology fellows stayed at Duke as faculty colleagues, and I watched with pride as they progressed through their careers. I was thankful that I didn't need to say goodbye to them, at least until my retirement in 2020.

For many years, I found ways to honor and celebrate our graduating Rheumatology fellows, whether they were leaving Duke or staying on our faculty. I often photographed our fellow groups at the end of the academic year and presented each one with a framed print. To each graduating fellow, I gave one of my favorite framed photographs along with a handwritten note of gratitude for their hard work and care of patients. This way, I marked their successful completion of fellowship and said goodbye to those who were leaving Duke.

I also enjoyed inviting trainees, students, and their families to our home for brunch, dinner, or an afternoon of fun for them. I did this annually when I was Clinical Fellowship Director for 12 years early in my career and occasionally in my later faculty years. The last event I hosted for Rheumatology faculty, trainees, and their families occurred in February 2020, timed with the annual Great Backyard Bird Count. For the party, I assembled snacks, drinks, children's toys, binoculars, and bird identification guides. Since this happy event took place a few short weeks before the start of the Covid-19 lockdown and four months before my planned retirement date, I didn't realize I was saying a more lasting face-to-face goodbye to those colleagues and their families.

LESSONS LEARNED

- Acknowledge the benefits of meeting many new residents, fellows, students, staff, and colleagues.
- Enjoy teaching, learning from, and mentoring them.
- Honor and celebrate them when they leave; say goodbye with a personalized gift, note, and/or social event.
- Keep in touch with former trainees and colleagues.

SAYING GOODBYE TO OUR OWN FAMILY MEMBERS

As a clinician and faculty member at Duke for more than four decades, aspects of my personal and professional lives intertwined or collided almost every day. The term "work–life balance" means something different to each of us and changes over time. There was little to no balance on the personal side while I was an intern on call every other night on most rotations and five nights out of seven on others. On one of my rare weekends "off," my parents visited my husband and me. Having fixed a nice dinner, I promptly fell asleep at the table, my head next to the soup bowl. Of course, Mom and Dad felt sorry for me. I'm sure I woke up to say, "I'm sorry" and "Goodnight" before I went upstairs.

My early faculty years were also busy with long days and frequent night and weekend calls. Then I managed a twin pregnancy and found that life became even more complicated. What a joy to raise children, participate in their school and extra-curricular events, take vacations that excite them, and share the journey with other families. Those of us who are parents know the challenges too—of finding child-care, of the child's illnesses or injuries requiring trips to the clinic or emergency room, of separation from our children due to our own work and travel obligations. We had many opportunities to say goodbye, some more momentous than others. Think of starting back to work after parental leave, putting your children on the bus on the first day of kindergarten or sending them off to camp or college. Even though we prepare them for independence, were we ready to live apart from them? I did my best to anticipate how I would feel; the children helped during their high school senior year by hardly being home unless they were asleep. In 2023, author and journalist Mary Louise Kelly's beautiful chronology of her son's last year at home before college resonated with my own experiences [1].

My mother, younger sister, and father passed away in 2010, 2015, and 2017, respectively (Figure 25.3). These were difficult times for me personally, and I was fortunate to have colleagues and staff to help manage my practice so I could focus on family. I admit that for years I was saddened by thinking about the day when I would need to say goodbye to a close family member. When my mother suffered the combination of a COPD flare, pneumonia, and a pulmonary embolus, I spent as much time as possible with her in those last six days of her life. My knowledge of medicine helped my family members understand her situation. I prepared myself to say goodbye. On the night before her death, I stayed awake in her quiet, darkened hospice room and started writing memories of her life. In the morning, I held her hand and said,

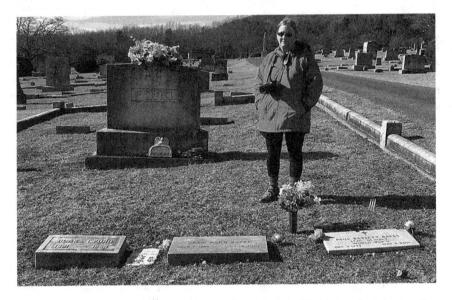

Figure 25.3 Author at Fairview Cemetery, Buchanan, Virginia, where her mother, father, and Nana are buried.

(Source: Photo by Barry Allen [2018].)

"Goodbye, Mom. I love you" before I left to take a nap. She died peacefully a few hours later, with my father, younger sister, niece, and nephew at her bedside.

When I observed one of our aging pets struggling with ambulation, climbing stairs, or eating, I turned my anticipatory grief into home hospice pet care. One of my constant companions during the pandemic and my retirement is a now 13-year-old Weimaraner named Atlas. He is in the room with me as I write this chapter and brings me comfort and inspiration. I know he has lived longer than other dogs of his breed, and I am grateful for that. But I am already preparing myself for the loss, while doing my best to keep him active and healthy for as long as possible before we say a final goodbye.

LESSONS LEARNED

- Take time to be with family members at end of life.

- Grieve the deaths of your close relatives and friends.

- Ask for help from colleagues and friends; offer help when they have their own losses.

SAYING GOODBYE AT RETIREMENT: To Patients, Colleagues, and Career

Many of you reading this chapter are years away from retirement. You are busy, as I was, balancing the many aspects of your career and your life. You work hard, contribute to your retirement accounts, and perhaps dream about what you will do in retirement. You may be in the sandwich phase of life, caring for children and parents, a time when you may be prioritizing how you wish to live your own later years. I thought about retirement periodically throughout my career but seriously started looking ahead when I was in my mid-sixties.

I am a planner. I think of what's ahead, sometimes far off in the future. For several years, patients would ask me or a staff member if I was retiring soon, as they dreaded that day. I felt anxious about concluding my long career and saying goodbye to patients. When I settled on a retirement date (June 30, 2020) in 2018, I started modifying my clinical and other professional responsibilities and discussing care transition plans with my patients. Both my patients and I needed time to adjust to the idea. At clinic visits, I would often introduce the patient to their future Duke provider. If the patient wished to move their care closer to home, I offered suggestions of locations and providers. I preferred this approach to the impersonal boilerplate letter stating, "Your provider is leaving Duke on such-and-such a date in 90 days," with little time or opportunity for real goodbyes or meaningful transition plans. I personalized my retirement letter and mailed it out one week before the Covid-19 lockdown when our practices changed completely. Included here are key excerpts of my letter:

"Dear Patient:

As most of you know, I have been planning my retirement over the past year or so. I have now set **6/30/2020** as my retirement date. . .

I have had a wonderful 42-year career here, including clinical care, teaching, research and a variety of administrative roles in the medical center and the university. In all areas, my goals were to do the best I can in each domain and to make Duke a better place. . .

As I wind down my practice, I may have already said **goodbye** to some of you in recent months. We mutually agreed upon appropriate transition of your care. . . If you have an upcoming scheduled appointment with me in the next few months, we will discuss your transition options at that time. . .

I want to take this opportunity to **thank you** – for your trust in me and in Duke, for your willingness to share your medical concerns and take an active partnership role in your health care and for, perhaps most of all, being a valued friend. It is bittersweet for me to **say goodbye** as I look forward to having new adventures. I wish you the best for the future.

Sincerely,
Nancy Bates Allen, MD"

Even though I planned my retirement, I did not anticipate the Covid-19 pandemic. As most of us experienced, our clinics abruptly transitioned from in-person visits to telehealth in March 2020, coinciding with my last three months of scheduled clinics. Saying goodbye to patients over the telephone while sitting alone in my office brought on a degree of sadness, I admit. Since I knew my patients so well due to the length of our relationships, I could envision them in front of me, and that made it a little easier. We took care of the important details of current symptoms, questions and concerns, prescriptions, follow-up care. We then shared memories and gratitude for our long relationship and eventually said goodbye for a last time.

At the time of my retirement in 2020, I looked back with gratitude, joy, and pride in my accomplishments, especially the long-term care of patients, some of whom I had seen for more than 35 years. While wrapping up my long career, I realized the importance of reviewing my experiences and considering my legacy. My husband gave me a wonderful, lasting gift of a professionally produced video-interview of me discussing the highlights of my career and personal life. *The Rheumatologist* ran a profile of me in 2020 [2].

While preparing my application for professor emeritus status, I wrote a career summary, highlighting aspects of my work related to clinical care, education, research, administration, and advocacy for women and diversity. This task helped me appreciate the wonderful variety of experiences I had had during my four decades at

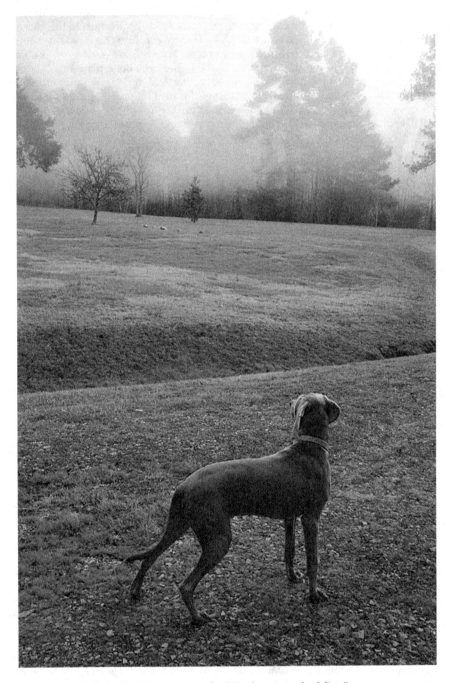

Figure 25.4 "Atlas Looking across the Meadow into the Mist."
(Photo by Nancy Bates Allen [2018].)

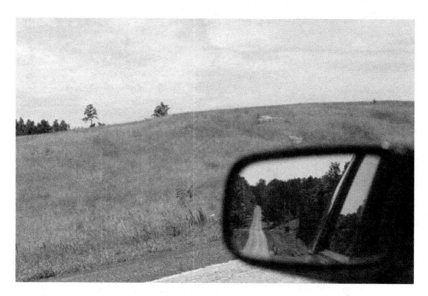

Figure 25.5 "Where I've Been."

(Photo by Nancy Bates Allen [2006].)

Duke: so many patients, so many friends and colleagues, so much accomplished. I then felt free to say goodbye to my professional roles—as well as to celebrate giving up the obligations and demands of the ever-changing electronic medical record.

My retirement party, held over Zoom due to the pandemic, turned out better than I expected. My rheumatology colleagues were very kind in recalling aspects of my career and our interactions. My older sister and my son surprised me on the call with a PowerPoint slide show of my life—as a baby, toddler, majorette in high school (twirling fire!), homecoming queen, photographer, our wedding, family, children. Those on the call learned some new facts about me just as I was retiring (Figures 25.4 and 25.5).

At present, I maintain professor emeritus status and continue to interact with members of the Duke Rheumatology and broader medical community through conferences, phone calls, and occasional visits to the clinic. I also keep in touch with former fellows and colleagues. I said goodbye to many but still appreciate knowing how and what they are doing. And I am enjoying photography, landscaping, projects at home, learning stained glass techniques, baking sourdough bread, more time with family and friends, long walks in the woods with our dog, Atlas. Saying goodbye to one's career opens new possibilities in retirement life.

LESSONS LEARNED

- Prepare yourself, your patients, staff, and colleagues for your retirement.
- Create your legacy; prepare a career summary.
- Share your gratitude, especially related to the relationships with patients, family, and colleagues.

REFERENCES

1. Mary Louise Kelly. *It Goes So Fast. The Year of No Do-Overs*. Henry Holt and Co., 2023.
2. Gretchen Henkel. "Nancy Bates Allen MD in the Spotlight". *The Rheumatologist*. 2020; 14(9):36–37.

Printed in the United States
by Baker & Taylor Publisher Services